TIPS AND TRICKS IN PROCEDURAL DERMATOLOGY

Efficient and Effective Approaches to Achieving Optimal Diagnostic and Therapeutic Results

Celebrating 50

Passion, Quality and Innovation In Healthcare Publishing

TIPS AND TRICKS IN PROCEDURAL DERMATOLOGY

Efficient and Effective Approaches to Achieving Optimal Diagnostic and Therapeutic Results

Editors

Robert T Brodell MD
Professor and Chair
Department of Dermatology
Professor and Interim Chair of Pathology
University of Mississippi Medical Center
Jackson, Mississippi, USA
Instructor in Dermatology
University of Rochester School of Medicine and Dentistry
Rochester, New York, USA

Stephen E Helms MD
Professor
Department of Dermatology
University of Mississippi Medical Center
Jackson, Mississippi, USA

Jeremy D Jackson MD
Associate Professor
Department of Dermatology
University of Mississippi Medical Center
Jackson, Mississippi, USA

Michael T Cosulich MD
Instructor
Department of Dermatology
University of Mississippi Medical Center
Jackson, Mississippi, USA

William Abramovits MD FAAD
Assistant Clinical Professor
Baylor University Medical Center
The University of Texas
Southwestern Medical School
Dallas, Texas, USA

Ashish C Bhatia MD
Associate Professor of Clinical Dermatology
Northwestern University, Feinberg School of Medicine
Chicago, Illinois, USA

Jennifer Schulmeier MD
Clinician Educator
University of Mississippi Medical Center
Jackson, Mississippi, USA

Foreword
Marc D Brown MD

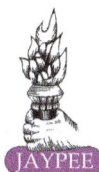

JAYPEE

JAYPEE BROTHERS MEDICAL PUBLISHERS
The Health Sciences Publisher
New Delhi | London | Panama

Jaypee Brothers Medical Publishers (P) Ltd

Headquarters
Jaypee Brothers Medical Publishers (P) Ltd.
4838/24, Ansari Road, Daryaganj
New Delhi 110 002, India
Phone: +91-11-43574357
Fax: +91-11-43574314
E-mail: jaypee@jaypeebrothers.com

Overseas Offices
JP Medical Ltd.
83, Victoria Street, London
SW1H 0HW (UK)
Phone: +44-20 3170 8910
Fax: +44(0)20 3008 6180
E-mail: info@jpmedpub.com

Jaypee Brothers Medical Publishers (P) Ltd.
17/1-B, Babar Road, Block-B, Shyamoli
Mohammadpur, Dhaka-1207
Bangladesh
Mobile: +08801912003485
E-mail: jaypeedhaka@gmail.com

Jaypee-Highlights Medical Publishers Inc.
City of Knowledge, Bld. 235, 2nd Floor, Clayton
Panama City, Panama
Phone: +1 507-301-0496
Fax: +1 507-301-0499
E-mail: cservice@jphmedical.com

Jaypee Brothers Medical Publishers (P) Ltd.
Bhotahity, Kathmandu, Nepal
Phone: +977-9741283608
E-mail: kathmandu@jaypeebrothers.com

Website: www.jaypeebrothers.com
Website: www.jaypeedigital.com

Tips and Tricks in Procedural Dermatology: Efficient and Effective Approaches to Achieving Optimal Diagnostic and Therapeutic Results

First Edition: 2019

ISBN: 978-93-86107-04-6

Dedication

Tips and Tricks in Procedural Dermatology is dedicated to our families who permitted us to devote the time required to write and edit this book

The medical students who motivate everything we do; and, the mentors who taught us the tips and tricks upon which we built our careers. These individuals include: Murad Alam MD; Kenneth Arndt MD; Philip Bailin MD; Eugene Bauer MD; Wilma Bergfeld MD; David R Bickers MD; Bob Brodell MD; George Cohen MD; Thomas Cropley MD; Vincent Derbes MD; Jeffrey Dover MD; Arthur Z Eisen MD; Boni E Elewski MD; Algin Garret MD; Leon Goldman MD; J Blake Goslen MD; Kenneth E Greer MD; Michael Kaminer MD; Arash Koochek MD, MPH; John Lenox MD; Michael Midgen MD; Christopher J Miller MD; William L Morgan MD; Eliot Mostow MD; Nancy Nieland MD; Tom Rohrer MD; Peter Rosenbaum MD; Daniel Santa Cruz MD; Meredith Sellers MD; Ken Tomecki MD; Douglas Torre MD; Allison Vidimos MD; Kimberly Dawn Vincent MD; and J Hutchison Williams MD; John Marion Yarborough MD; Simon Yoo MD and Setrag Zacarian MD.
Dr William Abramovits added his wish to dedicate his work to the United States and to his mother, brother, and sister living in Venezuela and his sons Andy and Alain and granddaughter Eliana. He wishes to deliver special thanks to the citizens of the United States who fight for human rights and understand the limits of socialism.

Contributors

William Abramovits MD FAAD
Assistant Clinical Professor
Baylor University Medical Center
The University of Texas
Southwestern Medical School
Dallas, Texas, USA

Hannah R Badon BS
Medical Student
University of Mississippi Medical Center
Jackson, Mississippi, USA

Ashish C Bhatia MD
Associate Professor of Clinical Dermatology
Northwestern University
Feinberg School of Medicine
Chicago, Illinois, USA

Robert T Brodell MD
Professor and Chair
Department of Dermatology
Professor and Interim Chair of Pathology
University of Mississippi Medical Center
Jackson, Mississippi
Instructor in Dermatology
University of Rochester School of Medicine and
Dentistry
Rochester, New York, USA

Patrick C Carr MD
Resident
Department of Dermatology
University of Virginia Medical Center
Charlottesville, Virginia, USA

Kathleen Casamiquela MD
Zena Medical
Newport Beach, California, USA

Michael T Cosulich MD
Instructor
Department of Dermatology
University of Mississippi Medical Center
Jackson, Mississippi, USA

Lauren M Craig MD FAAD
Chief Resident
Department of Dermatology
University of Mississippi Medical Center
Jackson, Mississippi, USA

Allison R Cruse MD
Chief Resident
Department of Dermatology
University of Mississippi Medical Center
Jackson, Mississippi, USA

Ashton B Davis MD
Resident
Department of Dermatology
University of Mississippi Medical Center
Jackson, Mississippi, USA

Jeremy R Etzkorn MD
Assistant Professor
Department of Dermatology
University of Pennsylvania
Philadelphia, Pennsylvania, USA

Amy E Flischel MD FAAD
Clinical Instructor of Dermatology
University of Illinois College of Medicine at Chicago
Chicago, Illinois, USA

Daniel P Friedmann MD FAAD
Associate
Westlake Dermatology and Cosmetic Surgery
Clinical Research Director
Westlake Dermatology Clinical Research Center
Diplomate of the American Board of Venous and
Lymphatic Medicine
Austin, Texas, USA

Dee Anna Glaser MD
Professor
Department of Dermatology
Saint Louis University School of Medicine
St Louis, Missouri, USA

Jacqueline Graham MD
Resident
Department of Dermatology
Geisinger Medical Center
Danville, Pennsylvania, USA

Ira Daniel Harber MD
Resident
Department of Dermatology
University of Mississippi Medical Center
Jackson, Mississippi, USA

Dylan Harrell MD
Dermatology Resident
University of Texas
Austin-Dell Dermatology
Austin, Texas, USA

Stephen E Helms MD
Professor
Department of Dermatology
University of Mississippi Medical Center
Jackson, Mississippi, USA

Derek Hsu MD
Resident
Department of Dermatology
Northwestern University
Feinberg School of Medicine
Chicago, Illinois, USA

Jeremy D Jackson MD
Associate Professor
Department of Dermatology
University of Mississippi Medical Center
Jackson, Mississippi, USA

Shilpi Khetarpal MD
Associate Professor of Dermatology
Cleveland Clinic Lerner College of Medicine
Cleveland Clinic Foundation
Cleveland, Ohio, USA

Joy Fen King MD PhD
Department of Pathology
University of Mississippi Medical Center
Jackson, Mississippi, USA

Madelyn King MD
Resident
Department of Dermatology
University of Mississippi Medical Center
Jackson, Mississippi, USA

Aleksandar L Krunic MD PhD
Health System Clinician
Department of Dermatology
Northwestern University
Feinberg School of Medicine
Chicago, Illinois, USA

Elaine Kunzler BS
4th Year Medical Student
Northeast Ohio Medical University
Rootstown, Ohio, USA

Anastasia Kurta DO
Resident
Department of Dermatology
Saint Louis University School of Medicine
St Louis, Missouri, USA

Lucette Teel Liddell MD
Resident
Department of Dermatology
Vanderbilt University
Nashville, Tennessee, USA

Ilya Lim MD
Assistant Professor
Department of Dermatology
University of Pennsylvania
Philadelphia, Pennsylvania, USA

Ronald Lubritz MD FAAD FACP
Clinical Professor of Dermatology
Tulane Medical Center
New Orleans, Louisiana, USA

Jennifer Lucas MD
Associate Professor
Department of Dermatology
Cleveland Clinic Foundation
Cleveland, Ohio, USA

Elizabeth I McBurney MD
Clinical Professor of Dermatology
Tulane University School of Medicine
Louisiana Health Science Center
New Orleans, Louisiana
Dermasurgery Center
Lafayette, Louisiana, USA

Ardalan Minokadeh MD PhD
Cosmetic Dermatologic Surgery Fellow
Skin Care and Laser Physicians of Beverly Hills
Los Angeles, California, USA

Vineet Mishra MD
Director of Mohs Surgery and Procedural Dermatology
Assistant Professor of Dermatology
Division of Dermatology and Cutaneous Surgery
University of Texas Health Science Center
San Antonio, Texas, USA

Ashley Nault MD
Resident
Department of Dermatology
Mayo Clinic
Rochester, Minnesota, USA

Maureen Offiah MD
Chief Resident
Department of Dermatology
University of Mississippi Medical Center
Jackson, Mississippi, USA

Hamad Patel BS
University of Texas at Dallas
Richardson, Texas, USA

Michael W Pelster MD
Micrographic Surgery and
Dermatologic Oncology Fellow
Department of Dermatology
Saint Louis University School of Medicine
St Louis, Missouri, USA

Kristen N Ramey MD
Resident
Department of Pediatrics
Monroe Carell Jr Children's Hospital at Vanderbilt
Nashville, Tennessee, USA

Caitlyn Reed MD
Resident
Department of Dermatology
University of Mississippi Medical Center
Jackson, Mississippi, USA

Lara E Rosenbaum MD MHS
Clinical Assistant Professor
University of Arizona College of Medicine
Phoenix, Arizona, USA

Jess (Logan) Rush MD
Resident
Department of Dermatology
University of Arkansas Health Sciences Center
Little Rock, Arkansas, USA

Jennifer Schulmeier MD
Clinician Educator
Department of Dermatology
University of Mississippi Medical Center
Jackson, Mississippi, USA

Natalie Semchyshyn MD
Assistant Professor
Saint Louis University School of Medicine
St Louis, Missouri, USA

Thuzar M Shin MD PhD
Assistant Professor
Department of Dermatology
University of Pennsylvania
Philadelphia, Pennsylvania, USA

Evan Stiegel MD
Resident
Department of Dermatology
Cleveland Clinic Lerner College of Medicine
Cleveland Clinic Foundation
Cleveland, Ohio, USA

Sreya Talasila MD
Resident
Department of Dermatology
Northwestern University
Feinberg School of Medicine
Chicago, Illinois, USA

Michelle B Tarbox MD
Assistant Professor of Dermatology
Texas Tech University Health Sciences
Center School of Medicine
Lubbock, Texas, USA

Jessica Tran BBA
Medical Student
Baylor College of Medicine
Houston, Texas, USA

Brittany L Vieira MD
Resident
Department of Plastic Surgery
Brigham and Women's Hospital
Boston, Massachusetts, USA

Kimberly Dawn Vincent MD FAAD
Belle Meade Dermatology
Nashville, Tennessee, USA

Anna Wile MD
Chief Resident
Department of Dermatology
University of Mississippi Medical Center
Jackson, Mississippi, USA

Shuai "Steve" Xu MD
Instructor
Department of Dermatology
Northwestern University
Feinberg School of Medicine
Chicago, Illinois, USA

Simon Yoo MD
Associate Professor
Department of Dermatology
Northwestern University
Feinberg School of Medicine
Chicago, Illinois, USA

Foreword

Why would we possibly want another book pertaining to dermatology surgery? On my office shelf, I have a number of excellent dermatology surgery textbooks (including my own) and several major textbooks of dermatology with outstanding surgery chapters. I would recommend *Tips and Tricks in Procedural Dermatology: Efficient and Effective Approaches to Achieving Optimal Diagnostic and Therapeutic Results* because it takes a different, unique, and creative approach to procedural dermatology. This book is not just about surgery per se, but other types of dermatologic procedures, including office dermatologic testing, light based procedures, cryotherapy, photodynamic therapy, as well as the "bread and butter" techniques of biopsies, elliptical excisions, curettage, and suturing. The concept is to teach efficiency, simplicity, effectiveness, and consistency. It is about achieving a practical approach to dermatological procedures that can be performed during a busy day in a dermatologist's office.

Dermatologic surgery textbooks are typically edited and written by fellowship training procedural dermatologists. Dr Brodell is not, which makes this textbook all the more interesting and creative. I have known Dr Brodell since we were medical residents together and have watched him become a well-known and prominent medical dermatologist and dermatopathologist. The last book I ever expected Bob to write or edit would be about dermatologic surgery and procedures, but this is exactly what makes this book truly unique; it is approached not from a Mohs surgeon's point of view, but from that of a forward thinking dermatology department chair who brought together ideas from around the country and then centered it in a growing new program in Jackson, Mississippi, USA.

I really enjoyed this book. It is appropriate for primary care doctors, advanced practice practitioners, medical students, dermatology residents, and even the dermatologists who have been in practice for many years. After 30 years as a busy Mohs surgeon, I thought I knew everything about surgery and procedures, but even I learned several new "tips and tricks". I congratulate Bob, his editors, and all the authors on a well-written, thoughtful and refreshing textbook on dermatologic procedures. It is practical, educational, and will serve as a frequent resource for anyone performing office-based dermatologic procedures.

Marc D Brown MD
Professor of Dermatology and Oncology
Chair of the Division of Mohs Surgery and Cutaneous Oncology
Department of Dermatology, University of Rochester
School of Medicine and Dentistry
Rochester, New York, USA

Preface

Knowledge in the field of dermatology is expanding at an almost exponential rate. In the era of electronic medical records and government and third party intrusion on the practice of medicine, it is increasingly difficult to find time to keep up! Sometimes, simple pearls that could improve the efficiency and effectiveness of our work are adopted into practice long after they are introduced because they are lost in the morass of new information. This was the motivation behind *Tips and Tricks in Procedural Dermatology: Efficient and Effective Approaches to Achieving Optimal Diagnostic and Therapeutic Results.* The book is organized by procedure and referenced to support the concepts that are presented. The authors are all excellent teachers whose organized approach to their topic will be immediately appreciated by the reader. There is information here that will help every healthcare provider who performs dermatologic procedures. The book is designed, however, to help even fully-trained dermatologists identify practical variations to their routine techniques that can be introduced immediately and will prove to be invaluable in their daily clinical work.

Robert T Brodell MD

Acknowledgments

I appreciate the constant support and encouragement of Shri Jitendar P Vij (Group Chairman) and Mr Ankit Vij (Managing Director) of Jaypee Brothers Medical Publishers, New Delhi, India in helping to publish this textbook and particularly Ms Chetna Malhotra Vohra (Associate Director—Content Strategy) and Ms Nikita Chauhan (Senior Development Editor) who have been prompt, efficient and most helpful.

Contents

Part 1: Diagnostic Tips and Tricks

Section - A: Tips and Tricks: Office Dermatologic Testing
Stephen E Helms

1. The KOH Preparation   **3**

Madelyn King, Joy Fen King, Stephen E Helms, Amy E Flischel

- History   *3*
- When to Utilize Potassium Hydroxide   *3*
- Materials Needed   *5*
- Obtaining an Adequate Sample   *5*
- Preparation Methods   *6*
- Interpretation and Microscopic Features   *9*

2. The Scabies Preparation   **12**

Ira Daniel Harber, Kathleen Casamiquela, Stephen E Helms

- History and Clinical Findings   *12*
- Procedures Utilized to Confirm the Diagnosis of Scabies   *14*
- Materials   *14*
- Recommended Procedure   *15*
- Benefits Compared to Alternative Approaches   *17*
- Risks and Limitations   *19*

3. The Tzanck Preparation   **21**

Ashton B Davis, Maureen Offiah, Joy Fen King, Stephen E Helms

- History   *21*
- Procedure   *21*
- Techniques for Staining and Fixation   *21*
- Utility of Tzanck Smear in Cytodiagnosis and the Associated Cytological Findings   *22*
- Using Tzanck Smear to Narrow a Differential Diagnosis   *26*
- Benefits Compared to Alternative Approaches   *26*
- Risks and Limitations   *26*

Section - B: Tips and Tricks: Biopsy—The Right Spot!
Jennifer Schulmeier, Caitlyn Reed

4. Biopsy Techniques in Dermatology: Maximizing Diagnostic Yield   **31**

Caitlyn Reed, Jennifer Schulmeier, Jeremy D Jackson, Robert T Brodell

- History   *31*
- Subepidermal Blistering Diseases   *31*
- Alopecia   *33*
- Porokeratosis   *34*
- Discoid Lupus   *35*
- Pigmented Lesions of the Palm or Sole   *36*
- Biopsy of Other Conditions   *36*

Section - C: Tips and Tricks: Basic Procedural Techniques
Michael T Cosulich

5. Shave and Saucerization Techniques   41
Lucette Teel Liddell, Michael T Cosulich, Anna Wile

- History and Overview *41*
- Procedure *41*
- Benefits *47*
- Risks and Limitations *48*

6. Punch Biopsies and Other Uses for the Punch Tool   51
Michael T Cosulich, Anna Wile

- History/Overview *51*
- Standard Punch Biopsy Technique *51*
- Special Uses for a Punch *54*
- Risks/Limitations *59*

7. Curettage   62
Jess (Logan) Rush, Lauren M Craig

- History *62*
- Procedures *62*
- Risks and Limitations *68*
- Other Uses for Curettes *68*

8. Suturing   70
Jeremy R Etzkorn, Ilya Lim, Thuzar M Shin

- History/Overview *70*
- Selection of Suturing Materials *70*
- Suturing Technique *76*
- Troubleshooting High-tension Wounds *81*
- Benefits Compared to Alternatives *83*
- Risks/Limitations *84*

Part 2: Tips and Tricks: Chemical Destruction of Skin Lesions
Robert T Brodell

9. Dichloroacetic Acid in Dermatology   87
Jacqueline Graham, Elaine Kunzler, Kristen N Ramey, Robert T Brodell

- History *87*
- Description of Procedure *87*
- Benefits Compared to Alternative Approaches *95*
- Risks and Limitations *96*
- Appendix 1 *97*

Part 3: Tips and Tricks: Complex Surgical Procedures
Ashish C Bhatia

10. Mohs Surgery   101
Brittany L Vieira, Lara E Rosenbaum, Ashish C Bhatia

- History *101*

■ Description of Procedure Highlighting Tips and Tricks   *101*
■ Benefits Compared to Alternative Approaches   *104*
■ Risks and Limitations   *106*

11. Elliptical Excision   109

Derek Hsu, Lara E Rosenbaum, Ashish C Bhatia

■ History   *109*
■ Description of Procedure   *109*
■ Comparison to Various Procedures   *113*
■ Complications   *113*

12. Nail Procedures: Tips and Tricks   115

Ashley Nault, Sreya Talasila, Shuai "Steve" Xu, Simon Yoo, Aleksandar L Krunic

■ History of Nail Procedures   *115*
■ Instrumentation: Tools of the Trade   *115*
■ Anesthesia Techniques   *116*
■ Common Nail Procedures   *117*
■ Anatomical Danger Zones   *122*
■ Wound Care   *122*
■ Avoiding Complications   *123*

13. Flaps and Grafts   125

Michael W Pelster, Ashish C Bhatia

■ History   *125*
■ Description of Procedures   *125*
■ Risks and Limitations   *133*

Part 4: Tips and Tricks: Cryosurgery and Cryotherapy

William Abramovits

14. Cryotherapy and Cryosurgery   139

William Abramovits, Hannah R Badon, Kimberly Dawn Vincent,
Hamad Patel, Stephen E Helms, Ronald Lubritz

■ History of Cryosurgery   *140*
■ Principles behind Cryosurgery   *140*
■ Clinical Decision-making in Cryosurgery   *143*
■ Management   *149*
■ Failures   *149*

Part 5: Tips and Tricks: Light-based Procedures

Robert T Brodell

155

15. Vascular Lesion Lasers

Natalie Semchyshyn, Anastasia Kurta, Dee Anna Glaser

■ History   *155*
■ Procedure   *155*
■ Port-Wine Stain Birthmarks   *156*
■ Hemangiomas   *158*
■ Cherry Angiomas and Spider Angiomas   *159*

- Telangiectasia: Rosacea, Poikiloderma of Civatte, Sun Damage   *160*
- Striae Distensae   *162*
- Scars   *162*
- Postprocedural Ecchymosis   *163*

16. Fractionated CO₂ Laser   166

Ardalan Minokadeh, Elizabeth I McBurney

- History   *166*
- Description of Procedure   *166*
- Benefits Compared to Alternative Approaches   *173*
- Risks and Limitations   *173*

17. Pigmented Lesion Lasers   174

Evan Stiegel, Shilpi Khetarpal, Michelle B Tarbox, Jennifer Lucas

- History   *174*
- Procedure   *175*
- Additional Tattoo Removal Treatment Tips   *180*
- Benefits Compared to Other Approaches   *181*
- Risks/Limitations   *183*

18. Intense Pulsed Light   186

Jessica Tran, Daniel P Friedmann, Vineet Mishra

- History   *186*
- Mechanism of Action   *186*
- Indications   *187*
- Contraindications   *187*
- Preoperative Considerations   *187*
- Treatment   *188*
- Benefits Compared to Alternative Approaches   *191*
- Risks/Limitations   *192*

Part 6: Tips and Tricks: Photodynamic Therapy

Allison R Cruse, Dylan Harrell, Jeremy D Jackson

19. Photodynamic Therapy   197

Allison R Cruse, Patrick C Carr, Dylan Harrell, Jeremy D Jackson

- History of Photodynamic Therapy   *197*
- Mechanism   *197*
- Actinic Keratoses   *198*
- Decreasing Adverse Side Effects   *201*
- Other Uses of Photodynamic Therapy   *202*
- Less Common Uses   *203*

Index   *205*

Introduction

The Times They Are A-Changin'

—**Bob Dylan**

The world of medicine is rapidly changing. Scientific knowledge grows exponentially, electronic medical records are becoming the norm, it seems that our clinical work is being evaluated by just about everyone, and medicine is being practiced by teams. In fact, the healthcare system is changing faster than at any time since Abraham Flexner's report on medical education in the North America in 1910. This led to scientific reforms in the education of physicians that spread across the United States, Canada, Europe, and the world. Of course, some things stay the same. The ethical tenets of our profession require physicians continue to put the interests of each patient ahead of their own.

And so it is that dermatologists are required to sift through reams of information in a continuing quest to validate the information they have been taught and make improvements based on evolving scientific and technical knowledge. The steady march of progress confirms that medicine is not perfect. Unfortunately, it often takes well over a decade for new, scientifically valid information to be widely utilized by physicians.[1] Healthy skepticism may be a good thing as physicians try to "do no harm", but in the case of many procedural tips and tricks, the time to introduction could be markedly reduced if: (1) the changes are based on sound concepts; (2) the introduction of the tip requires only a variation of commonly accepted approaches; (3) once tried, the advantages are obvious; (4) the information about the value of new approaches is efficiently disseminated to physicians.

To the extent that the improvements are simple and easy to adapt to standard practice, offer little risk (almost fail-safe) and work the vast majority of the time "as advertised", there is little reason NOT to adopt. In other words, physicians should not wait for expensive clinical trials for many important procedures that work safely nearly every time. Still, physicians strive to provide scientific support for the effectiveness and safety of their procedures when they can and this scientific support helps us overcome the resistance to change.

The editors encourage a cautious approach. The dictum, "See one, do one, teach one" encourages the reader to find a mentor that can demonstrate a technique. Sometimes this is not possible. In such cases, test the new technique or variation on one lesion even though the patient may have 20 similar lesions. If the results are "as advertised" repetition will breed confidence and allow you to better educate the patient about risks and benefits of procedures performed with your hands.

It is our hope that every dermatologist, primary care physician, resident physician or medical student who reads this book will validate many of their current approaches and identify at least one or two variations in their clinical practice that will improve efficiency or outcomes leading to significant benefits for the patients we serve. Consider sending me your own tips and tricks to include in the second edition of this book!

Robert T Brodell MD

REFERENCE

1. Morris ZS, Wooding S, Grant J. The answer is 17 years, what is the question: understanding time lags in translational research. JR Soc Med. 2011;104(12):510-20.

PART 1

Diagnostic Tips and Tricks

SECTION - A

Tips and Tricks:
Office Dermatologic Testing

—*Stephen E Helms*

"Never go to battle and then try to win the war. Win the war first, and then go into battle"
—General Yu, 2000 BC

CHAPTER 1

The KOH Preparation

Madelyn King, Joy Fen King, Stephen E Helms, Amy E Flischel

HISTORY

Potassium hydroxide (KOH) preparations have been used to diagnose superficial fungal infections, known as dermatophytoses, for more than a hundred years. This bedside test has stood the test of time because it provides a rapid and accurate diagnosis in clinical settings where the diagnosis is in doubt. The precise origin of the KOH examination remains unclear.[1] However, some of the earliest accounts describe the use of "potash" to help visualize *Trichophyton tonsurans* in the late 19th century.[2,3] Raymond Sabouraud is credited for publicizing the utility of KOH in microscopic examination of dermatophytes in his 1894 piece Le Trichophyties Humaines.[1,4] His careful description of technique solidified the importance of KOH in eliciting dermatophytic diagnoses.

> After 100 years, KOH preparations remain an essential tool for evaluating papulosquamous dermatoses that could represent superficial fungal infections.

By the 20th century, the benefit of the KOH examination was firmly established. Physicians began experimenting with variations of technique and specimen preparation. The KOH preparation was taught to generations of medical students in the fashion of an apprenticeship. Certain mid-century innovations to the KOH examination are still commonly employed today, such as the addition of dimethyl sulfoxide (DMSO) to KOH solution. This variation clears keratin more quickly than KOH at room temperature that requires 10–30 minutes or more before the sample can most effectively be examined.[5] The KOH examination continues to be taught in clinical settings with physicians passing along their own personal nuances to specimen collection and preparation. The sensitivity of KOH preparation has been reported to be as high as 87–91% highlighting KOH as a necessary diagnostic tool that should be mastered by all physicians treating dermatological problems.[6]

WHEN TO UTILIZE POTASSIUM HYDROXIDE

Potassium hydroxide preparation is an essential tool for the diagnosis of superficial fungal infections. This test is cost-effective and has a high sensitivity when performed by an experienced individual. However, to save time or because they have not developed this skill, some practitioners do not perform KOH preparations preferring empiric antifungal therapy. Unfortunately, this causes a delay in diagnosis and the majority of papulosquamous conditions that are clinically similar to tinea will not respond to antifungal creams.[7] Other clinicians eschew KOH preparation in favor of using a combination of a corticosteroid/azole antifungal agent. The anti-inflammatory effect of topical steroids, however, decreases the effectiveness of the antifungal cream component and most patients with tinea will not clear.

Superficial dermatophyte infections are classified by their location on the body because of tinea's distinctive clinical features at each site. Examples include tinea pedis which often presents subtly as scaling and maceration between the toes, and tinea cruris, also known as 'jock itch', which presents as erythematous moist and/

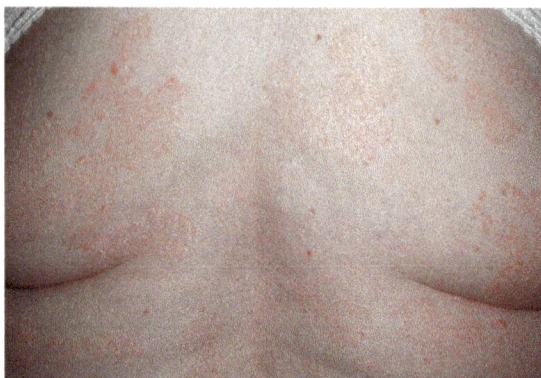

Fig. 1: *Tinea corporis*: Large patches of subtle scaling most marked at the periphery. This is a very common appearance of tinea corporis.

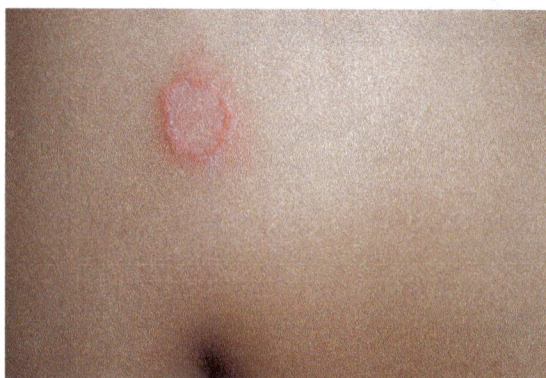

Fig. 2: *Tinea corporis*. This 4 cm patch of scaling shows more marked scaling at the periphery than noted in Figure 1.

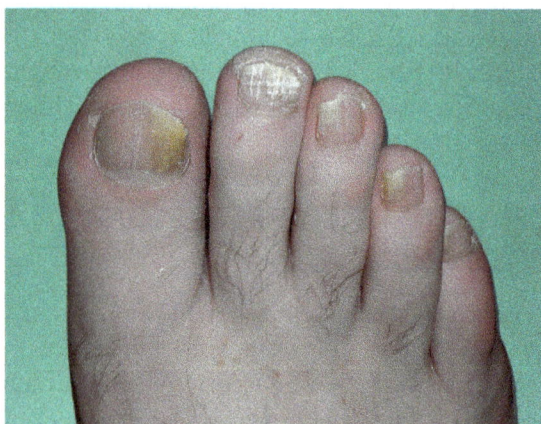

Fig. 3: Onychomycosis. The great toe, third and fourth tonails show distal subungual onychomycosis with yellowing and thickening of the toenails and lifting of the distal nail (onycholysis). The second toe shows white friable changes typical of superficial white onychomycosis.

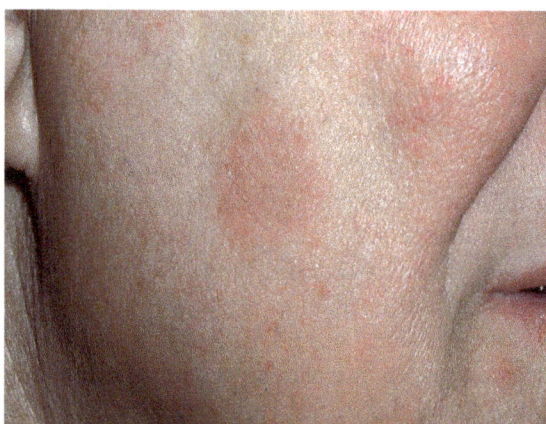

Fig. 4: Tinea faciei. An erythematous patch with slight scaling is present on the cheek of an elderly man. The classic scaly advancing margin of superficial fungal infections is not present in this case. A potassium hydroxide (KOH) preparation showed septate hyphae confirming the correct diagnosis.

or scaly patches involving the medial thighs and may spread to involve the pubic area and lower medial buttocks. Tinea corporis has a similar scaling annular appearance but presents on the trunk or extremities (Figs. 1 and 2), while tinea faciei involves the face. Tinea capitis may show little erythema and only scaly patches of alopecia but can less commonly present with boggy inflammatory papulopustules or nodules on the scalp. Onychomycosis, or tinea unguium, is a fungal infection of the nails, which may present as distal thickening and dystrophic changes (distal subungual onychomycosis) or opaque, friable, whitish superficial spots on the nail plate (superficial white onycho-mycosis) (Fig. 3). In some cases, an erythematous minimally scaly patch may show no accentuation at the periphery. This is why a KOH preparation should be considered in any scaly patch (Fig. 4).

Many other cutaneous disorders show similar clinical morphology. Psoriasis, various forms of eczema, and pityriasis rosea should be included in the differential diagnosis and can quickly be ruled out by a positive KOH, thus negating the need for a biopsy in many cases. Other entities that can be mistaken for superficial fungal infections include erythema annulare centrifugum, lichen planus, cutaneous T-cell lymphoma, and parapsoriasis.[8]

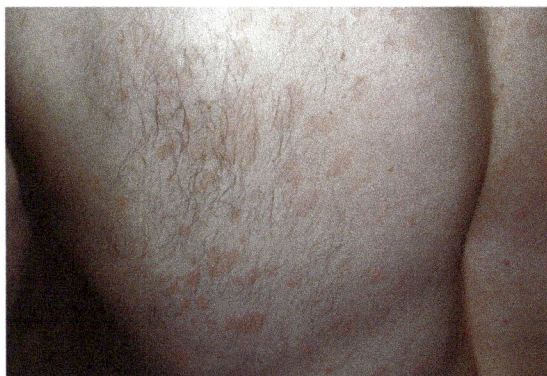

Fig. 5: Pityriasis versicolor. Superficial scaly, mildly erythematous patches are present on the trunk.

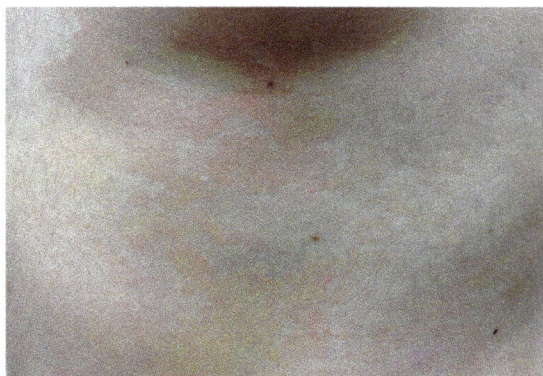

Fig. 6: Pityriasis versicolor. Extensive tan, confluent patches with fine scaling are present on the trunk.

> Potassium hydroxide preparations are a relatively easy-to-learn bedside test that may quickly aid the practitioner in making a correct diagnosis of superficial fungal infection.

Yeast organisms, such as *Malassezia furfur* and *Candida albicans*, also can cause superficial fungal infections. *M. furfur* is the etiologic agent of "tinea" versicolor (pityriasis versicolor). It presents with tan hyperpigmented and/or hypopigmented macules and patches with overlying scale that is most often found on the trunk and proximal extremities (Figs. 5 and 6). Some patients have associated pruritus. Due to its variable appearance, it can be mistaken for pityriasis alba or occasionally vitiligo. *Candida albicans* is responsible for a myriad of clinical infections, including thrush, perleche/angular cheilitis, intertriginous dermatitis, vulvovaginitis, and balanitis. It is imperative to perform a KOH examination on any rash suspicious for superficial fungal infection to ensure a prompt and accurate diagnosis, thus avoiding unnecessary delays and proper therapy.

MATERIALS NEEDED

Materials required include:
- Microscope slide and cover slip
- Number 15 scalpel blade
- A 10–20% KOH solution combined with contrast dye of choice (KOH with DMSO [Dimethyl Sulfoxide] optional)
- Methanol burner or match/lighter (optional)
- Microscope

OBTAINING AN ADEQUATE SAMPLE

Where

It is best to obtain sample material from specific areas of rash to ensure the highest diagnostic yield. In suspected dermatophytic infections, procuring scale from the active outer border of the lesion is more likely to garner a positive result compared with material obtained from the center of the lesion.[8,9] For cases of possible Malassezia, sampling the characteristic diffuse scale of the patches is appropriate. In suspected superficial candidal infections it is best to obtain specimen from the moist, macerated, caseous matter.

For nail sampling, one should target the white or yellow, crumbly areas, as these regions are most likely to consist of active infection.[10] If no single apparent area is present, sampling from the distal subungual debris is appropriate with an attempt to get material from the most proximal area of involvement preferred. If concerned about paronychia, a candidal skin infection affecting the periungual skin, obtain pus from underneath the nail fold for microscopic examination, either by compression or incision with a number 11 scalpel blade of the inflamed tissue.

When considering tinea capitis, obtain scale scrapings from the base of the broken hair and the affected scalp. *Trichophyton tonsurans* is the most

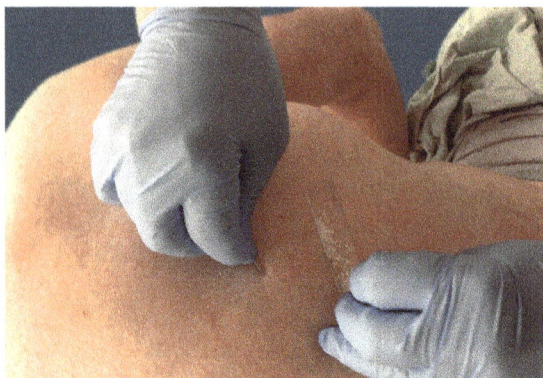

Fig. 7: Proper scraping technique. The advancing margin of this scaling patch was selected to obtain a sample. The skin is gently scraped with a number 15 scalpel blade. The sharp edge of the blade trails behind to avoid lacerating the skin.

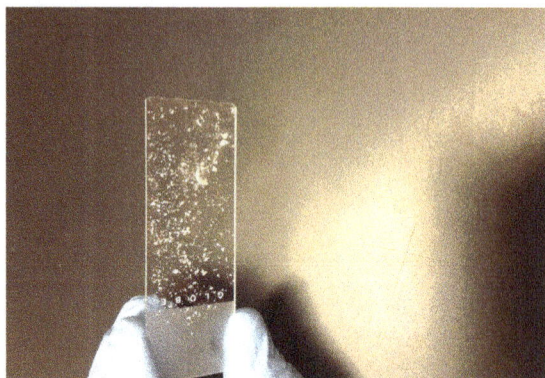

Fig. 8: Proper scraping technique. A large amount of scale is collected to increase the sensitivity of the potassium hydroxide (KOH) preparation.

common cause of tinea capitis in children and is referred to as the "black dot ringworm" with short dark broken hairs giving the appearance of black dots. It is important to sample and examine these hairs for endothrix spores. Specimen can be easily obtained with gentle scraping as outlined below. Occasionally, only scaly patches mimicking seborrheic dermatitis or psoriasis of the scalp may be seen.

How

After a suitable area has been selected, clean the area gently with an alcohol pad. The moisture from the pad will facilitate scale collection by causing the scale to stick more readily to the scraping device.[7] Alternatively, a dampened gauze can be used to moisten the dry scale to help with specimen collection. A number 15 blade is most commonly used to obtain scale. Hold the slide perpendicular to the skin of the affected area and begin scraping with the sharp end of the blade "trailing behind", so as not to lacerate the skin (Fig. 7). When collecting samples for KOH preparation it is important to remember two key facts. First, and very importantly, a large amount of scale must be collected in order to maximize the chance of visualizing any superficial fungus that may be present (Fig. 8).[11,12] Second, each microscopic slide should be immediately covered with a cover slip to ensure that collected specimen is not lost (blown off by the air) while transferring

the slide from the examination room to the microscope. In patients who will not remain still, a microscope slide, a curette, or even a toothbrush have been used in place of the sharp blade.[9]

> Potassium hydroxide yield is enhanced by collecting a generous amount of scraped material.

PREPARATION METHODS

Staining/Ink

In order to accurately view the specimen a clearing agent must be added to digest the keratin. KOH serves as the most commonly used agent.[7,8,13] However the standard KOH preparation lacks color contrast. This deficit may make it difficult for individuals to differentiate between keratinocytes (walls) and fungal elements. The addition of contrast dyes that stain the fungal spores and hyphae facilitate visualization and increase sensitivity (Figs. 9 and 10). A number of KOH solutions with contrast dyes are commercially available. Studies of these solutions demonstrate varying sensitivities (Table 1).[14,15] Our experience with any of the contrast dyes shows much higher sensitivity than reported with Parker Super Quink` ink (Helms, Brodell).[16,17]

Applying the clearing solution is best performed as follows: draw up KOH/ink solution in an eye dropper and place one to two drops on each side of the cover slip allowing the solution

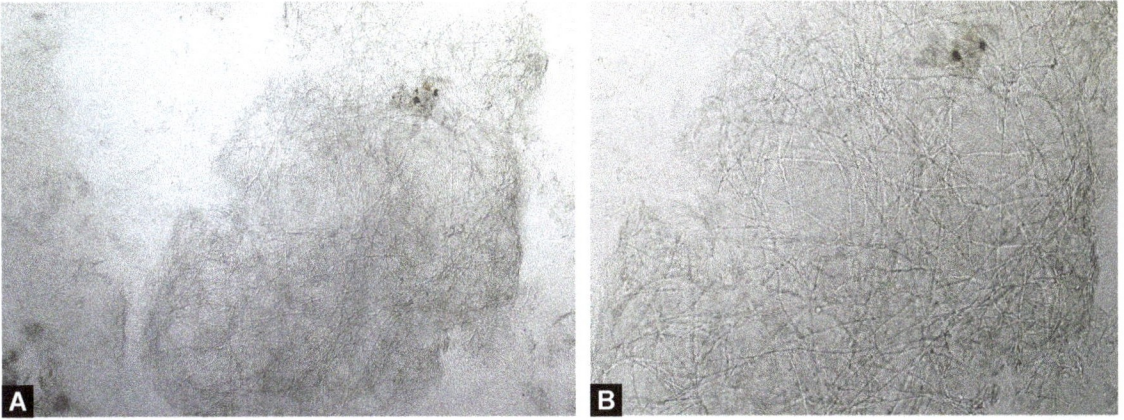

Figs. 9A and B: (A) Potassium hydroxide (KOH) preparation without stain. A preparation using KOH with dimethyl sulfoxide (DMSO) demonstrates hyphae that blend in with the walls of background keratinocytes (100X). (B) KOH preparation closer view of hyphae demonstrates similarity of hyphae and cell walls (400X).

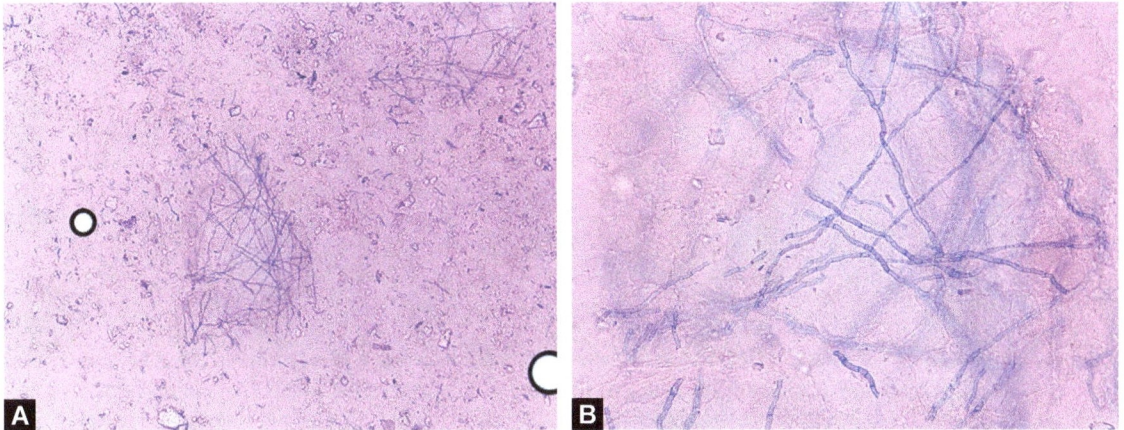

Figs. 10A and B: (A) Potassium hydroxide (KOH) preparation with stain. Chicago blue stains hyphal walls blue to differentiate them from cell walls (100X). (B) KOH preparation with stain. Blue hyphae are easily seen on higher power when compared to unstained keratinocyte walls (400X).

Table 1: Commercially available stains.[14]		
Stain	Appearance	Sensitivity and specificity
Parker® ink	Fungal elements appear clear against a clear/brown background	Sensitivity 48%, specificity 96%
Chlorazole black	Fungal elements appear grey against a grey/clear background	Sensitivity 63%, specificity 97% *Possibly carcinogenic requiring special handling[15]
Chicago blue®	Fungal elements appear blue against a purplish background	Sensitivity 78%, specificity 96%

to diffuse through capillary action beneath the slide (Figs. 11A and B).[9] To further facilitate diffusion, press lightly on the cover slip and employ a side-to-side technique to flatten out the layer of scale and to mobilize excess solution to the edge[7] (Fig. 12A). In scrapings from patients with tinea capitis, care must be taken to avoid exerting too much pressure on the slide as this can express the spores from within the hair shaft altering the "typical picture" seen with the spores neatly in line inside the hair shaft.[8] Excess solution can be gently blotted away with a paper towel, lens paper or tissue[7,9] (Figs. 12B and C).

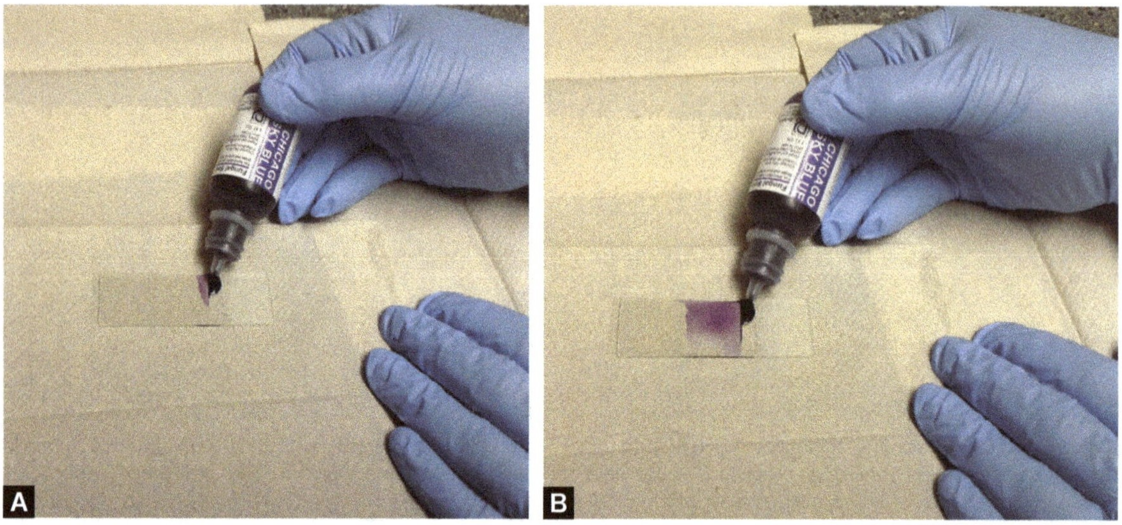

Figs. 11A and B: (A) Application of potassium hydroxide (KOH) solution to slide. KOH solution is applied at the edge of the cover slip. (B) Application of KOH solution to slide. Capillary action moves the KOH solution underneath the cover slip.

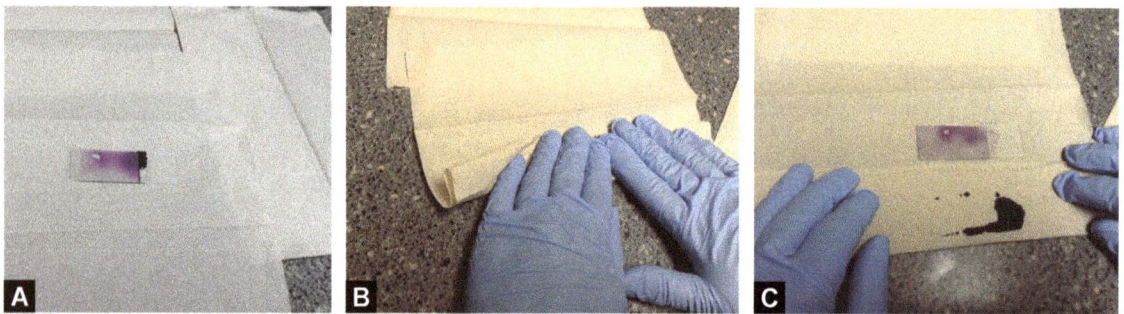

Figs. 12A to C: Removing excess potassium hydroxide (KOH) solution. (A) Inked KOH is evenly distributed under the entire cover slip. (B) A paper towel is folded over the slide and pressed gently to remove excess liquid and flatten clumps of cells. (C) The towel is unfolded and the slide is ready for viewing under the microscope.

> Patients who shower frequently may wash away superficial spores making them more difficult to identify on KOH exam. This is particularly seen in pityriasis versicolor since the yeast elements are very superficial and patients may wash the thin scale off leaving only a few hyphal elements and spores to be seen when collecting the material for a KOH examination.

Heat/Time

Prior to microscopic visualization, the utilization of a heat source is often used to accelerate keratinocyte digestion when using KOH. A methanol burner can be used, but care must be taken to not heat the specimen to boiling as this can promote KOH crystallization and cause artifact.[8] Sampling from the hair and nails may require more heating to digest the thicker keratinous material. Another chemical that may be used to clear keratin is DMSO which eliminates the need for heating KOH solution to quickly clear keratin.[18] Commercial preparations are available that contain KOH and DMSO, and one contains KOH, DMSO, with a dye (Chlorazol Black E⁻). Although it is common to immediately examine the slide after heating when using KOH alone, waiting 5–15 minutes or longer before viewing is most ideal to allow adequate keratinocyte digestion and maximize sensitivity. Finally, KOH with DMSO can be mixed with Chicago Sky Blue™ by adding one drop of each to

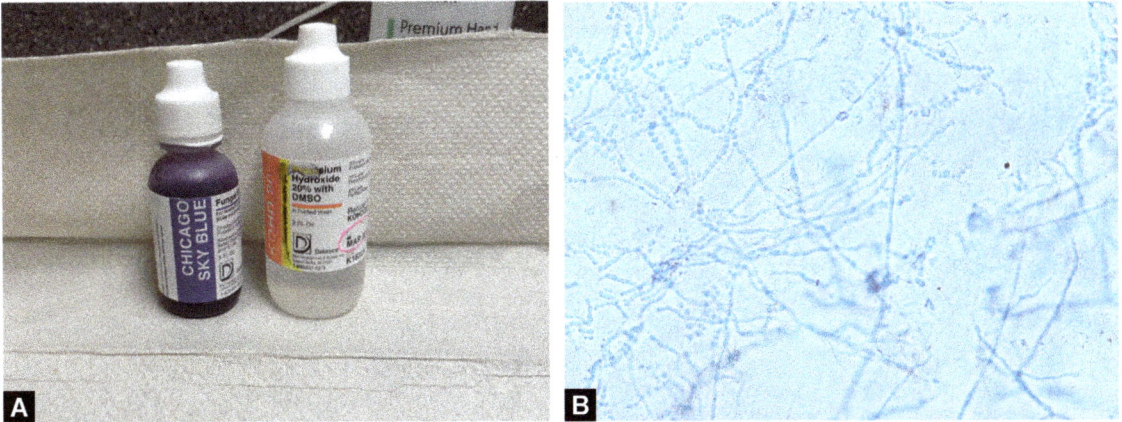

Figs. 13A and B: (A) Bottles showing Chicago sky blue stain 1% with 8% KOH and a bottle of KOH 20% containing dimethyl sulfoxide (DMSO). The Chicago sky blue stain is very dark when used alone. Chicago sky blue (CSB) stain can be added to the routine potassium hydroxide (KOH) wet-mount to provide a color contrast and facilitate the diagnosis of dermatomycoses. (B) Potassium hydroxide (KOH) option favored by authors. One drop of Chicago blue KOH may be dropped onto the slide with one drop of a commercially available KOH 20% with DMSO to make a solution with a lighter background coloration. The use of the DMSO also leads to more clearing of keratin.

the slide which will aid in rapid clearing without heating and at the same time allow inked hyphae to be more easily identified (Figs. 13A and B).

> Heating the KOH after applying the coverslip on the slide clears keratin and makes hyphae and spores more easily visualized.

> Inks and stains are added to KOH solution to highlight hyphae and spores and differentiate them from keratinocyte cell walls.

Table 2: Microscopic features of different fungal elements.

Fungal type	Microscopic feature
Dermatophyte infection	Long branching mycelia with septae or cross-walls
Candidiasis	Pseudohyphae (non-septate hyphae) and round to oval yeast bodies
Tinea versicolor	Clusters of short hyphae and spores; referred to as "spaghetti and meat-balls"
Tinea capitis infection	May show either endothrix pattern in which spores are seen in the hair shaft or ectothrix pattern where spores are also seen on the external surface of the hair shaft

INTERPRETATION AND MICROSCOPIC FEATURES

To best visualize a KOH preparation, adjust the microscope, so that the condenser is as far down as possible and adjust to a lower intensity of lighting. Limiting the light better emphasizes the contrast between keratinocytes and the fungal spores and hyphae.[8] It is important to be comfortable in recognizing the microscopic features of characteristic fungal elements (Table 2). You likely will have to increase the amount of light as you move to higher powers to confirm what appear to be fungal elements.

Hyphae and spores can also be seen in hematoxylin and eosin (H&E) stained biopsy specimens. However, they are much more easily iden-

tified when periodic acid-Schiff (PAS)-diastase staining is used (Fig. 14). This also demonstrates why scraping of superficial fungal infections show fungal elements.

Benefits to Alternative Therapies

Potassium hydroxide is a rapid, cost-effective technique for diagnosing superficial fungal infections. The sensitivity of KOH is dependent on the examiner's skill and expertise.[7,19] It has been reported that obtaining a positive laboratory test prior to initiating antifungal therapy is more cost-effective than beginning empiric antifungal therapy without a confirmatory diagnosis.[18] As a multitude of clinical entities can present similarly

Fig. 14: Skin biopsy demonstrating hyphal elements in stratum corneum with periodic acid-Schiff (PAS) stain.

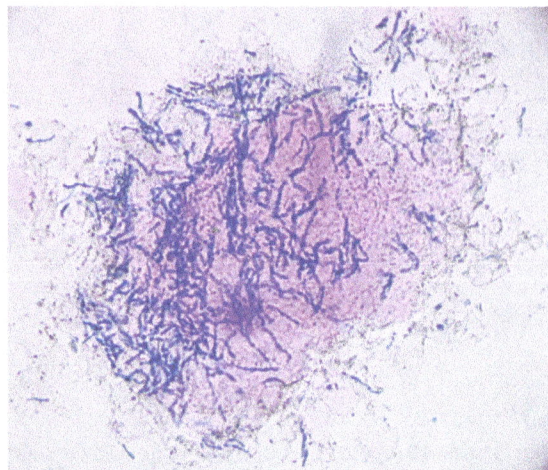

Fig. 15: Hyphal elements and spores typical of tinea versicolor stained with KOH and Parker Super Quink ink (400X). *Courtesy*: Adam Byrd, MD

to superficial fungal infections, utilizing empiric antifungal therapy in place of laboratory testing can delay diagnosis and increase overall costs.

Periodic acid-Schiff staining of a biopsy specimen has the highest sensitivity of superficial fungal diagnostic tests (Fig. 14).[6] However its high cost makes it a less attractive test when compared to KOH preparation. KOH is also as a screening test to fungal culture because of its increase sensitivity.[19] In addition, fungal culture is much more time intensive and expensive when compared to the rapid in-office results of KOH.[19] It is particularly important to perform a KOH when tinea versicolor is suspected. This yeast cannot be cultured on regular fungal media but has a characteristic picture under the microscope often referred to as "spaghetti and meatballs" with short hyphal elements and many small round spores (Fig. 15).

Combining KOH with calcofluor-white, a fluorescent dye, has been described as a sensitive method for evaluating potential superficial infections. However, there are disadvantages to this process since it requires the use of a fluorescence microscope. In addition, it has been shown to have a higher false-negative rate when compared to KOH preparation with ink.[6]

The benefits of utilizing KOH preparation to diagnose superficial infections are, therefore, multifactorial. The test is highly sensitive at detecting infection, timely and cost-effective, and relatively easily mastered without an extensive amount of training.

Limitations

The primary limitation of KOH preparation is its dependence on operator's expertise. There is a positive correlation between examiner's skill and the sensitivity of KOH preparation with or without stains or ink.[7] Examiners unfamiliar with microscopic interpretation and the steps that produce an adequate KOH preparation may misinterpret the test as a false-negative or false-positive result. Multiple tips and tricks described in this chapter should help alleviate operator-dependent errors.

Causes of false-negative results may also include previous treatment with antifungals and the collection of inadequate samples. Therefore, a strong clinical suspicion for superficial fungal infection in the presence of a negative KOH test should prompt repetition of KOH and possibly a fungal culture. Only on a rare occasion should empiric therapy be indicated, if the clinical picture is so clearly suggestive of fungal infection.[8]

False-positive results, although less common, can occur. These are typically attributed to observation error by the examiner. Intercellular spaces, especially with overlapping cell walls, and artifacts, such as hair, clothing fibers, lipids, or KOH crystals caused by overheating can all be misinterpreted as hyphae or spores. These errors tend to be alleviated with experience.

Conflict of Interest

Madelyn King, Amy Flischel, Joy King, and Stephen Helms have no conflicts of interest.

REFERENCES

1. Dasgupta T, Sahu J. Origins of the KOH technique. Clin Dermatol. 2012;30(2):238-41.
2. Fox T. On ringworm of the head, and its management. Lancet. 1877;110:719-22.
3. Thin G. Contributions to the pathology of parasitic diseases of the skin. Br Med J. 1982;2(1129):301-5.
4. Sabouraud R. Les Trichophyties Humaines. Paris, France: Rueff & Cie; 1894.
5. Zaias N, Taplin D. Improved preparation for the diagnosis of mycologic diseases. Arch Dermatol. 1966;93(5):608-9.
6. Lily KK, Koshnick RL, Grill JP, et al. Cost-effectiveness of diagnostic tests for toenail onychomycosis: a repeated-measure, single-blinded, cross-sectional evaluation of 7 diagnostic tests. J Am Acad Dermatol. 2006;55(4):620-6.
7. Wilkison BD, Sperling LC, Spillane AP, et al. How to teach the potassium hydroxide preparation: a disappearing clinical art form. Cutis. 2015;96(2):109-12.
8. Brodell RT, Helms SH, Snelson ME. Office dermatologic testing: the KOH preparation. Am Fam Physician. 1991;43(6):2061-5.
9. Bronfenbrener R. Stains and smears: resident guide to bedside diagnostic testing. Cutis. 2014;94(6):E29-30.
10. Shelley WB, Wood MG. The white spot target for microscopic examination of nails for fungi. J Am Acad Dermatol. 1982;6(1):92-6.
11. Merrill N, Mallory SB. Superficial fungal infections in children. J Ark Med Soc. 1987;84(6):235-8.
12. McBurney EI. Diagnostic dermatologic methods. Pediatr Clin North Am. 1983;30(3):419-34.
13. Swartz JH, Lamkins BE. A rapid, simple stain for fungi in skin, nail scrapings, and hairs. Arch Dermatol. 1964;89:89-94.
14. Tambosis E, Lim C. A comparison of the contrast stains, Chicago blue, chlorazole black, and Parker ink, for the rapid diagnosis of skin and nail infections. Int J Dermatol. 2012;51(8):935-8.
15. Sigma-Aldrich. (2017). Safety Data Sheets Version 4.1. [online] Available from www.sigmaaldrich.com/united-kingdom/technical-services/material-safety-data.html. [Accessed March, 2017].
16. Levitt JO, Levitt BH, Akhavan A, et al. The sensitivity and specificity of potassium hydroxide smear and fungal culture relative to clinical assessment in the evaluation of tinea pedis: a pooled analysis. Dermatology Research Practice. Volume 2010(2010), Article ID 764843, 8 pages. http://dx.doi.org/10.1155/2010/764843.
17. Prakash R, Prashanth HV, Ragunatha S, et al. Comparative study of efficacy, rapidity of detection, and cost-effectiveness of potassium hydroxide, calcofluor white, and Chicago sky blue stains in the diagnosis of dermatophytoses. Int J Dermatol. 2016;55(4):e172-5.
18. James WD, Berger T, Elston D. Andrew's Diseases of the Skin: Clinical Dermatology, 11th edition. New York, NY, USA: Elsevier-Saunders; 2011.
19. Mehregan DR, Gee SL. The cost effectiveness of testing for onychomycosis versus empiric treatment of onychodystrophies with oral antifungal agents. Cutis. 1999;64(6):407-10.

CHAPTER 2

The Scabies Preparation

Ira Daniel Harber, Kathleen Casamiquela, Stephen E Helms

INTRODUCTION

Sarcoptes scabiei infestation can present a diagnostic challenge to even the most experienced clinician because of its ability to mimic other diseases of the skin including multiple eczematous conditions, impetigo, bullous pemphigoid, varicella, dermatitis herpetiformis, irritant or allergic contact dermatitis, seborrheic dermatitis or arthropod bites. Scabies requires specific treatment and the infestation is exacerbated and further masked by the incorrect use of topical and systemic corticosteroids. Furthermore, the nature of scabies infestation predisposes both patient and practitioner to doubt the effectiveness of antiscabetic treatment because the intense itching and rash may take several weeks to subside after appropriate therapy. For all of these reasons, it is important to confirm the diagnosis of scabies when the patient first presents whenever this is possible. This chapter presents a modified scabies preparation designed to maximize the yield of skin scrapings in patients with scabies.

HISTORY AND CLINICAL FINDINGS

The human itch mite, *Sarcoptes scabiei,* was first described in scientific letters over 300 years ago.[1] A definitive diagnosis is often difficult to make on clinical grounds. In fact, scabies has been called the 'Great Imitator'[2] since it can manifest with a myriad of primary and secondary lesions including vesicles, erythematous papules, eczematous papules or patches, nodules, pustules, urticarial papules and patches and, very frequently, excoriated papules.[3-6]

Scabies has been called "the Great Imitator".

Thus, it can mimic a variety of eczematous conditions including atopic eczema, irritant or allergic contact dermatitis, seborrheic dermatitis as well as impetigo, papular urticaria, arthropod bites, folliculitis, animal scabies, varicella, drug eruption, and dermatitis herpetiformis (Figs. 1 to 3).[7,8] The diagnosis of scabies may be even more difficult in patients whose pruritus has been treated with topical or systemic steroids for prolonged periods of time. This alters the clinical signs and symptoms of this infestation, thus producing "sca-

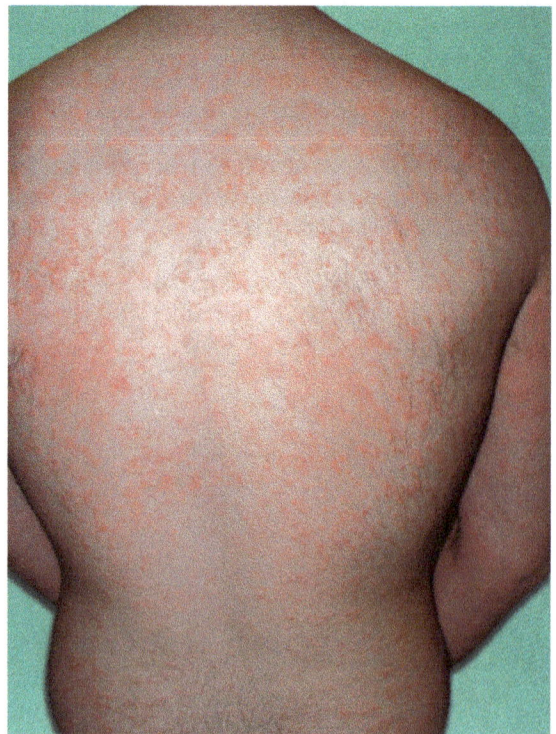

Fig. 1: Diffuse eczematous papules, patches and auto-eczematization in a patient with scabies previously treated with topical corticosteroids.

Fig. 2: Rarely, scabies may present with vesicles or bullae. *Courtesy*: Gary Bolton, MD.

Fig. 3: Scabies presenting with multiple nodules and impetiginized papules in a typical flexural location.

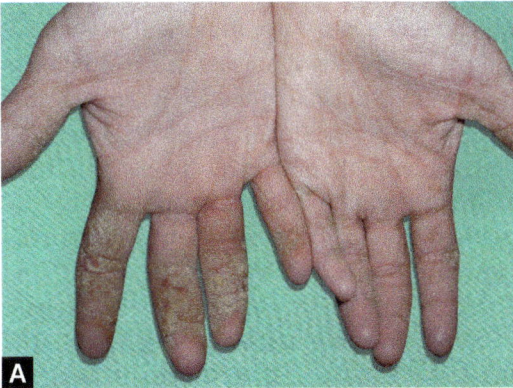

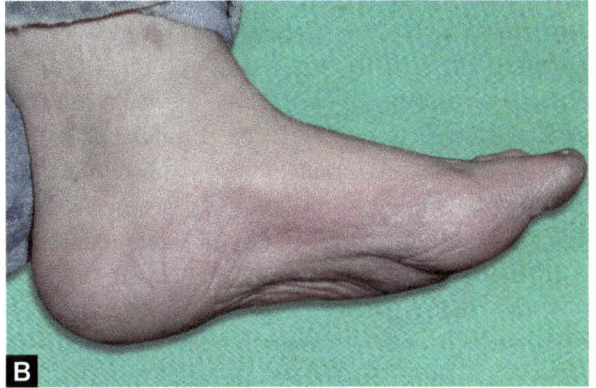

Figs. 4A and B: Hyperkeratosis of palms and soles in crusted scabies may resemble psoriasis or other hyperkeratotic disorders.

bies incognito".[9] Crusted scabies, formerly known as Norwegian scabies, is a severe variant that presents with widespread hyperkeratotic plaques that harbor thousands to millions of mites.[10]

> Crusted scabies harbors thousands to millions of mites

It occurs predominantly in immunocompromised individuals, such as those with HIV, or otherwise debilitated patients (Figs. 4A and B).[10] The unusual clinical features of crusted scabies often delay making the diagnosis. This delay, in combination with the extreme contagiousness of crusted scabies, sets the stage for outbreaks in institutions and multimember homes. Scores of staff members and patients can be infected from one patient with crusted scabies.[11,12]

The clinical course of scabies is variable. Most patients experience a steadily worsening rash with pruritus that is particularly intense at night. Pruritus and visible rash, however, may not be present immediately after exposure. A 4–6 week incubation period is common.[13] Subsequent infestations become symptomatic as early as 1–3 days after exposure, since the host's immune system has been previously sensitized to mite antigens.[14]

Considering the importance of early diagnosis and prompt treatment to each patient and to prevent spread, scabies should be included in the differential diagnosis of any persistent pruritic eruption.

PROCEDURES UTILIZED TO CONFIRM THE DIAGNOSIS OF SCABIES

Between 1888 and 1928, the burrow ink test (BIT) was introduced to diagnose scabies. The procedure was passed along by word of mouth through generations of French dermatologists. In 1981, a formal study was performed which, for the first time, clearly established its diagnostic accuracy and utility.[15] Clinically, it can be difficult to observe the signal marker of scabies, the burrow, with the naked eye. Hebra, in 1869, reported that the classically described scabietic burrows could be appreciated more readily after altering their appearance with dirt or dyes.[16] Perhaps a cleaner patient population has made it more difficult to observe the burrows with the naked eye, as successive studies from the 1940s through 1970s described a decreasing incidence of observable burrows in patients with confirmed scabies.[17-19] The identification of a burrow by an experienced dermatologist correlated with the classic history and clinical picture is sufficient for the presumptive diagnosis of scabies in many instances. However, demonstration of a mite or its products under power of a microscope remains the gold standard for diagnosis of scabies in the United States.[20]

> An inked burrow may be considered confirmatory by some clinicians

Recognizing the difficulty in obtaining a positive scabies preparation in some patients suffering from scabies, it is best to combine the BIT to select "high yield" lesions that can be sampled using the standard scrape method of microscopic inspection of skin debris.[21] This maximizes the likelihood of finding evidence of infestation and minimizing the time, cost, and patient discomfort related to extended searches with unguided sampling.[21]

It is not uncommon for dermatologists to treat patients with the presumptive diagnosis of scabies without performing a confirmatory test. A patient is treated for scabies the same way whether a scabies preparation is performed or not, however, when a nonresponding patient with a confirmed positive scabies preparation returns to the office for a follow-up visit, the explanations are few:

- The patient did not fill their prescription (primary nonadherence)
- Lack of adherence to the treatment regimen, e.g. failure to treat every inch of the skin from the neck down
- Treatment failure
- Reinfection

On the other hand, a patient treated for presumed scabies without a confirmatory test could be suffering from a host of other conditions in addition to the situations noted above. Presumptive therapy for scabies is also confounded by the nature of the disease. Successful antiscabietic treatment against live mites and larvae usually does not quickly eradicate the symptoms of hypersensitivity reactions to the mite antigen, and pruritus often persists for one to several weeks following therapy. Without microscopic confirmation of the scabietic infestation one might begin to doubt the initial diagnosis when symptoms fail to improve immediately after treatment and embark on unnecessary diagnostic or treatment adventures. In summary, since the treatment of scabies is unique and quite different from the approach taken for other papulosquamous diseases, performing a test to make a definitive diagnosis is imperative.[22,23]

MATERIALS

Ink

While full-strength fountain pen ink is commonly used for the BIT, we favor diluting the ink to decrease its viscosity and allow it to more easily seep into burrows (1–3 mL ink in 10 mL water). At the same time, diluted ink is more easily removed by alcohol when the test is completed, leaving less staining. Of course, viscosity may vary between ink manufacturers. To determine, if the mixture is thin enough, place a drop onto the dorsum of

Fig. 5: Barely visible papule prior to application of ink.

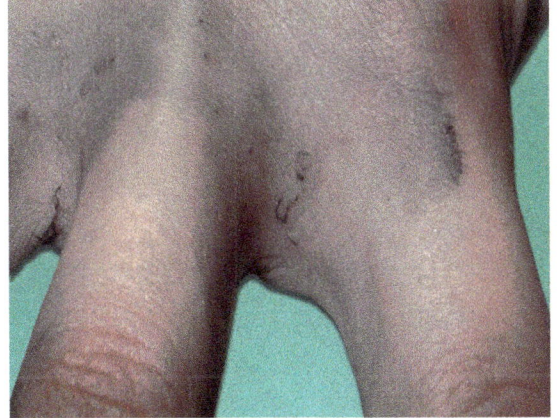

Fig. 6: After inking, a small, thread-like burrow is easily visualized in the web-space.

a gloved hand; a 15-degree tilt will allow the drop to descend across the back of the hand due to the effects of gravity.

"Materials to perform Scabies Preparations"

- #15 scalpel blade (small curette optional)
- Mineral oil
- Glass slide and cover slip
- Rubbing alcohol
- Microscope.

RECOMMENDED PROCEDURE

- Blue or black ink and water mixture is applied with a cotton-tipped applicator liberally over commonly affected areas demonstrating rashing, focusing especially on the finger webs, wrists (palms/soles in young children), hypothenar eminence, axillary folds, and peri-umbilical areas as these often provide the best results.[21] When patients can direct the health care provider to the areas which have most recently become itchy, intact, nonexcoriated burrows are more likely to be found. Warn the patient that slight darkening of ink-treated areas may persist for a few days despite cleaning off the ink with alcohol.
- Try to get enough ink onto the skin so that a small puddle is formed. Avoid the temptation to ink only skin with active inflammation; instead focus on seemingly lesion-free skin adjacent to these areas since the burrows may be found up to a centimeter or two away from papules and vesicles (Fig. 5). The ink is left in place for 20–30 seconds to allow it to be pulled into the burrow by capillary action.
- Alcohol wipes and gauze are used to remove ink from the skin's surface, leaving behind ink that has seeped into and highlighted burrows. An important point is that burrows are not distinguishable from the background of inked skin until wiping with alcohol provides the contrast necessary to appreciate them. Most often, a burrow is found in the first three or four sample areas, but occasionally a more extensive search is necessary. Of note, inked burrows are less obvious in Fitzpatrick V or VI skin, but the BIT is still valuable in many cases.

Burrows appear as slightly elevated, thread-like, zig-zagged structures on the skin's surface, some of which may have small holes in their roofs produced by larvae that have pierced through after hatching within.[15] Inked lesions may range from as small as 1 millimeter to several centimeters.[15] A helpful distinction between scabietic burrows and excoriations is that the burrows cross skin lines and typically are not linear (Fig. 6). In most cases, an ink-filled burrow is readily apparent and discernible from any other structure one might otherwise find in the skin.

> Ink-stained burrows are more easily visualized

Special attention should be paid to the ends of the burrow; one end may have a round, discrete dot that appears deeper in the skin than the rest of

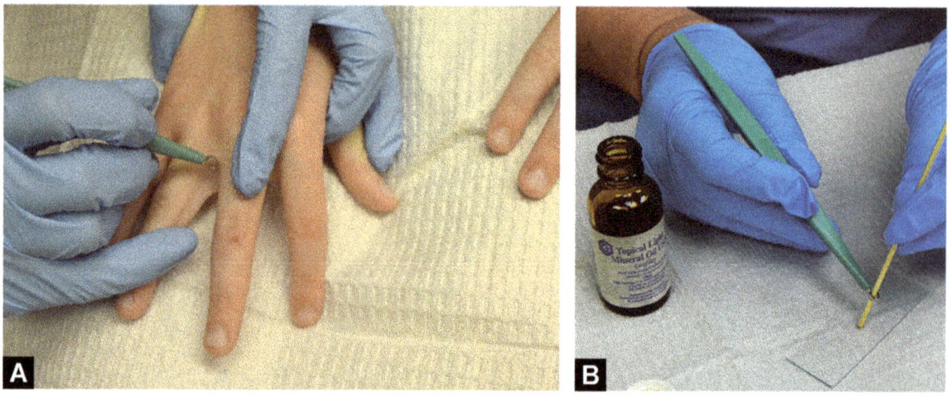

Figs. 7A and B: Instead of a scalpel blade, a 3 mm disposable curette may be utilized in children. Insert wood end of Q-tip to remove epidermis from curette onto a small drop of oil on the slide.
Courtesy: Stephanie Jacks, MD.

the burrow. This is the mite itself.[16] Dermoscopy is used by some clinicians to identify the burrows and contents.[24]

• A drop of oil is placed on the skin over an ink-filled burrow with a Q-tip or applied gently with a moistened piece of gauze.

• Multiple burrows are "scraped," collecting oil, scale, and debris for inspection later. A No. 15 scalpel blade is used to unroof the stratum corneum above the burrow removing its contents. It may be necessary to "scrape" several times to remove portions of epidermis and obtain adequate debris. Minute bleeding may occur when the epidermis is denuded and blood vessels in the papillary dermis are penetrated, however, since burrows are formed in the outermost layer of the epidermis, in the stratum corneum, scraping deeply is unnecessary and will not improve yield. Patients should experience only minor discomfort. Avoid scraping vesicles and excoriations since these lesions are historically "low-yield,"[15] and increasing the risk of secondary bacterial infection of opened vesicles is unnecessary. Skipping the first three steps outlined above and scraping the skin for mites without the guide of the BIT has a lower yield.

In the presence of children, the word "tickle" or rub is used instead of the frightening word "scrape" to explain the procedure. Special care must be taken to restrain children to prevent a quick movement that could lead to a laceration. Instead of a scalpel blade, a 3 mm disposable curette may be utilized with a gentle scooping motion. After scooping a thin layer of epidermis the material inside the curette may be placed onto the slide containing a drop of mineral oil by inserting the wood end of a Q-tip through the curette. This provides a safer option in pediatric patients who sometimes move without warning (Figs. 7A and B).[25] This also reduces anxiety experienced by children and their mothers when a scalpel blade is used.[25]

Oil and debris are collected onto a glass slide, covered with a cover slip, and observed initially under a scanning power moving to higher power to confirm positive findings. *Sarcoptes scabiei* mites have eight total legs, a set of two anterior legs on both sides of a clearly visible head at the rostral end and four legs at the caudal end (Fig. 8). The female scabies mite is 0.33–0.40 mm long and the male mite is half this size.[18] Some experience is required to interpret variations in the appearance of scabies mites under magnification. The "scraping" process can distort its appearance, and dead or decomposing mites begin to lose some of their features. Familiarity with the mite's appearance can also help one appreciate a portion of the mite if the rest of it has been cut away. Eggs appear as smooth, brown ovals, and scybala (feces) appear as dark, round, clustered structures that are roughly one-tenth the size of an egg (Fig. 9). Newly hatched nymphs are about the size of an egg.[20] Identification of the mite and its products is not difficult since they vary significantly in appearance from other structures normally found in the skin, but it is possible for scale or skin

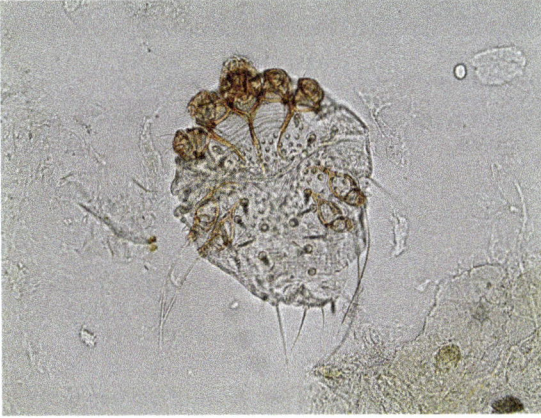

Fig. 8: A scabies mite visualized in an oil prep (100X).

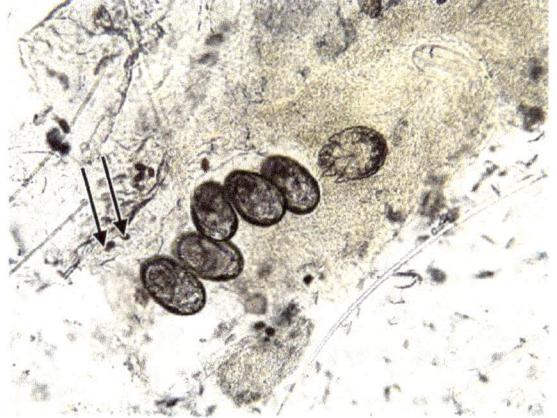

Fig. 9: A scabies mite, eggs and scybala (arrows) are demonstrated in this oil prep (40X).

debris to cover the mite from view. It is important to carefully scan the entire field at a lower power for evidence of infestation.

> Scrapings may reveal mites, eggs and/or feces

Sometimes no BIT-positive lesions can be identified in patients where there is a high index of suspicion for scabies despite a diligent search. In such cases, a scraping of nonspecific lesions in high-yield areas like the wrists, upper medial buttocks, periumbilical area, and finger webs will sometimes produce a mite, egg, or feces.

Special Sites

Subungual areas: In patients with clinical evidence of scabies, subungual scaling should always be sampled. This area commonly harbors mites.[26]

Scabietic nodules: The mite at the center of these nodules may be intradermal and, therefore, "scraping" these lesions may be less likely to produce a mite when compared to scraping burrows.[27] A punch biopsy can be helpful here, but it may be necessary to examine many sections before a mite is identified.[27]

Scaling plaques of crusted scabies: Inking crusted scabies is not necessary. These plaques contain hundreds and thousands of mites that are easily identified in a scraping after oil application.

Diagnosis Leads to Preventive Measures and Treatment

Once the definitive diagnosis has been made, the patient and family must understand the impor-

tance of treating close contacts and household members who may also be infested. Effective treatment is dependent on simultaneous elimination of the mites in all contacts through concurrent treatment, even if symptoms are not present in all household contacts.[28] Bedding, clothing, etc. should be washed with hot water and machine-dried using the hot cycle. Materials that would require dry cleaning may be quarantined in plastic bags for 5–10 days to avoid the expense of professional dry-cleaning. Scabies mites are not expected to live away from human skin for more than several days, and fumigation of the home is not necessary.[29] Treatment is summarized in Table 1.[30-36]

BENEFITS COMPARED TO ALTERNATIVE APPROACHES

In 1981, Woodley et al. published their work assessing the diagnostic validity of the BIT. They found at least one positive BIT lesion in all subjects, though thorough searching up to 30 minutes was occasionally required. In addition, microscopic evidence of scabietic infestation was present in 100% of BIT-positive lesions, thus formally confirming the diagnostic utility of the test in their hands.[15] Although some dermatologists believe a positive BIT is sufficient evidence for the diagnosis of scabies, a certain diagnosis rests on demonstrating a mite or its products using a microscope. The BIT guides the physician to the best area to find evidence of infestation. Thus, BIT plus scrap-

Table 1: Treatment of scabies.

Drug	Classic scabies[12,29]	Crusted scabies recommendation 1[12]	Crusted scabies recommendation 2[29]
5% Permethrin cream	Apply cream to entire body surface and leave on for 8–14 hours (i.e. apply at bedtime and wash off in morning). Repeat above treatment 8–14 days later.	Apply cream every 2–3 days for 1–2 weeks	Apply cream daily for 7 days, then twice weekly until resolution of rash. May substitute 5% benzoyl benzoate cream
Oral Ivermectin* (not recommended for pregnant women or children <15 kg)[29,35]	200 µg/kg with food, another dose 8–15 days later	200 µg/kg/dose for 3 doses (days 1,2,8), 5 doses (add days 9 and 15), or 7 doses (days 22 and 29) depending on severity	200 µg/kg/dose for 5 doses (days 1, 2, 8, 9 and 15) or 7 doses (add days 22 and 29)
Comments	A thin vinyl or rubber glove makes application of cream easier. Two doses of oral ivermectin given a week apart have similar efficacy as a single application of permethrin, though symptoms of infestation resolve quicker in those treated with permethrin cream.[36]		

*Not currently FDA-approved for treatment of scabies.

ing and microscopic examination represents a simple, low cost bedside test which utilizes readily available equipment with immediate confirmation of the diagnosis.

Dermoscopy has also been studied to determine its utility in the diagnosis of scabies. The "delta glider-shaped" dark anterior portion of the mite in vivo can be visualized with reported sensitivities of 83–91% and specificities of 46–86%.[24,30] The vast majority of dermatology residents are now trained in using dermoscopy,[31] though the novice dermoscopist will of course be less successful in accurately identifying a mite in vivo.[24] While the gold standard of diagnosis remains demonstrating evidence of infestation using a microscope, dermoscopy in experienced hands may be an especially useful tool in resource poor areas where a microscope is not available.[30] Thus, the best use of dermoscopy is to direct the clinician to likely locations where a scabies preparation can be performed to make a definitive diagnosis.

Dermoscopy may have special utility in skin of color. Some studies have suggested it is difficult or impossible to detect dark-appearing mites in pigmented skin. Other authors claim the efficacy of dermoscopy is unimpeded by pigmented skin.[24,32]

There are several significant disadvantages of dermoscopy. False positive results can occur when debris, scabs, excoriations, or specs of blood are confused for mites. In addition, the dermoscopy device necessitates the observer's eyes be in close proximity to the patient's skin and presents challenges to patient and physician comfort and modesty when lesions are near the genitals. Finally, careful disinfection of dermoscopy devices is required to avoid dissemination of infestation among subsequent patients.

> Histopathologic examination of a biopsy specimen often does not reveal the scabies mites or burrows that are necessary for a definitive diagnosis of scabies.

Though a shave or punch biopsy in patients with scabies will provide evidence of a hypersensitivity phenomenon, it is not possible to distinguish scabies from other insect bites, allergic contact dermatitis, spongiotic drug eruption and eczematous forms of pemphigoid unless mites or burrows are visualized in the tissue examined. Since many patients with scabies may only have a dozen mites or less over their entire cutaneous surface, the potential of identifying a mite in a 4 micron section of skin is small. In addition, biopsy procedures are more expensive, more painful, take additional time to perform, and there is an inherent delay in diagnosis equal to the time required to deliver the specimen to the laboratory, prepare a hematoxylin and eosin stain (H&E) slide, and have it examined by a dermatopathologist.

RISKS AND LIMITATIONS

Two recent reviews of diagnostic standards for diagnosing scabies have omitted the BIT, an important portion of the scabies preparation discussed in this chapter. One review suggested that the sensitivity and specificity for BIT could not be calculated from the Woodley 1981 study because it was not known whether all patients in the study had BIT-positive lesions, when in fact the Woodley 1981 paper reported "at least one BIT-positive lesion in all of the subjects."[15,33] Another study did not include BIT because of the difficulty identifying a burrow in pigmented skin and citing Katsumata and Katsumata 2006 as reporting that a burrow is not necessarily inhabited by a mite.[30,34] The Katsumata article does not concern the presence or absence of mites in burrows; in fact, the word "burrow" is not even used in their article. It is unfortunate these studies did not include the BIT because in our hands it increases the yield of skin scrapings. The results reported for skin scraping in studies not using BIT are skewed when the yield is not maximized. As a result, there are no side-by-side statistical studies evaluating the efficacy of the BIT directed scabies preparation compared to other proposed methods for diagnosing scabies. Additionally, recognizing that a prolonged search and repeated "scrapings" may be required to make a definitive diagnosis, some cases reported to be negative for scabies may be false negatives.

Conflict of Interest

Ira Harber, Kathleen Casamiquela, and Stephen Helms have no conflicts of interest. There was no financial support for the preparation of this manuscript.

REFERENCES

1. Lane JE. Bonomo's letter to Redi: important document in the history of scabies. Arch Dermatol Syph. 1928;18:1-25.
2. Richey HK, Fenske NA, Cohen LE. Scabies: diagnosis and management. Hosp Pract [Off] 1986; 21:124A-C,H,K-L.
3. Shelley WB, Shelley ED. Scanning electron microscopy of the scabies burrow and its contents, with special reference to the *Sarcoptes scabiei* egg. J Am Acad Dermatol. 1983;9:673-9.
4. Shelley WB, Wood MG. Larval papule as a sign of scabies. JAMA 1976;236:1144-5.
5. Gurevitch AW. Scabies and lice. Pediatr Clin North Am. 1985;32:987-1018.
6. Conley BE. Toxic effects of technical benzene hexachloride and its principle isomers. JAMA. 1951; 147:571-4.
7. Alexander JO. Scabies in children. Clin Pediatr. 1969;8:73-85.
8. Ackerman AB, Stewart R, Stillman M. Scabies masquerading as dermatitis herpetiformis. JAMA. 1975;233:53-4.
9. Orkin M, Maibach HI. Current concepts in parasitology. This scabies epidemic. N Engl J Med. 1978;298:496-8.
10. Chosidow O. Scabies and pediculosis. Lancet. 2000;355:819-26.
11. Degelau J. Scabies in long-term care facilities. Infect Control Hosp Epidemiol. 1992;13:421-5.
12. Currie BJ, McCarthy JS. Permethrin and ivermectin for scabies. N Engl J Med. 2010;362:717-25.
13. Walton SF, Oprescu FI. Immunology of scabies and translational outcomes: identifying the missing links. Curr Opin Infect Dis. 2013;26:116-22.
14. Walton SF. The immunology of susceptibility and resistance to scabies. Parasite Immunol. 2010; 32:532-40.
15. Woodley D, Saurat JH. The burrow ink test and the scabies mite. J Am Acad Dermatol. 1981;4:715-22.
16. Hebra F. Traité des maladies de la peau. In: Traduit et annoté par (Doyon A). Paris: Victor Masson et Fils; 1869.pp. 588-681.
17. Johnson CG, Mellanby K. The parasitology of human scabies. Parasitology. 1942;34:285-94.
18. Heilesen B. Studies on acarus scabie and scabies. Acta Derm Venereol. 1946;26:1-370.
19. Sehgal VN, Rao TL, Rege VL, et al. Scabies: a study of incidence and a treatment method. Int J Dermatol. 1972;11:106-11.
20. Martin WE, Wheeler CE Jr. Diagnosis of human scabies by epidermal shave biopsy. J Am Acad Dermatol. 1979;1:335-7.
21. Brodell RT, Helms SE. Office dermatologic testing: the scabies preparation. Am Fam Phys. 1991; 44:505-8.
22. Feldman YM, Nikitas JA. Scabies. Cutis. 1984; 33; 266,270-4,284.
23. Taplin D, Meinking TL, Porcelain SL, et al. Permethrin 5% dermal cream: a new treatment for scabies. J Am Acad Dermatol. 1986;15(5 Pt 1):995-1001.
24. Dupuy A, Dehen L, Bourrat E, et al. Accuracy of standard dermoscopy for diagnosing scabies. J Am Acad Dermatol. 2007;56:1:53-62.
25. Jacks SK, Lewis EA, Witman PM. The curette prep: a modification of the traditional scabies preparation. Pediatr Dermatol. 2012;29:544-5.
26. Witkowski JA, Parish LC. Scabies. Subungual areas harbor mites. JAMA. 1984;252:1318-9.

27. Tesner B, Williams NO, Brodell RT. The patho-physiologic basis of scabietic nodules. J Am Acad Dermatol. 2007;57:S56-7.

28. Chambliss ML. Treating asymptomatic bodily contacts of patients with scabies. Arch Fam Med. 2000;9:473-4.

29. Workowski KA, Bolan GA, Gail A. Sexually transmitted diseases treatment guidelines, 2015. MMWR Recomm Rep. 2015;64:1-137.

30. Walter B, Heukelbach J, Fengler G, et al. Comparison of dermoscopy, skin scraping, and the adhesive tape test for the diagnosis of scabies in a resource-poor setting. Arch Dermatol. 2011; 147:468-73.

31. Marghoob AA. Current status of dermoscopy in the diagnosis of dermatologic disease. J Am Acad Dermatol. 2013;69:814-5.

32. Feldmeier H. Diagnosis of parasitic skin diseases. In: Maibach H, Gorouhni F (Eds). Evidence-Based Dermatology, 2nd edition. Oak Park, IL: PMPH-USA; 2010.

33. Leung V, Miller M. Detection of scabies: A systematic review of diagnostic methods. Can J Infect Dis Med Microbiol. 2011;22:143-6.

34. Katsumata K, Katsumata K. Simple method of detecting *Sarcoptes scabiei var hominis* mites among bedridden elderly patients suffering from severe scabies infestation using adhesive tape. Intern Med. 2006;45:857-9.

35. Briggs GC, Freeman RK, Yaffe SJ. Drugs in Pregnancy and Lactation, 9th edition. Philadelphia, PA: Lippincott Williams & Wilkins; 2011.

36. Usha V, Gopalakrishna Nair TV. A comparative study of oral ivermectin and topical permethrin cream in the treatment of scabies. J Am Acad Dermatol. 2000;42:236-40.

CHAPTER 3

The Tzanck Preparation

Ashton B Davis, Maureen Offiah, Joy Fen King, Stephen E Helms

HISTORY

In 1947, French dermatologist, Arnault Tzanck (1886–1954), first described a technique to cytopathologically examine the walls and contents of blisters.[1] The "Tzanck smear" has since remained a reliable and useful tool in the evaluation of vesicular, bullous, erosive and pustular dermatoses (Figs. 1A to D) Although the most widely known application is in the evaluation and diagnosis of herpes virus infections, the Tzanck smear has been used in the evaluation of other categories of dermatologic diseases as listed in Table 1. Most studies, however, have focused on the diagnostic value of the Tzanck smear as it relates to herpetic infections, pemphigus, cutaneous leishmaniasis, and cutaneous neoplasms, especially basal cell carcinoma.[2]

PROCEDURE

The Tzanck preparation is a rapid and relatively simple test requiring little specialized equipment. The basic materials required include an alcohol swab, No. 15 scalpel blade, glass slide and coverslip, the stain of choice, syringe, immersion oil, and microscope.[3] Irrespective of the specific staining technique utilized, the step-by-step process of obtaining the sample is the same (Figs. 2A and B). This approach begins with identification of an intact primary lesion whenever possible or a noncrusted erosion, if no primary lesions are seen. Then, the area is gently cleansed with an alcohol swab.

> A better yield is obtained by scraping the floor and roof of an opened early vesicular primary lesion.

The vesicle, bulla or pustule is then unroofed and the base, roof, and sides scraped using either a No. 15 scalpel blade, tongue blade for young children or uncooperative patients or spatula in certain mucosal surfaces to avoid inadvertent laceration of the skin. However, it may be impossible to avoid a small amount of bleeding which should not inhibit the observation of blue staining nuclei in multinucleated giant cells. A thin layer of the resultant material is applied to a glass slide, and allowed to dry.

> Carefully unroof the lesion and scrape the base, roof, and sides with a #15 scalpel blade then apply fluid and material onto the slide. Minimal bleeding will not prevent visualization of the blue staining nuclei in multinucleated giant cells

The specimen is fixed with a preservative and then stained by one of the methods described below.

TECHNIQUES FOR STAINING AND FIXATION

The staining methods used for Tzanck preparation all stain nuclei blue. Three of these approaches are detailed in Table 2.[4-6]

> The modified test is easier, quicker, and utilizes fewer supplies than the traditional test.

The choice of stain depends on the sample, diagnostic possibilities, and tester preference. For a modified, quick Tzanck smear, Cyto Prep spray fixative and Sedi-Stain™ may be used. Most

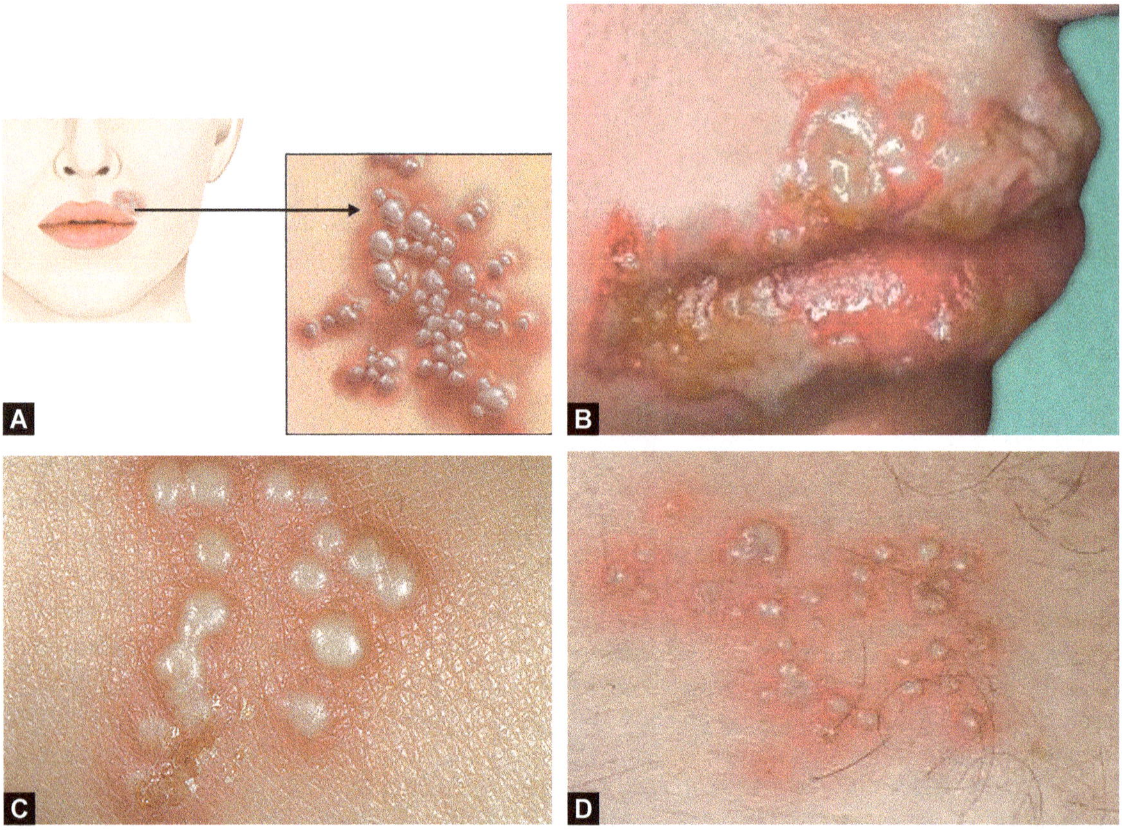

Figs. 1A to D: The evaluation of vesicular, bullous, erosive and pustular dermatoses. (A) herpes simplex vesicopustules; (B) herpes simplex of lips; (C) herpes-simplex cluster of vesicopustules; and (D) vesicopustules demonstrating delling or umbilication typical of viral lesions.

Table 1: Tzanck smear in dermatologic practice.
- Infectious diseases
- Spongiotic dermatitis
- Immune disorders
- Tumors
- Genodermatoses
- Pigmented skin lesions

commonly, 95% methanol, distilled water, and Giemsa, Wright's, or Hansel stains have been the chosen method. One of the simplest and most readily available stains is the Diff-Quik Differential Staining Set (American Scientific Products, McGaw Park, Ill.).

After staining, a drop of immersion oil is placed on the glass slide, which is then covered with a cover slip and viewed under the microscope.

UTILITY OF TZANCK SMEAR IN CYTODIAGNOSIS AND THE ASSOCIATED CYTOLOGICAL FINDINGS

A number of diseases that present with cutaneous lesions have specific cytological characteristics that can be demonstrated by a simple Tzanck smear. These cytological differences can aid a physician in narrowing a differential diagnosis, and, in some cases, making the diagnosis. Table 3 delineates the characteristic cytological findings that are diagnostic for or suggestive of the listed dermatological diseases.[2,7,8] The most important finding is the multinucleated giant cell seen in Herpes infections (Fig. 3) obtained from primary lesions as demonstrated by this immunocompromised patient with disseminated *H. zoster* when multiple diagnoses must be considered

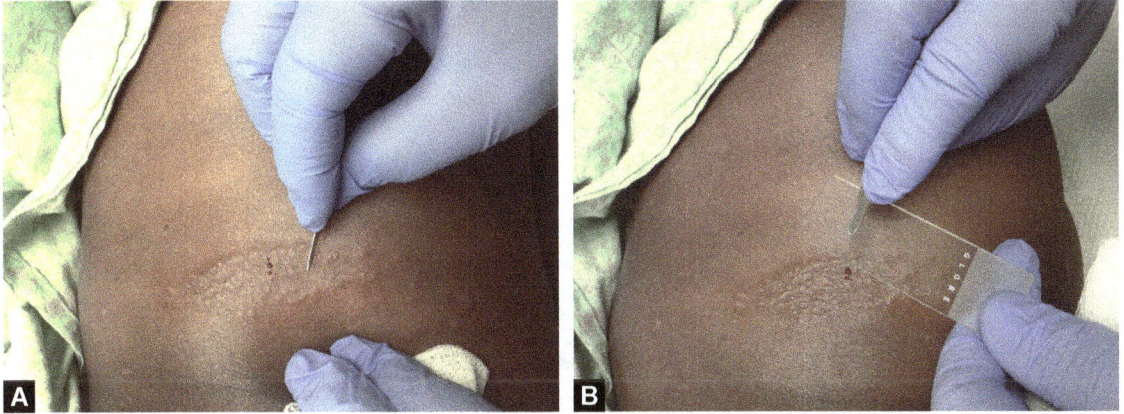

Figs. 2A and B: (A) Using universal precautions, a #15 blade is used to incise a blister or blisters then scraped across the affected area with the sharp edge "trailing" attempting to not lacerate the skin. However, as seen here, it is sometimes impossible to not nick the skin resulting in a small amount of superficial bleeding. (b) The material is horizontally applied in a thin smear onto a glass slide ready for fixation and staining.

Table 2: Tzanck preparation techniques.

- Modified Tzanck test:
  - Immediately fix with Cyto Prep and air dry 5–10 minutes.
  - Flood slide with Sedi-Stain for 30–60 seconds, rinse gently with tap water, and air dry.
- Routine staining:
  - Fix specimen by flooding slide with 95% methanol for 5 seconds, air dry 1–2 minutes.
  - Flood slide with nuclear stain (Wright's, May-Grünwald-Giemsa, or Hansel stain) 30–60 seconds.
  - Add distilled water to slide for 30 seconds, immediately flood with distilled water to remove any remaining stain.
  - Flood slide again with 95% methanol, if Hansel stain is used.
  - Air-dry without blotting.
- Diff-Quik:®
  - Allow material on the slide to air dry.
  - Apply several drops of Quik-Fix fixative for 5 seconds, allow to run off.
  - Apply Quik-Fix solution I for 5 seconds, allow to run off.
  - Apply Quik-Fix solution II for 3–5 seconds, carefully rinse slide with tap water.

Table 3: Typical cytological findings of various skin diseases.

Skin disease	Cytologic findings
Infectious diseases	
• Herpes simplex	Acantholytic and multinucleated giant cells
• Varicella zoster	
Molluscum contagiosum	Henderson-Patterson bodies
Hand-foot-mouth disease	Cells with syncytial nuclei
Orf	Guarnieri bodies
Bullous impetigo	Dyskeratotic, acantholytic cells and cocci
Staphylococcal scalded skin syndrome (SSSS)	Subcorneal cleavage with viable epidermis; normal sometimes acantholytic keratinocytes without inflammatory cells
Leprosy	Acid-fast bacilli
Tuberculosis	Acid-fast bacilli

Contd...

Contd...

Candidiasis	Pseudohyphae and spores
Aspergillosis	Septate hyphae with parallel walls, Dichotomous branching at 45° angle, and Aspergillus heads
Blastomycosis	Budding spores
Mucormycosis	Broad, nonseptate, ribbon-like, often distorted hyphae with nonparallel walls
Botryomycosis	Balls of coccal or bacillary bacterial colonies
Leishmaniasis (early stage only)	Leishman-Donovan bodies in "swarm of bees" pattern within cytoplasm of large macrophages
Spongiotic dermatitis	
Allergic contact dermatitis	Tadpole cells and lymphocyte predominance
Irritant contact dermatitis	Tadpole cells and neutrophil predominance
Immune disorders	
Pemphigus vulgaris, pemphigus foliaceus, and pemphigus herpetiformis	Acantholytic or "mourning-edged" or Tzanck cells; streptocytes; Sertoli rosettes
Bullous pemphigoid	Lack of acantholytic cells; eosinophils
Erythema multiforme	Absence of acantholytic cells; necrotic cells, leukocytes
Erosive lichen planus	Lack of acantholytic cells; nonspecific with leukocytes, fibrin filaments, altered or necrotic epitheliocytes and rare fibroblasts
Stevens-Johnson syndrome/Toxic epidermal necrolysis (TEN)	Lack of acantholytic cells; subepidermal splitting with full-thickness necrosis of epidermis; necrotic keratinocytes with lymphocytes and fibroblasts
Tumors	
Sebaceous adenoma	Groups of mature sebocytes with large cytoplasmic vacuoles, basal-type germinative cells, and transitional cells with only initial sebaceous differentiation
Mastocytoma	Mast cells with metachromatically stained, reddish purple, cytoplasmic granules
Basal cell carcinoma	Basaloid cells
Squamous cell carcinoma	Atypical squamous cells with dysplastic nuclei and irregularly stained cytoplasm
Erythroplasia of Queyrat	Poikilokaryosis, naked, and clumped nuclei
Paget disease	Paget cells (using special stains: mucicarmine and periodic acid-Schiff)
Histiocytosis X	Atypical Langerhans cells with microvacuolated or granular cytoplasm, and large, convoluted, reniform, indented nucleus
Genodermatoses	
Hailey-Hailey disease	Acantholytic cells with deeply stained nucleolated nucleus
Darier disease	Acantholytic, mantle cells and corps ronds and grains
Pigmented skin lesions	
Melanocytic	
Melanocytic nevi	Epidermal and dermal-type nevoid cells
Melanoma	Epithelioid or spindle-type atypical nevoid cells
Benign nonmelanocytic	
Seborrheic keratosis	Horny cysts, pigmented keratinocytes, hyperkeratosis
Warts	Koilocytes
Dermatofibroma	Spindle-shaped fibroblasts with collagenized stroma
Malignant nonmelanocytic	
Pigmented basal cell carcinoma	Clusters of basaloid cells containing pigment granules
Pigmented mammary Paget disease	Clusters of round to ovoid Paget cells
Metastatic carcinoma	Atypical (nonkeratinocytic and nonnevoid) cells

Fig. 3: This multinucleated giant cell was identified in a Tzanck preparation from a grouped-blister on the penis and confirmed the presence of a Herpes infection (H&E, 1000X). *Courtesy*: Thanks to Joy King, MD, and Elizabeth Chastain, MD, University of Mississippi, Department of Pathology for taking this photomicrograph.

Fig. 4: This 32-year-old immunocompromised patient presented with widespread erythematous papules and vesicles on the trunk and extremities. The differential diagnosis included erythema multiforme, blistering drug eruption, and disseminated Herpes simplex. Multinucleated giant cells were identified on Tzanck preparation and systemic antivirals were started immediately. Herpes polymerase chain reaction (PCR) studies confirmed the diagnosis of Herpes simplex the next day.

in the differential diagnosis (Fig. 4). The presence of multinucleated giant cells within intact vesicles and attached to the vesicle floor and roof in hematoxylin and eosin-stained sections

(Figs. 5A to C) demonstrates why this technique yields multinucleated giant cells in Tzanck preparations of herpetic blisters.

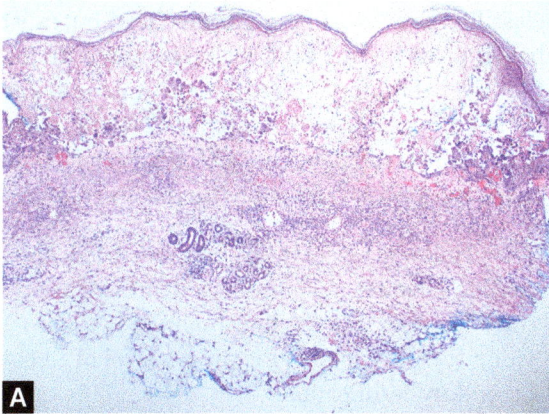

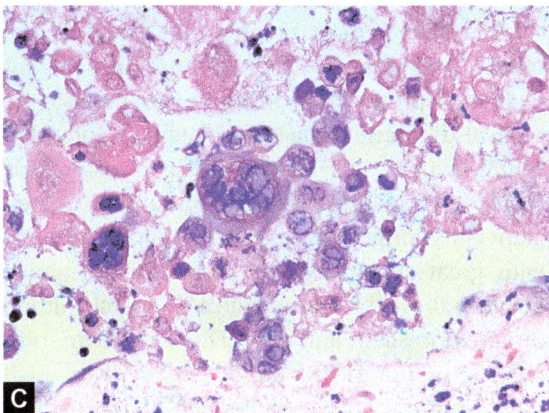

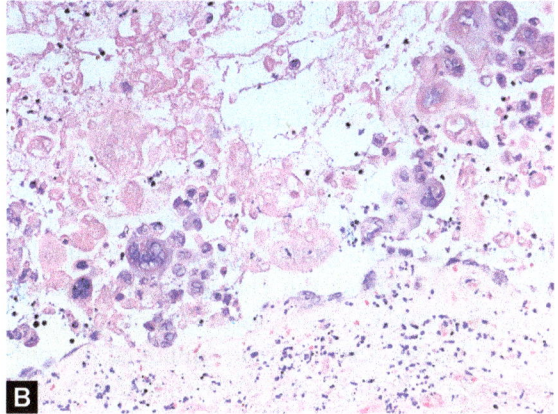

Figs. 5A to C: An intraepidermal blister shows inflammatory cells within the blister fluid (H&E, 40X); (B) One edge of the blister shows several multinucleated giant cells at the floor of the blister and within the blister fluid (H&E, 100X); and (C) A closer view shows multinucleated giant cells and the classic steel-gray coloration and margination of chromatin around the periphery of keratinocyte nuclei (H&E, 400X).

USING TZANCK SMEAR TO NARROW A DIFFERENTIAL DIAGNOSIS

While the Tzanck findings of the numerous conditions listed above have been reported, the clinical utility of the Tzanck preparation is focused on distinguishing between several pairs of diagnoses that are clinically similar. For instance, the presence of necrotic keratinocytes on Tzanck smear in toxic epidermal necrolysis (TEN) could distinguish it from staphylococcal scalded skin syndrome (SSSS). More commonly, however, a frozen section of a punch biopsy specimen might be chosen to show the characteristic subcorneal cleavage with a viable appearing epidermis and no inflammatory cells in SSSS versus the subepidermal splitting with full-thickness necrosis of the epidermis in TEN[2]. Similarly, the Tzanck smear can be helpful in confirming a diagnosis of oral pemphigus vulgaris that shows acantholytic cells and differentiates it from bullous pemphigoid, erosive lichen planus, and Stevens-Johnson syndrome all of which may mimic oral pemphigus clinically.[9] In the same manner, Hailey-Hailey disease demonstrates acantholytic cells on Tzanck preparations and can be helpful when considering flexural irritant or allergic contact dermatitis, flexural psoriasis, or intertrigo in the clinical differential diagnosis.[9]

The most common use of the Tzanck preparation, however, is in distinguishing herpes infections from other blistering processes. This is accomplished by identifying the classic multinucleated giant cells (MGC) of herpes infections. Disseminated herpes zoster or disseminated herpes simplex requires immediate systemic antiviral treatment, but the clinical differential diagnosis includes drug eruptions, erythema multiforme, and perhaps graft-vs-host disease. MGCs are visible in biopsy specimens attached to the roof or floor of the blister, and within the blister fluid. This is why they are so easily obtained with appropriate sampling in a Tzanck Prep.

BENEFITS COMPARED TO ALTERNATIVE APPROACHES

There are several benefits of performing a Tzanck smear in comparison to other alternative procedures. The Tzanck smear is a quick and simple test, requiring little specialized equipment. Another significant benefit of the Tzanck smear is that it is a relatively inexpensive test. Because it is superficial and noninvasive, a Tzanck smear is especially well tolerated by most patients, producing little patient discomfort. For this same reason, a simple Tzanck smear is more likely to be tolerated by children. A Tzanck smear may also be preferred over a biopsy in more sensitive areas, such as the lips, oral mucosa and genitalia. Cosmetically, results are more esthetically pleasing to patients. A typical Tzanck smear takes no more than 25–30 minutes to perform, making for a faster diagnosis and therefore an earlier initiation of treatment. A biopsy may be relatively quick and easy to perform but the specimen would require much more time to process in the laboratory than the Tzanck smear.

RISKS AND LIMITATIONS

There may be a slight risk of bleeding and discomfort, but this is rare. An important limitation of the Tzanck smear is that in the United States, it is not classified as a "provider performed test" but must be performed only by those who comply with the Clinical Laboratory Improvement Amendments of 1988 (CLIA '88), which establish the minimum performance standards for all laboratory testing, including specific regulations for quality control.[10]

> A specimen may safely be collected, dried, and fixed in the office then processed through a certified laboratory in a timely manner, Wif a provider does not possess the proper level of CLIA laboratory certification.

The Tzanck preparation is not useful in certain clinical situations. For instance, in a patient with widespread "dew drops on rose petals", the clinical differential diagnosis might include disseminated HSV-1, HSV-2 or varicella zoster virus (chickenpox). The presence of multinucleated giant cells confirms that a herpes virus is present with great specificity but does not distinguish between these three possibilites.[9,11] A viral culture, direct fluorescent antibody (DFA) or polymerase chain reaction (PCR) study would distinguish these entities.[9] Of these, the DFA or PCR results may be available within hours depending upon the ability of your laboratory to receive the specimen and perform the test. The diagnostic utility of the Tzanck smear is also influenced by the stage of the lesion. A newly erupted, intact vesicle is more likely to result in a positive Tzanck smear than an eroded or crusted ulcer.[12] Finally, the sensitivity and specificity of the Tzanck smear is dependent upon the skill of the health care provider at the bedside or the pathologist reading the test. Errors can occur in the preparation of the slide or interpretation of the cytology.

CONCLUSION

While cytodiagnosis is not a substitute for histopathology, viral cultures, PCR and other standard diagnostic techniques, it does represent a practical, simple, quick, and reliable method to establish a precise preliminary clinical diagnosis in certain skin conditions.[13] It is relatively inexpensive and rarely causes any discomfort to the patient. It is ideal when a rapid diagnosis is required and in instances where a skin biopsy is not easily performed, e.g. in newborns, infants or very young children, where anatomic locations are limited, or where esthetic issues may arise. The tips and tricks in this chapter increase the reliability of the Tzanck smear in arriving at an accurate diagnosis.

Conflict of Interest

Ira Harber, Kathleen Casamiquela, and Stephen Helms have no conflicts of interest. There was no financial support for the preparation of this manuscript.

REFERENCES

1. Schneider WH. Pioneers and Pathfinders: Arnault Tzanck (1886–1954). Transfus Med Rev. 2010;24(2):147-50.
2. Durdu M, Baba M, Seçkin D. The value of Tzanck smear test in diagnosis of erosive, vesicular, bullous, and pustular skin lesions. J Am Acad Dermatol. 2008;59(6):958-64.
3. Bolognia JL, Jorizzo JL, Schaffer JV (Eds). Dermatology, 3rd edition. Philadelphia (PA): Elsevier Limited; 2012. pp. 1345-65.
4. Olansky AJ. A better stain for Tzanck smears. Am Acad Dermatol. 1983;8(6):908.
5. Goldstein BG, Goldstein AO. Dermatologic procedures. In: Post TW (Ed). UpToDate. Waltham, MA: UpToDate Inc; 2016. p. 81.
6. Brodell RT, Helms SE, Devine M. Office Dermatologic Testing: The Tzanck Preparation. Am Fam Phys. 1991;44(3):857-60.
7. Durdu M, Baba M, Seçkin D. More experiences with the Tzanck smear test: Cytologic findings in cutaneous granulomatous disorders. Am Acad Dermatol. 2009;61(3):441-50.
8. Durdu M, Baba M, Seçkin D. Dermatoscopy versus Tzanck smear test: A comparison of the value of two tests in the diagnosis of pigmented skin lesions. Am Acad Dermatol. 2011;65(5):972-82.
9. Ruocco E, Baroni A, Donnarumma G, et al. Diagnostic Procedures in Dermatology. Clin Dermatol. 2011;29:548-56.
10. US Department of Health and Human Services. Medicare, Medicaid and CLIA programs: Regulations implementing the Clinical Laboratory Improvement Amendments of 1988 (CLIA). Final rule. Fed Regist. 1992;57:7002-186.
11. James WD, Berger TG, Elston DM (Eds). Andrews' Diseases of the Skin, 11th edition. Philadelphia (PA): Elsevier; 2011. pp. 359-417.
12. Gupta LK, Singhi MK. Tzanck Smear: A useful Diagnostic Tool. Indian J Dermatol Venereol Leprol. 2005;71:295-9.
13. Ruocco V, Ruocco E. Tzanck smear, an old test for the new millennium: when and how. Int J Dermatol. 1999;38(11):830-4.

PART 1

Diagnostic Tips and Tricks

SECTION - B

Tips and Tricks:
Biopsy – The Right Spot!

—Jennifer Schulmeier, Caitlyn Reed

Biopsy Techniques in Dermatology: Maximizing Diagnostic Yield

Caitlyn Reed, Jennifer Schulmeier, Jeremy D Jackson, Robert T Brodell

> *"A skin biopsy of the right type from the right place will eventuate in the right histopathologic diagnosis"*
>
> —Robert T Brodell

HISTORY

The field of cutaneous surgery is continuously evolving as clinicians develop methods to accomplish therapeutic and diagnostic goals while minimizing cosmetic defects. Unfortunately, the laudable concern for cosmesis can have unintended consequences, including a tendency toward increasingly smaller biopsies which may be inadequate for pathologic interpretation.[1] In some cases, a specimen is not obtained from an optimal site or is not properly prepared at the bedside; and occasionally, clinicians provide historical information that is inadequate for proper clinical-pathologic correlation.[2] These shortcomings may result in everything from the dermatopathologist's request for additional tissue to a pathologic diagnosis that correlates poorly with the clinical presentation to a significant error in diagnosis.

> This chapter stresses the need for clinicians to "think pathologically."

This chapter stresses the need for clinicians to "think pathologically." For example, selection of the correct biopsy site is often directed by both a good working diagnosis and knowledge of the histopathology of the disease processes entertained. In some cases, bedside "grossing" maximizes the information that can be gleaned from a tissue specimen while minimizing harm to the patient. Providing the laboratory with an abstracted history and physical examination and any requests for special specimen handling will help ensure the best possible pathologic diagnosis.[3] We will discuss optimal biopsy sites for a few selected disease processes and some directed bedside biopsy and "grossing" techniques that will help lead to correct histopathologic diagnoses.

SUBEPIDERMAL BLISTERING DISEASES

Subepidermal blistering diseases include bullous pemphigoid (BP), epidermolysis bullosa acquisita (EBA), dermatitis herpetiformis (DH), linear IgA bullous dermatosis (LABD) and porphyria cutanea tarda (PCT). Each of these conditions presents with tense bullae.

Traditionally, the diagnosis of these conditions is confirmed by obtaining two punch biopsies: one from perilesional skin for direct immunofluorescence (DIF) and the other from lesional skin for hematoxylin and eosin (H&E) light microscopy.[4-6] A biopsy of perilesional skin is required because the epidermis must be attached for successful DIF studies.[7] A more efficient approach requires only one punch biopsy used for both H&E and DIF studies. This punch may be obtained in one of two ways (Figs. 1A to D), both methods yielding an ideal specimen for diagnosis.[8]

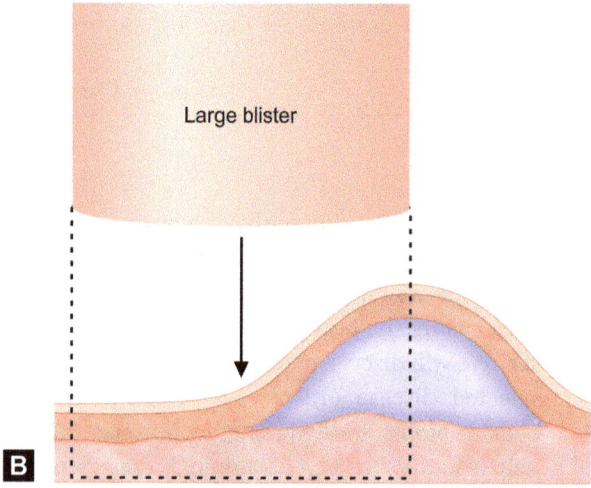

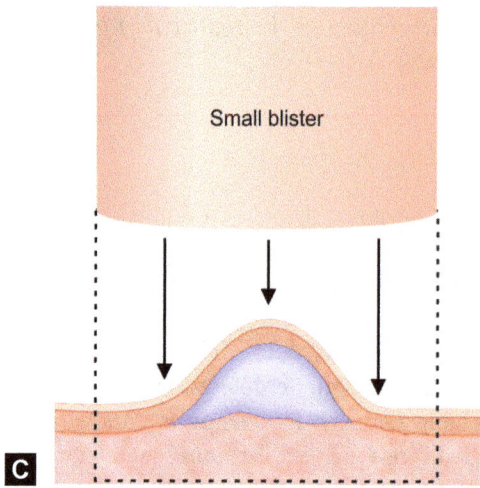

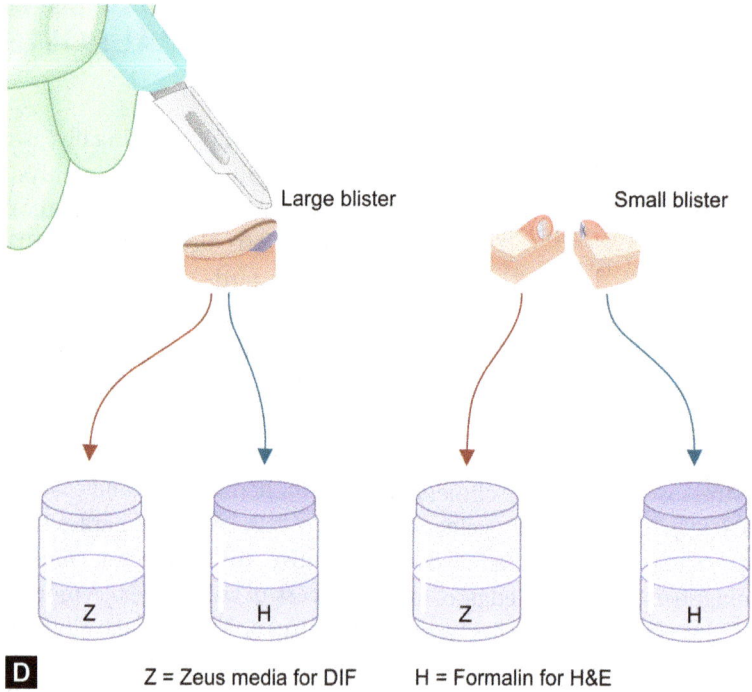

Figs. 1A to D: An efficient approach for obtaining maximal information from the biopsy of a tense blister.
Source: Adapted from reference 9.

A more efficient approach requires only one punch biopsy used for both H&E and DIF studies.

To biopsy an entire blister, choose a small 1–2 mm tense blister. Anesthetize the area with 1% lidocaine with epinephrine. Using an 8-mm punch, center the blister under the punch. This will include at least 3 mm of perilesional skin all the way around the blister. Using a number 15 blade and holding the specimen with a pair of forceps, bisect the specimen with a sawing motion.

For the second approach, any intact blister may be chosen. First clean the skin with an alcohol pad. Then draw a line from the apex of the blister onto the adjacent perilesional skin. Anesthetize the area with 1% lidocaine with epinephrine. Using an 8-mm punch, take a biopsy, centered on the line, to include 75% perilesional skin and 25% blister. Bisect the specimen along the line using a number 15 blade with a sawing motion, stabilizing the specimen with a pair of forceps.

With each technique, one-half of the specimens is submitted in formalin for H&E and one-half in Zeus (or Michel's) medium for DIF. If the selected blister is located in an area that may be difficult to close after a deep punch biopsy, such as the anterior shins, a saucerization biopsy may be preferable. The biopsy should still be taken to include the blister "take-off point" as well as perilesional skin, but there is no need to include subcutaneous tissue.

Including the "take-off point" of the blister in the DIF specimen makes it possible to determine if the immunoprecipitants are decorating the roof or on the floor of the blister. This provides much the same information as a "salt-split skin" specimen, without having to perform this additional, expensive procedure. Since perilesional skin is also included in the DIF specimen, the dermatopathologist will also distinguish immunoprecipitants at the dermoepidermal junction versus papillary dermis of nonblistered skin.[5,6]

ALOPECIA

Biopsies of the scalp are often performed for the evaluation of alopecia. Again, biopsy site selec-

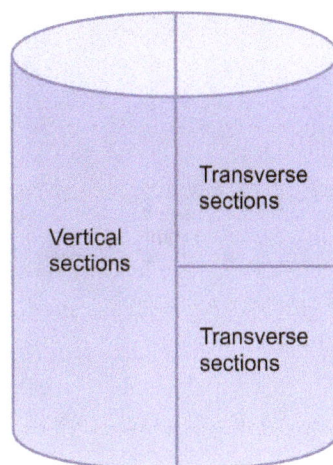

Fig. 2: The Tyler technique for efficient punch biopsy sampling of scalp alopecia.
Source: Adapted from reference 12.

tion is one of the most important steps in the process, though this is often challenging. While sampling the center of a lesion from a nonscarring process may yield helpful information, the active margin of a cicatricial alopecia usually is a better choice. Submission of two 4 mm punch biopsies, each extending into peribulbar fat, is recommended, so that one biopsy may be submitted for vertical sectioning, while the other is submitted for transverse sectioning.[9] The horizontal sections allow the pathologist to evaluate the density of hair follicles as well as the morphology of multiple follicles in a single section. For disease processes, such as lupus erythematosus (LE), vertical sections are ideal for evaluation of the dermoepidermal junction.[10]

Alternatively, there are two grossing techniques that allow both horizontal and vertical sections to be obtained from a single punch biopsy. The Tyler technique involves bisecting a punch biopsy vertically, then bisecting one of the two resulting halves transversely.[11] The vertical section is then submitted with the two transverse sections side-by-side in a single block with their new cut edges embedded down (Fig. 2). Each resulting slide level shows both progressively deeper and more superficial transverse sections alongside a vertical section. This technique is especially useful when the differential diagnosis includes entities that may require visualization

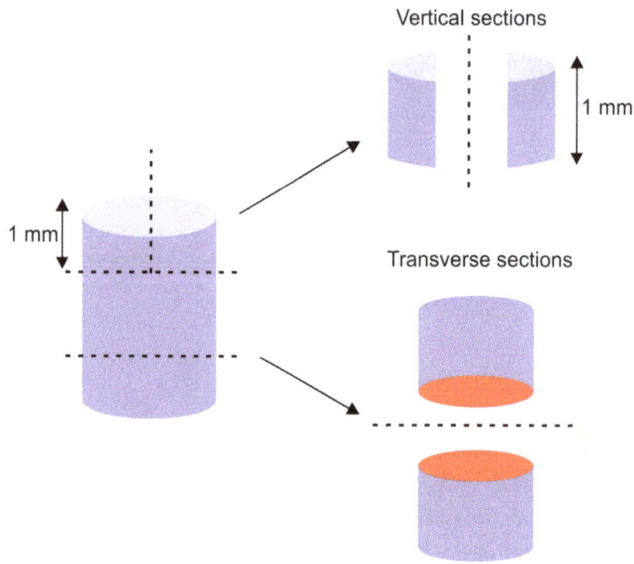

Fig. 3: The HoVert technique for efficient punch biopsy sampling of scalp alopecia.
Source: Adapted from reference 13.

of deep peribulbar fat as well as both vertical and transverse sections for diagnosis.

> There are two grossing techniques which allow both horizontal and vertical sections to be obtained from a single punch biopsy: the Tyler and HoVert techniques.

The HoVert technique of preparing a punch biopsy is a three-step process (Fig. 3).[12] First, the most superficial 1 mm of the punch is removed, creating an "epidermal disk". The deep surface of the epidermal disk is inked, then the disk is bisected vertically and embedded for vertical sectioning. One-half of the epidermal disk may also be submitted for DIF studies, if needed. The lower portion of the biopsy is then bisected or trisected transversely and submitted for transverse sectioning. This method allows for vertical sections of the epidermis and upper dermis along with transverse sections of the lower dermis and peribulbar fat while minimizing the number of biopsies required.

POROKERATOSIS

Porokeratosis is a condition characterized by a small keratotic papule that slowly expands, producing plaques up to several centimeters in dia-

meter.[13,14] Because variable, nonspecific findings (atrophy, acanthosis, verrucous hyperplasia, a lichenoid tissue reaction) are present at the centers of patches of porokeratosis, it is critical to appropriately biopsy the raised margin (cornoid lamella).[15]

A three-step technique ensures proper orientation of the punch biopsy to maximize the potential for a correct diagnosis (Figs. 4A to C).[16] First, after blotting the skin with an alcohol swab, a line is drawn with a skin marker across and perpendicular to the margin of the patch (cornoid lamella). Then, a 6 mm punch biopsy is performed centered on the intersection of the line and the cornoid lamella. Last, the biopsy is bisected at bedside along the skin marker line using a number 15 blade and a sawing motion. The requisition sheet should include instructions for the laboratory technician to embed the specimen with the cut surfaces down so that cross-sections of the cornoid lamella will be visible.

> A critical step in this process is bisecting the punch biopsy specimen at the bedside.

A critical step in this process is bisecting the punch biopsy specimen at the bedside. The clinician cannot depend upon the laboratory to pro-

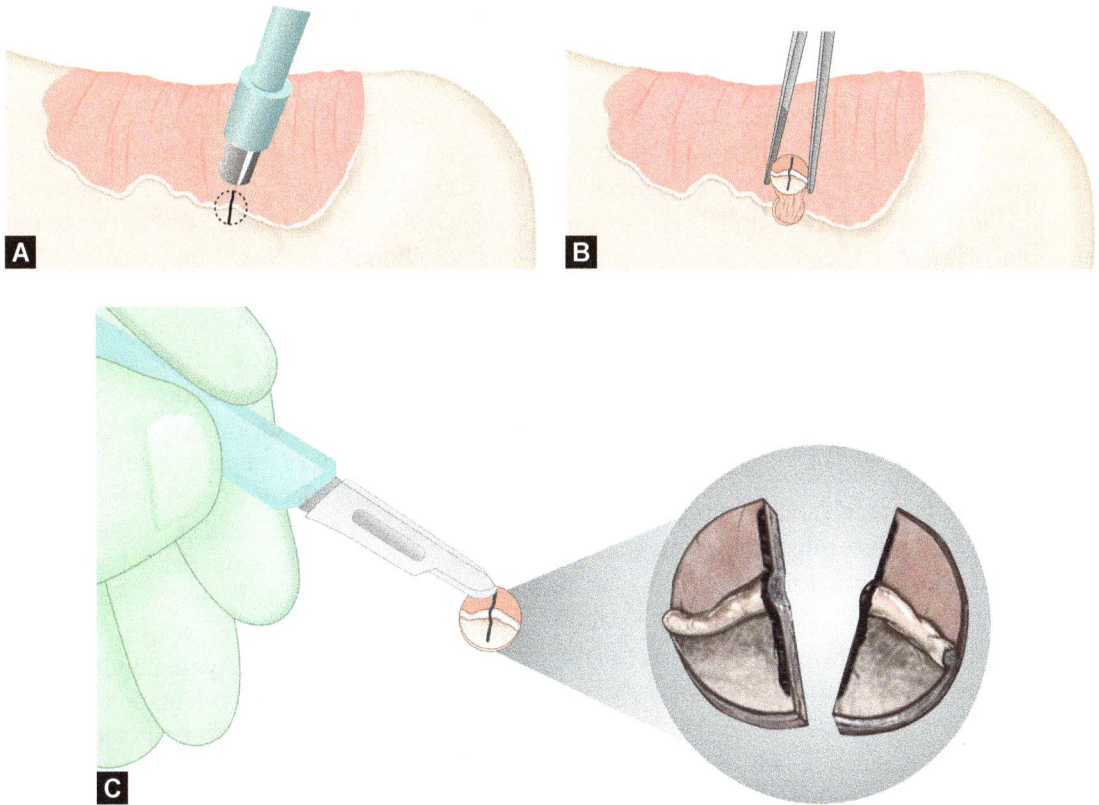

Figs. 4A to C: An efficient and effective approach to biopsy porokeratosis.
Source: Adapted from reference 17.

perly orient the punch specimen since it is likely the cornoid lamella will not be visible on the skin surface. Furthermore, a technician grossing the specimen may not be aware of the importance of properly oriented sectioning of the cornoid lamella.

DISCOID LUPUS

Lupus erythematosus is an autoimmune disease with myriad presentations affecting multiple organ systems. The disease may be limited to the skin, or it may lead to multiorgan dysfunction. Clinically, the disease is subdivided into systemic, subacute cutaneous, and discoid or chronic forms, each with its own characteristic skin manifestation. The diagnosis of systemic LE is made clinically, based on a well-established set of criteria.[10] However, the diagnosis of cutaneous LE may require the correlation of clinical findings with histopathology, occasionally with the aid of DIF.

Discoid LE is by far the most common form of cutaneous LE, representing up to 85% of cutaneous LE cases.[17] Classically, the lesions of discoid LE are well-circumscribed, erythematous plaques with thick, adherent scale and follicular plugging. Central scarring with hypopigmentation is characteristic of older lesions, while earlier lesions are erythematous due to active cutaneous inflammation.[18]

> The advancing margin of a scarred plaque is the optimal biopsy site for discoid LE.

The advancing margin of a scarred plaque is the optimal biopsy site for discoid LE.[19] This site is most likely to demonstrate active disease without nonspecific findings, such as scarring, which appear in the older, central areas of these lesions. Conversely, when submitting a specimen for DIF, the center of a scarred plaque will have the highest diagnostic yield, showing granular immunoglobulin G (IgG) deposition at the basement membrane.

PIGMENTED LESIONS OF THE PALM OR SOLE

Acral skin is distinct from other areas of the body. It is characterized by a thick and compact stratum corneum, numerous eccrine glands, and lack of pilosebaceous units.[20] It is also the only area of skin which contains dermatoglyphs. These distinctive features of acral skin lead to similarly distinctive patterns of pigment deposition in benign and malignant lesions.[21] Typical patterns of benign melanocytic nevi may be observed by dermoscopy and include: parallel-furrow pattern, lattice-like pattern, and fibrillar pattern.[22] These patterns result from melanocytic nests located in the furrows rather than ridges of dermatoglyphs. In contrast, malignant lesions, such as acral lentiginous melanoma, tend to exhibit a parallel-ridge pattern or irregular diffuse pigmentation with melanocytic nests at the ridges of dermatoglyphs.[23]

Because the distinction between benign and malignant acral pigmented lesions lies in visualization of melanocytic nests and their location relative to the ridges and furrows of dermatoglyphs, correct preparation of biopsies is essential. If the shave or saucerization biopsy is bisected longitudinally (parallel to dermatoglyphs) the histopathology is difficult to interpret. Subsequent sections may or may not be sufficient to view the location of nests. To ensure that the nests are present on histology in the correct orientation, the biopsy may be bisected at bedside perpendicular to the dermatoglyphs visualized dermatoscopically. The requisition should include a note to the histology technician that the specimen should be imbedded with the cut surfaces down.

BIOPSY OF OTHER CONDITIONS

A quick reference (Table 1)[24-26] includes the tips and tricks mentioned above and other recommended approaches organized by physical findings. These include suggestions for palpable purpura (possible leukocytoclastic vasculitis), subdermal nodules (possible panniculitis), pearly plaques (possible basal cell carcinoma), and crusted warty plaques (possible squamous cell carcinoma).

Benefits of Using these Biopsy Approaches

Conventionally, when submitting a biopsy for either subepidermal blistering disease or for alopecia, two biopsies were required. In the case of blistering diseases, perilesional skin and lesional skin ideally are inspected microscopically to make a diagnosis. For alopecias, both vertical and transverse sections may be needed. Alternative techniques which allow for all the required information to be obtained from a single biopsy which has several distinct advantages. First, a single biopsy can be performed more quickly in a busy outpatient setting. Second, a single biopsy offers a cosmetic advantage. Third, a single biopsy is more cost-effective since the patient is billed for only one biopsy instead of two.

In the case of porokeratosis or discoid LE, biopsy site selection is a key. Including the cornoid lamella in the correct orientation allows the diagnosis of porokeratosis to be made correctly virtually every time. If a biopsy is taken from the center of porokeratosis, or if it is not prepared correctly, the chances of making a correct histopathologic diagnosis are greatly reduced. Similarly, if a biopsy is taken from the center of a discoid LE plaque, H&E sections will show only nonspecific changes, while if the advancing margin is biopsied, active disease can be identified and the correct diagnosis made.

In all of the techniques presented in this chapter, "grossing" of the specimen is a key factor. Both the dermatologist taking the biopsy and the pathologist or technician preparing the specimen must know the steps and the correct orientation for imbedding the tissue. If the correct procedure is followed, the likelihood of making an accurate diagnosis is greatly increased.

Risks and Limitations of these Techniques

The main limitation associated with a new biopsy technique is incorrect handling of the specimen. Each specimen must be taken from the correct location, prepared in the correct way and embedded in the correct orientation. If any of these steps is performed incorrectly, the resultant

Table 1: Summary of skin biopsy tips and tricks.

Physical findings	Biopsy technique	Location	Comments
Tense blister	8 mm punch biopsy	Either an entire small (1–2 mm) blister or part of a large blister, including perilesional skin	See the above section
Flaccid blister	3 mm or 4 mm punch biopsy	Early, small blister	Take care to preserve the dermal-epidermal attachment; refrigerant spray may be used prior to biopsy[23]
Palpable purpura (possible leukocytoclastic vasculitis)	Deep punch biopsy including subcutaneous fat	Well-established lesion	A more acute lesion may be chosen for DIF evaluation[24]
Tender subdermal nodules (possible panniculitis)	Deep incisional biopsy or ≥6-mm punch biopsy	Nonulcerated area; subcutaneous fat must be included for the evaluation of panniculitis	If a necrotic focus is present, the edge of this focus should be submitted for culture and special stains
Scarred plaque	Punch biopsy	Active border of lesion for H&E; center of lesion for DIF, if LE is suspected	See the above section
Scarring alopecia	≥4 mm punch biopsy	Erythematous area with visible hair shafts	See above section; if an area of complete scarring is chosen, only nonspecific changes will be present on histopathology[25]
Nonscarring alopecia	≥4 mm punch biopsy	Established area for suspected telogen effluvium or pattern alopecia; newer area for suspected alopecia areata or syphilis[24]	See the above section; transverse sections are important in evaluating the anagen-to-telogen and terminal-to-vellus hair ratios[24]
Pearly eroded plaque (possible basal cell carcinoma)	Shave or punch biopsy	Entire lesion, if possible, or area without necrosis	A conservative excisional biopsy may be performed for evaluation of margins and invasion
Crusted warty plaque (possible squamous cell carcinoma)	Shave or punch biopsy	Entire lesion, if possible, or area without necrosis; if possible, sample base of lesion	A conservative excisional biopsy may be performed for evaluation of margins and possible invasive growth
Atypical pigmented lesion (possible melanoma)	Shave or saucerization	Entire lesion, if possible	A maximal view of the dermoepidermal junction aids in diagnosis and determination of Breslow depth requires sampling of the dermis below the lesion

(H&E: Hematoxylin and eosin; DIF: Direct immunofluorescence; LE: Lupus erythematosus).

histopathology may be nondiagnostic. Communication between all levels of providers—from the dermatologist to the laboratory technician to the dermatopathologist—is key.

Conflict of Interest

Robert T Brodell discloses the following potential conflicts of interest: honoraria have been received from presentations for Allergan, Galderma, and PharmaDerm, a division of Nycomed US Incorporation. Consultancy fees have been received from Galderma Laboratories, LP. Clinical trials have been performed for Genentech and Janssen Biotech, Incorporation. Jeremy Jeremy Jackson discloses the following potential conflicts of interest: honoraria have been received from presentations for Abbvie, Celgene, Actelion, and Sun Pharmaceuticals. Caitlyn Reed and Jennifer Schulmeier have no conflicts of interest.

REFERENCES

1. Fernandez EM, Helm T, Ioffreda M, et al. The vanishing biopsy: the trend toward smaller specimens. Cutis. 2005;76(5):335-9.
2. Comfere NI, Sokumbi O, Montori VM, et al. Provider-to-provider communication in dermatology

and implications of missing clinical information in skin biopsy requisition forms: a systematic review. Int J Dermatol. 2014;53(5):549-57.

3. Cockerell CJ. How can dermatologists help dermatopathologists work "smarter" for them? Cutis. 2015;95(4):190-1.

4. Mihai S, Sitaru C. Immunopathology and molecular diagnosis of autoimmune bullous diseases. J Cell Mol Med. 2007;11(3):462-81.

5. Yeh SW, Ahmed B, Sami N, et al. Blistering disorders: diagnosis and treatment. Dermatol Ther. 2003;16(3):214-23.

6. Habif TP. Vesicular and bullous diseases. In: Clinical Dermatology: A Color Guide to Diagnosis and Therapy, 5th edition. Edinburg, Scotland: Mosby; 2010. pp. 635-70.

7. High WA. Blistering diseases. In: Elston DM, Ferringer T (Eds). Requisites in Dermatology: Dermatopathology, 1st edition. Edinburgh, Scotland: Saunders-Elsevier; 2009. pp. 161-72.

8. Braswell MA, McCowan NK, Schulmeier JS, et al. High-yield biopsy technique for subepidermal blisters. Cutis. 2015;95(4):237-40.

9. Elston D, McCollough ML, Angeloni VL. Vertical and transverse sections of alopecia biopsy specimens: combining the two to maximize diagnostic yield. J Am Acad Dermatol. 1995;32(3):454-7.

10. Crowson AN, Magro C. The cutaneous pathology of lupus erythematosus: a review. J Cutan Pathol. 2001;28(1):1-23.

11. Elston D. The 'Tyler technique' for alopecia biopsies. J Cutan Pathol. 2012;39(2):306.

12. Nguyen JV, Hudacek K, Whitten JA, et al. The HoVert technique: a novel method for the sectioning of alopecia biopsies. J Cutan Pathol. 2011;38(5): 401-6.

13. Pierson D, Bandel C, Ehrig, et al. Benign epidermal tumors and proliferations. In: Bolognia J, Jorizzo J, Rapini R, Horn T, Mascaro J, Saurat J, Mancini A, Salasche S, Stingl G (Eds). Dermatology. Edinburgh, Scotland: Elsevier; 2003. pp. 1707-9.

14. Richard G, Irvine A, Traupe H, et al. Ichthyosis and disorders of other cornification. In: Schachenr L, Hansen R, Krafchik B, Lucky A, Paller A, Rogers M, Torrelo A (Eds). Pediatric Dermatology. Philadelphia, PA, USA: Elsevier; 2011. pp. 640-3.

15. De Simone C, Paradisi A, Massi G, et al. Giant verrucous porokeratosis of Mibelli mimicking psoriasis in a patient with psoriasis. J Am Acad Dermatol. 2007;57(4):665-8.

16. Reed C, Reddy R, Brodell RT. Diagnosing porokeratosis of Mibelli every time: a novel biopsy technique to maximize histopathologic confirmation. Cutis. 2016;97(3):188-90.

17. Bharti S, Dogra S, Saikia B, et al. Immunofluorescence profile of discoid lupus erythematosus. Indian J Pathol Microbiol. 2015;58(4):479-82.

18. Winfield H, Jaworsky C. Connective tissue diseases. In: Elder DE, Elenitas R, Murphy GF, Johnson BL, Xu X (Eds). Lever's Histopathology of the Skin, 10th edition. Philadelphia, PA, USA: Lippincott Williams & Watkins; 2009. pp. 329-64.

19. Sina B, Kao GF, Deng AC, et al. Skin biopsy for inflammatory and common neoplastic skin diseases: optimum time, best location and preferred techniques. A critical review. J Cutan Pathol. 2009; 36(5):505-10.

20. Lian CG, Murphy GF. Chapter 3. Histology of the skin. In: Elder DE, Elenitsas R, Rosenbach M, Murphy GF, Rubin AI, Xu X. Lever's Histopathology of the Skin, 11th edition. Philadelphia, PA, USA: Lippincott Williams & Wilkins; 2015. pp. 8-75.

21. Thomas L, Phan A, Pralong P, et al. Special locations dermoscopy: facial, acral, and nail. Derm Clin. 2013;31(4):615-24.

22. Saida T, Oguchi S, Ishihara Y. In vivo observation of magnified features of pigmented lesions on volar skin using videomicroscope: usefulness of epiluminescence technique in clinical diagnosis. Arch Dermatol. 1995;131:298-304.

23. Phan A, Dalle S, Touzet S, et al. Dermoscopic features o facral lentiginous melanoma in a large series of 110 cases in a white population. Br J Dermatol. 2010;162(4):765-71.

24. Wu H, Allan AE, Harrist TJ. Chapter 9. Noninfectious vesiculobullous and vesiculopustular diseases. In: Elder DE, Elenitsas R, Rosenbach M, Murphy GF, Rubin AI, Xu X. Lever's Histopathology of the Skin, 11th edition. Philadelphia, PA, USA: Lippincott Williams & Wilkins; 2015. pp. 276-328.

25. Elston DM, Stratman EJ, Miller SJ. Skin biopsy: Biopsy issues in specific diseases. J Am Acad Dermatol. 2016;74(1):1-16.

26. Elentsas R, Ming ME. Chapter 2. Biopsy techniques. In: Elder DE, Elenitsas R, Rosenbach M, Murphy GF, Rubin AI, Xu X. Lever's Histopathology of the Skin, 11th edition. Philadelphia, PA, USA: Lippincott Williams & Wilkins; 2015. pp. 6-7.

Diagnostic Tips and Tricks

SECTION - C

Tips and Tricks:
Basic Procedural Techniques

—*Michael T Cosulich*

CHAPTER 5

Shave and Saucerization Techniques

Lucette Teel Liddell, Michael T Cosulich, Anna Wile

HISTORY AND OVERVIEW

The shave biopsy is one of the most commonly utilized techniques by the dermatologist and primary care physicians. It is a simple procedure that can be performed rapidly. It samples the epidermis broadly and is primarily used to diagnose and eliminate epidermal proliferative processes, such as superficial skin cancers and exophytic benign lesions. Of course, shave procedures are not intended to sample the mid or deep dermis and are not appropriate for deep-seated lesions. For instance, a dermatofibroma is most commonly removed utilizing an elliptical excision or punch excision technique designed to completely remove the lesion. Excisional biopsy, however, is a more invasive and time-consuming procedure.

In the past, it has been suggested that pigmented lesions are removed by elliptical excision so that the lesion is not transected. This makes it difficult to accurately determine Breslow level if the lesion should prove to be an invasive melanoma.[1] Over the last 10 years, the variation of shave biopsy termed as "saucerization" biopsy has been accepted as an effective alternative to excisional biopsy for some pigmented lesions.[2] This approach provides acceptable cosmesis while avoiding unnecessarily invasive surgery.[3]

> The "saucerization" biopsy is an effective alternative to excisional biopsy for some pigmented lesions.

Initially proposed for biopsy of small, flat lesions no more than 1.5 cm in diameter, the saucerization or "scoop shave" provides an adequate histopathologic assessment of the horizontal architecture of the lesion as well as an intentionally deeper specimen than the traditional shave due to angulation of the blade at a 30–45° angle to the skin.[3-5] Like an excision, it allows histologic examination of the entire lesion, which improves diagnostic accuracy.[6] Should a pigmented lesion, that proves to be melanoma, be transected, adding the measurement of the original lesional depth to the deep margin and the depth of the re-excision remnant of melanoma can provide an estimation of the Breslow depth. Because the shave and saucerization techniques are simple and quick procedures, there is no reason to delay sampling a suspicious lesion in a busy practice-setting.

PROCEDURE

Prior to beginning the procedure, it is imperative to accurately document the exact biopsy site. Some lesions (e.g. basal cell carcinoma) may require further surgical intervention and the shave biopsy site may be hard to locate weeks later when the patient arrives at the dermatologic surgeon's office. Careful measurements using biangulation and triangulation from well-defined anatomical landmarks have traditionally been used to document biopsy sites. Zhang et al. confirmed that the rates of postponed surgeries were decreased and patient confidence in the surgical site selection was increased when the original shave biopsy site was documented by photography.[7] Furthermore, photodocumentation is quicker and easier than any other method when specific applications insert images seamlessly into the electronic medical record. Prior to taking the photograph, the authors recommend using a surgical marker or ink pen to draw an arrow on the skin, pointing out the lesion that will be removed. This prevents any

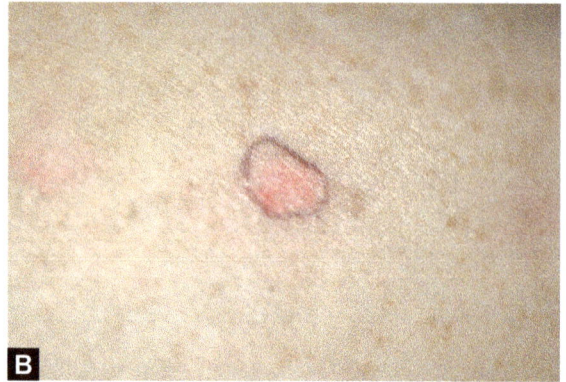

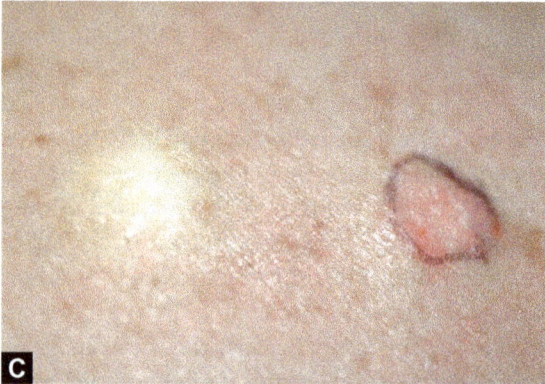

Figs. 1A to C: (A) Two 1 cm diameter erythematous, slightly scaled patches which proved to be superficial basal cell carcinomas are noted on the upper back; (B) One of these two lesions was marked with a pen to demonstrate the value of defining the boundaries before injecting a local anesthetic; (C) Lidocaine 1% with epinephrine was injected into each lesion. The boundaries of the unmarked lesion can no longer be defined.

confusion that could arise when a photograph contains several skin lesions. Drawing numbers or letters on the skin, depending on the preference of your dermatopathologist, can be helpful in documenting locations when more than one lesion are sampled. The frame of the photograph should be sufficiently large to include the nearby anatomical landmarks to ensure the biopsy site can be identified.

> Drawing numbers or letters on the skin can be helpful in documenting locations when more than one lesion is sampled.

The tools necessary for the biopsy—a blade, specimen container, and a hemostatic agent—should be autoclaved together in the same packet so that they can be quickly organized on a Mayo stand. The site should be prepared and anesthetized using a modified-sterile technique. The physician and assistant must wear gloves as required by universal precautions when the biopsy site is isolated and cleaned with 70% isopropyl alcohol.

A helpful tip is to outline the lesion using a skin marker or pen prior to injecting anesthesia.

Intradermal injections of anesthetic can blanche erythematous lesions making them harder to identify at the time of biopsy especially when it is combined with epinephrine (Figs. 1A to C). The authors recommend cleaning with an alcohol swab first and then marking the lesion so the ink does not smear.

> Outlining erythematous patches with a marker before injecting anesthesia will insure that the shave biopsy encompasses the entire lesion being targeted.

Lidocaine is routinely used for local anesthesia to do its quick onset of action. Buffering to a physiologic pH with sodium bicarbonate alleviates much of the burning sensation associated with lidocaine injections.[8] Choosing a smaller-gauged needle (30 gauge) and injecting slowly also reduces the pain associated with injection of anesthetic. It is helpful to use lidocaine with epinephrine to minimize bleeding. Waiting 15 minutes to permit maximum vasoconstriction is particularly helpful in highly vascular areas such as the face and scalp.[9]

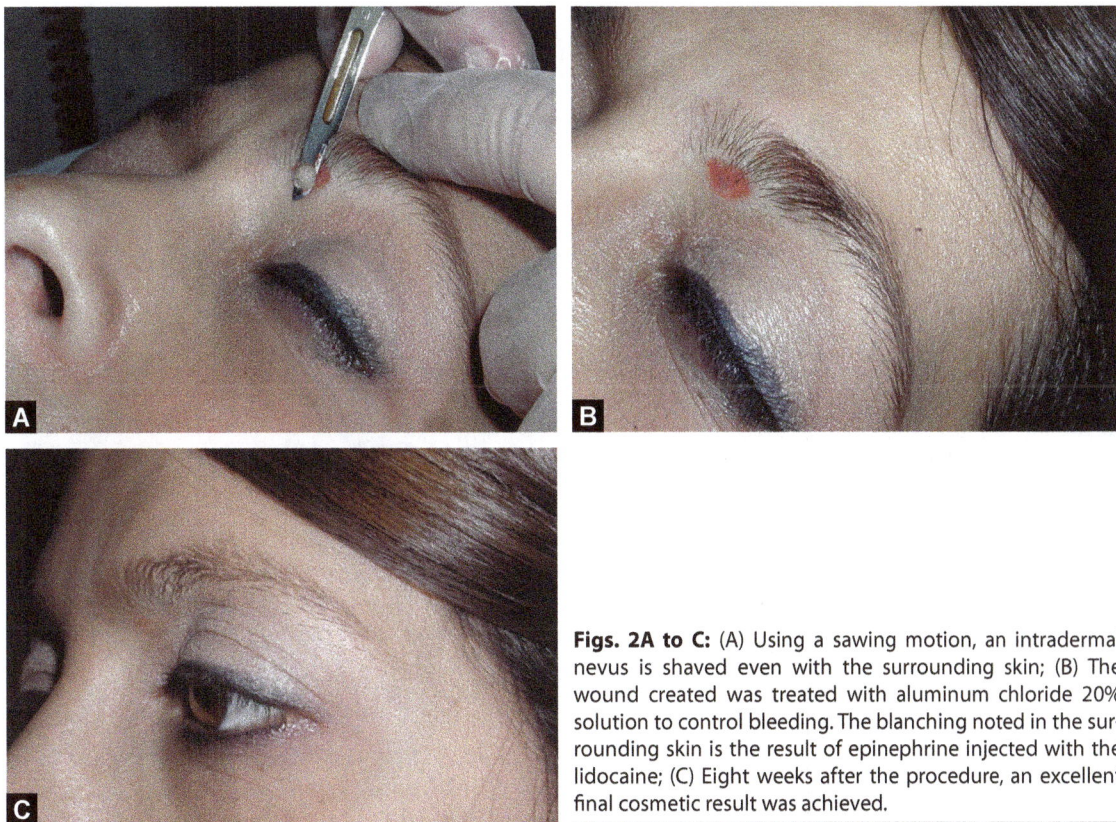

Figs. 2A to C: (A) Using a sawing motion, an intradermal nevus is shaved even with the surrounding skin; (B) The wound created was treated with aluminum chloride 20% solution to control bleeding. The blanching noted in the surrounding skin is the result of epinephrine injected with the lidocaine; (C) Eight weeks after the procedure, an excellent final cosmetic result was achieved.

Waiting 15 minutes after anesthetizing with lidocaine and epinephrine will minimize bleeding in highly vascular areas, such as the face and scalp.

When injecting anesthesia, producing a wheal under the lesion elevates it above the plane of surrounding skin.[10,11] This makes it easier to superficially shave the lesion.

The traditional shave biopsy is performed using a number 15 blade attached to a scalpel handle holding it like a pencil. The skin is cut almost parallel to the skin surface. Some skilled surgeons use only the blade without the blade handle but we recommend utilizing a handle for better control. Initially, the blade is held more vertically to incise through the epidermis and then the angle of the blade is transitioned to a horizontal position to complete removal of the specimen.[12] Once in the horizontal position, a sawing motion is used to remove the specimen (Figs. 2A to C). Forceps can be used to grip the specimen and provide traction. A toothed forceps minimizes

crush injury when compared to smooth or ridged forceps. The goal is a shallow defect and a single piece of tissue with smooth edges while avoiding fragmentation.[5] The specimen is then placed in the appropriate container: formaldehyde for H&E/Michel's media for direct immunofluorescence.

A recent innovation replaces the traditional scalpel or inflexible surgical blade with a versatile flexible blade bonded to a plastic grip: the DermaBlade® (Personna).[13] The design allows a dermatologist to easily transition from minimal to maximum flex as the blade is held between the thumb and index finger. The minimum flex position provides a nearly straight blade used to level a protuberant or pedunculated lesion even with the skin (Fig. 3A).

Flexible surgical blades permit transition from minimum to maximum flex while performing shave biopsies.

A more pronounced flex produces a bowed blade used for narrower, but deeper, sauceri-

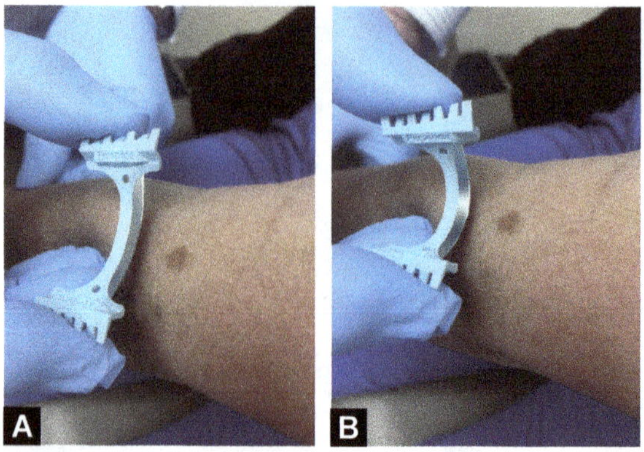

Figs. 3A and B: (A) Dermablade with minimum flex used in this position for superficial shave removals; (B) Using a more pronounced flex, the dermablade will produce a deeper "saucerization" specimen.

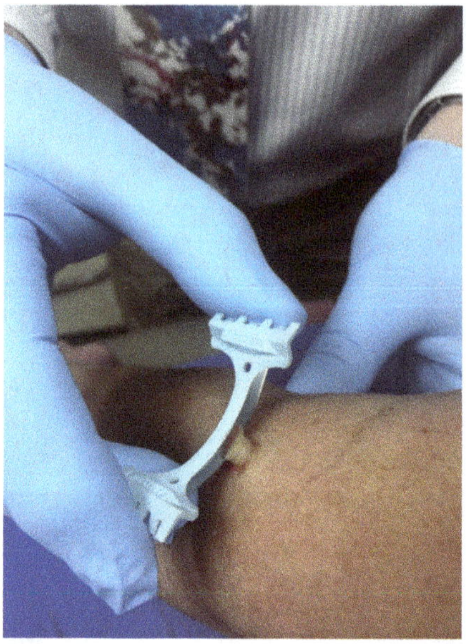

Fig. 4: When using the dermablade, a hinge is sometimes created just before the tissue is completely separated from the subjacent skin.

zation biopsies which reach a depth of 2–4 mm (Fig. 3B).[14,15] A gentle side-to-side slicing or sawing motion is recommended as the blade is advanced to scoop out the tissue including 1–2 mm of adjacent marginal skin.[13] Skin countertraction with the nondominant hand permits the blade to be advanced more easily, but care must be taken to avoid injury to the surgeon or assistant with this very sharp instrument. A common difficulty encountered when using the DermaBlade® is the creation of a skin hinge just before the biopsy is completed. The specimen can flip on this hinge, making it difficult to fully separate (Fig. 4). Light downward pressure to provide countertraction on the top of the specimen with a forceps or cotton-tipped applicator using the non-dominant hand just before finishing the shave or saucerization procedure prevents this problem (Figs. 5A to D). We do not recommend using the first and third digits to grip the DermaBlade® and the second digit to apply pressure to the flap. This method prevents hinging but risks cutting the glove or finger.

> Light downward pressure on the top of the specimen before finishing the shave or saucerization procedure can eliminate the development of a hinge flap that is difficult to separate from the underlying skin.

A common error is sampling the epidermis too superficially preventing a definitive pathologic diagnosis. We recommend visualizing the histopathology of the lesion in your mind's eye. If it is suspected that the lesion extends into the mid-dermis, a saucerization approach can be substituted for the more superficial shave technique. For optimal healing, care should be taken to avoid extending the defect into the subcutaneous fat.

> Increasing the bowing and convexity of the flexible surgical blade provides a deeper and narrower excision.

In many cases, the entire lesion is removed with this shave technique.[3] In the case of nevi, where residual pigment is seen in the dermis following a shave procedure, the defect may be shaved more deeply or if melanoma is suspected, the procedure can be converted to an elliptical excision with narrow margins around the original shave defect.[5] Another tip, crusting overlying a lesion should be removed prior to the biopsy to avoid submitting a specimen that may show only scale crusting.[2]

After the shave or saucerization biopsy is completed, there are several adjunctive techniques that may improve cosmetic outcomes.

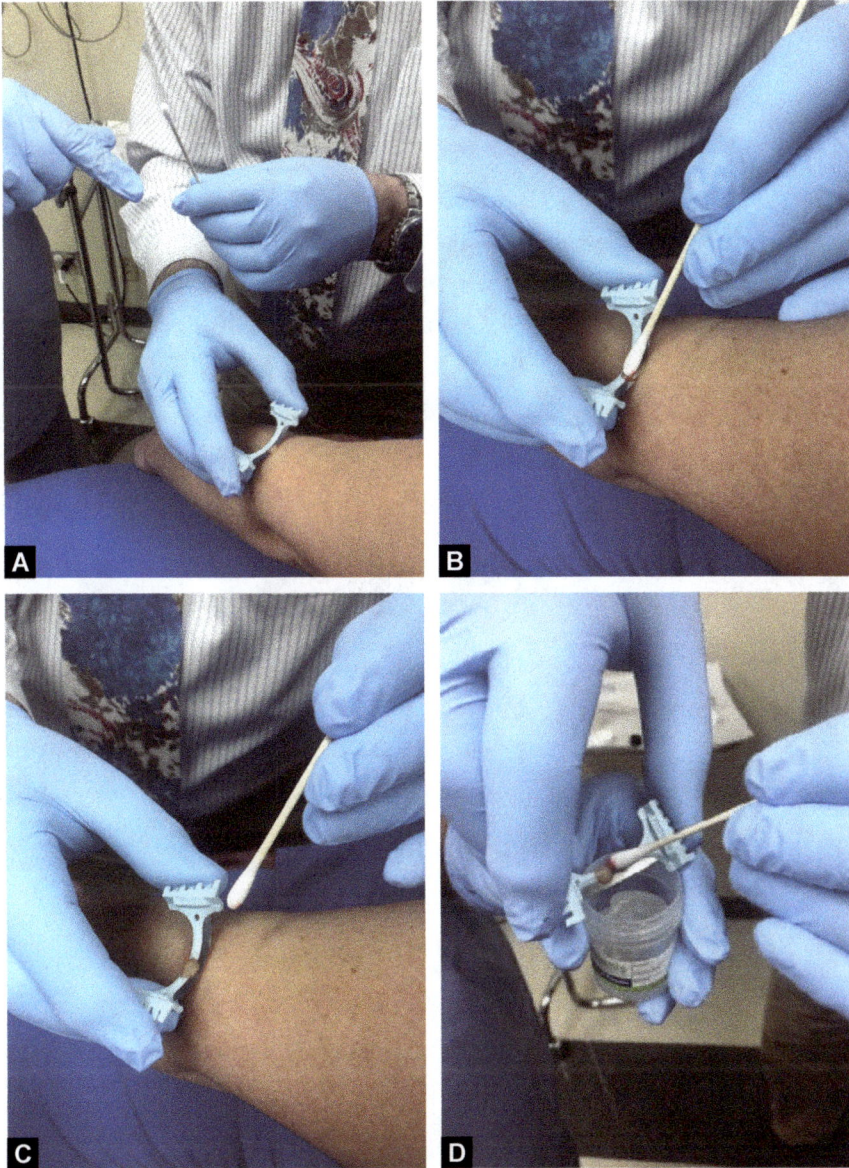

Figs. 5A to D: (A) An assistant passes you a cotton-tipped applicator just before completing the biopsy to help prevent the specimen from flipping over the hinge; (B) Downward pressure on the hinged tissue with a forceps allows the surgeon to easily complete the shave removal procedure; (C) The specimen is now sitting on the blade no longer attached to the skin; (D) The cotton-tipped applicator is used to push the specimen into a container containing formaldehyde keeping the operator's fingers out of harm's way.

This is particularly important for clinical benign lesions where it is anticipated that additional surgery will not be required. A curette can be used to remove any residual lesional tissue and to blend the biopsy site with surrounding skin by feathering the biopsy edges to minimize the potential for producing sharp demarcation lines at the edge of healing shave biopsy wounds (Figs. 6A to E).

A feathering technique is recommended to smoothen the biopsy edges and prevent "divot" scars and sharp demarcation lines at the edge of healing wounds.

The same technique can be accomplished with a DermaBlade® by forming an alternative "curette" as described by Peterson et al.[16,17] Holding the

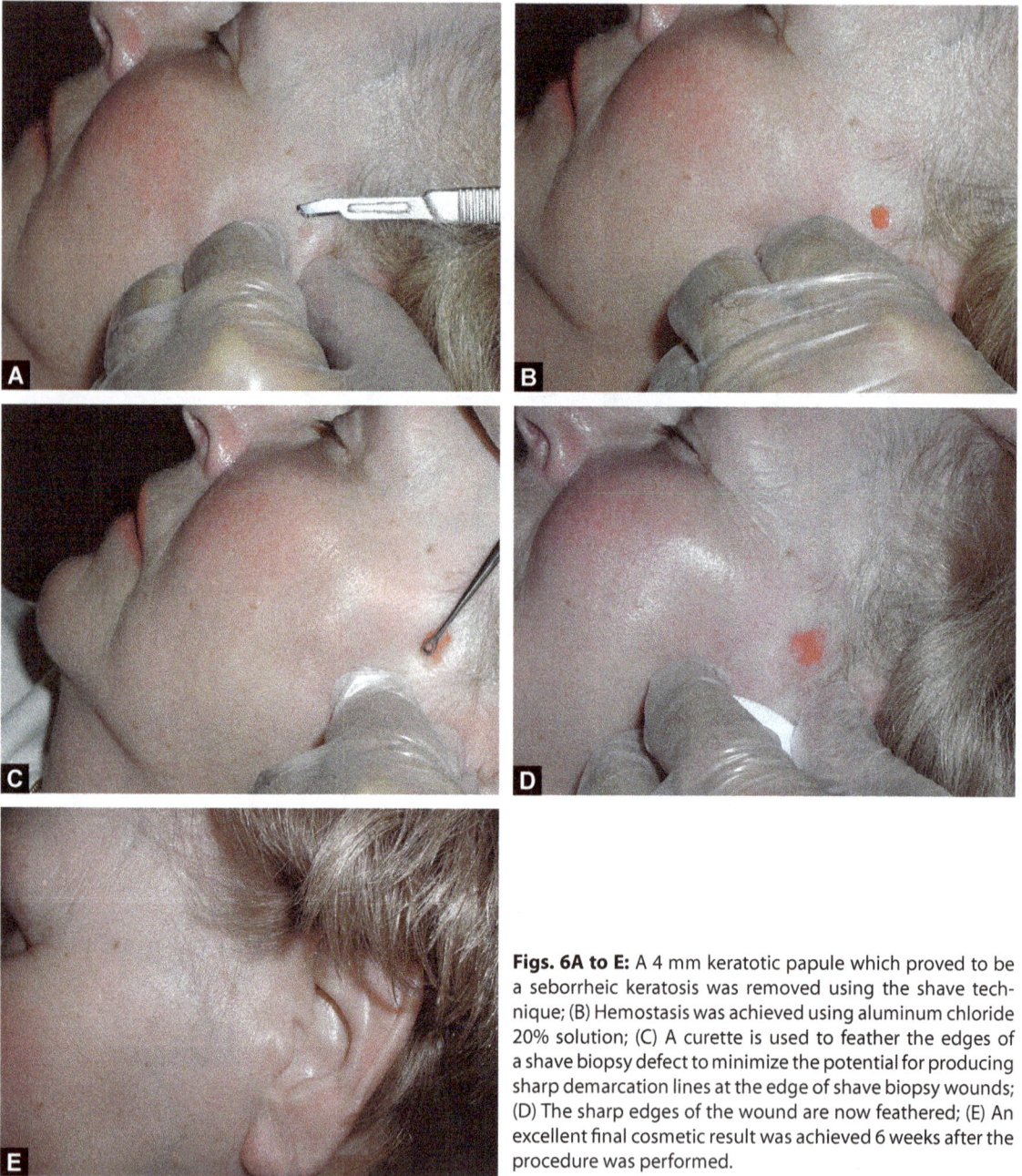

Figs. 6A to E: A 4 mm keratotic papule which proved to be a seborrheic keratosis was removed using the shave technique; (B) Hemostasis was achieved using aluminum chloride 20% solution; (C) A curette is used to feather the edges of a shave biopsy defect to minimize the potential for producing sharp demarcation lines at the edge of shave biopsy wounds; (D) The sharp edges of the wound are now feathered; (E) An excellent final cosmetic result was achieved 6 weeks after the procedure was performed.

DermaBlade® tightly between the index finger and the thumb creates a small, loop-like rounded blade that can be used to feather the margins like a traditional curette (Fig. 7). Alternatively, the number 15 blade used for the shave procedure can be used to perform "scalpel dermabrasion" feathering of wound edges.[16] The skin is stretched taunt with one hand while the number 15 blade is held perpendicular to the skin surface and scraped over the area in a back-and-forth motion in several directions to scrape while avoiding incising the skin.[16] This removes any remaining exophytic lesions without forming a divot and smoothen the transition into the surrounding skin, minimizing sharp lines of demarcation. When this technique is performed correctly, the epidermis is removed to the level of the superficial papillary dermis. This level is recognized when pinpoint bleeding is produced.

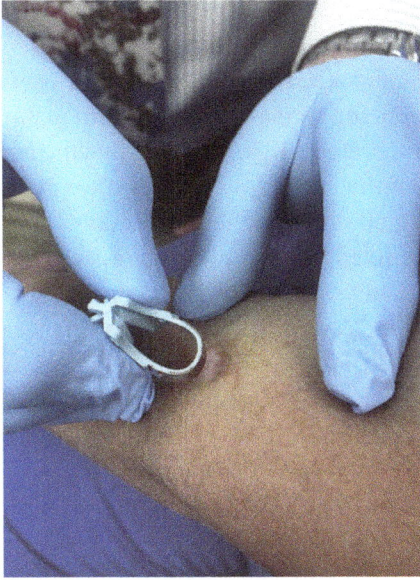

Fig. 7: A dermablade can be used as a curette after the biopsy is completed for a better cosmetic outcome.

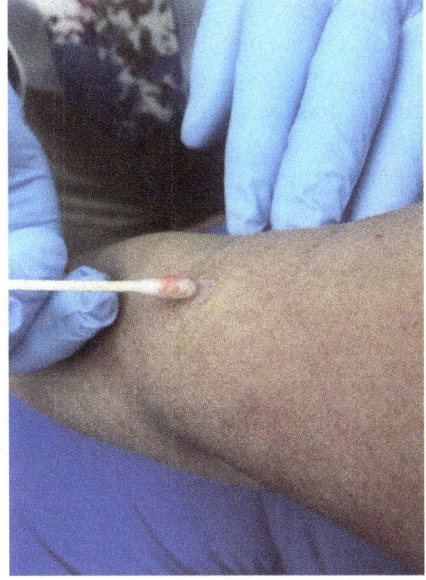

Fig. 8: Hemostasis is achieved using aluminum chloride 20% solution.

After completing the biopsy and any adjuvant cosmetic techniques, attention is turned to hemostasis. Hemostasis is traditionally achieved by chemical cautery using aluminum chloride 20% solution or Monsel's solution (ferric subsulfate 20%). Either solution is applied directly to the site with a cotton-tipped applicator. The aluminum chloride is favored because of the risk of tattooing of the skin with Monsel's solution secondary to iron deposition (Fig. 8).[18] Tattooing disfigures the patient, can confuse the clinician into believing that a pigmented lesion has recurred, and could potentially cause confusion histologically if the lesion were to be re-biopsied in the future. Additionally, Monsel's solution has been shown to decrease wound-healing through a direct cytotoxic effect.[19] Exuberant bleeding may require electrodesiciation for adequate control. Electrodesiciation can, however, interfere with pacemaker electronics and handheld electrocautery units are favored in these patients.

After stopping postoperative bleeding, petroleum jelly and a bandage should be applied. Wound care instructions include washing daily with soap and water and covering the wound with petroleum jelly to prevent scab formation which slows wound-healing. Antibiotic ointments were traditionally recommended after biopsies but a study comparing wound care with white petrolatum versus bacitracin ointment found no difference in infection rate.[20] Additionally, the rate of allergic contact dermatitis is much higher when antibiotic ointments are applied to wounds.

Chen and Mellette describe a useful way to master the shave and saucerization biopsy techniques by practicing on a tomato.[21] They argue that a firm tomato simulates various aspects of human skin better than a pig's feet. Notably, tomatoes have the advantage of being widely available and inexpensive. Practice-shaving "lesions" of various shapes, sizes, and depths on the tomato will hone skills of medical students and resident physicians.[22] This model is particularly useful in practice to avoid hinge flaps. The same model can be used to practice local anesthesia and curettage techniques.

> A firm tomtato simulates various aspects of human skin better than a pig's feet when practicing shave and saucerization techniques.

BENEFITS

While all biopsy techniques can be performed in the office-setting, both shave and saucerization biopsies offer several distinct advantages when compared to other biopsy approaches, e.g. elliptical excision and the punch biopsy. The tangential techniques do not require suturing and they are the quickest and least expensive biopsy approaches. Of note, the shave biopsy is an optimal method of sampling epidermal lesions including exophytic tumors. A saucerization biopsy, however, is also an efficient way to provide a broad view of broad lesions including lentigo maligna without concern for the sampling error that can be produced when a smaller portion of the lesion is sampled using the punch technique.[6,15] With regard to sampling pigmented lesions that are found to be malignant melanoma on histopathology, the reliability of saucerization has been demonstrated in several studies.[22] Pariser et al. determined that the quality of deep shave specimens was superior to punch and shave specimens, with the certainty of histologic diagnosis similar to that of excisions.[22-26] Mir et al. showed saucerization biopsies to accurately assess tumor stage in 99% of cases examined in their study.[2] Other studies have indicated that the saucerization technique produces specimens that can reliably be used to determine Breslow thickness and this approach does not negatively impact patient survival when compared to elliptical excision.[5] Saucerization biopsy is particularly useful when pigmented lesions are thought to be benign, but some uncertainty persists even after dermatoscopic examination. In such lesions, sensitivity is more important than specificity. The efficiency and low morbidity of the saucerization technique permit the prompt sampling of suspicious pigmented lesions in a busy practice setting without the need to reschedule patients for a separate appointment for elliptical excision. This further delays diagnosis and some patients may not return at all.[3] It also avoids more extensive and expensive surgery in a significant majority of cases when the benign nature of the questionable lesion is confirmed by histopathology. Still, if there is a high likelihood that a pigmented lesion is melanoma, elliptical excision of the entire lesion is still the preferred approach.[27-31]

> Saucerization technique allows the prompt sampling of suspicious pigmented lesions in a busy practice-setting without the need to reschedule patients.

Another distinct advantage of shave and saucerization biopsies is the simplicity of postoperative care. Because healing occurs by second intention, the patient need not return to the office for suture removal.[3] In the event that the resulting pathology necessitates a full thickness excision or lymph node biopsy, these procedures may then be scheduled. Pre-emptive, aggressive measures, which oblige additional follow-up appointments and wound care, are thus avoided with these techniques.[3] In fact, the patient may return to work the same day and is permitted to swim in a chlorinated pool, shower, and perform other activities without any special considerations.

Finally, the shave and saucerization biopsies provide excellent cosmetic outcomes coupled with a very short healing time, usually no more than 2 weeks. They leave a small, flat or depressed scar rather than a longer linear scar as seen after an elliptical excision.[3] This consideration is particularly significant in those patients with many suspicious pigmented lesions requiring biopsy, such as dysplastic nevi syndrome. In one study evaluating the cosmetic outcomes of 56 biopsy sites after 6 months, each patient reported a "good" or "excellent" result. The evaluating physicians were actually more stringent in their assessment, noting mild hypopigmentation, marginal hyperpigmentation, and erythema, with no significant differences in scarring when comparing various anatomic sites.[16]

RISKS AND LIMITATIONS

A considerable disadvantage of a shave or saucerization procedure is the potential for horizontal transection of a melanoma, which would complicate determination of the Breslow depth needed to gauge tumor stage and determine the prognosis.[3] However, this can be largely avoided by reserving the saucerization technique for flat or only slightly raised lesions and utilizing an elliptical excision technique for nodular lesions in which the Breslow depth may be significantly greater. Furthermore, in the rare instance of melanoma transection, the sum of the tumor depth can be calculated by adding the initial Breslow depth to that of the subsequent excision.[3]

Another complication following transection of a benign lesion with shave or saucerization is the development of a recurrent nevus, which, on clinical and histopathological examination, may be difficult to distinguish from junctional malignant melanoma in situ. Residual melanocytes grow into the scar, and atypical pigmented streaks may result in the dermatoscopic appearance of a melanoma. Without access to the original pathology report, it may be difficult to determine whether the lesion is a benign recurrent nevus, a dysplastic nevus, or a melanoma. In this case, however, an excision of the recurrent nevus will be curative.[3] While the concern for transection is noteworthy, Mir's study demonstrated that the transection of melanoma did not affect overall disease-free survival or mortality in the population studied. In addition, the rate of transection was not statistically different when compared with punch biopsy specimens.[5] The final disadvantage of shave and saucerization techniques is the longer healing time necessitated by secondary intention when compared to a linear excision. This is particularly important on the lower legs of mature individuals where healing by second intention may take weeks to months on the distal lower extremities, depending on the size of the lesion.[5]

Conflict of Interest

Drs Liddell, Cosulich and Wile have no conflicts of interest.

REFERENCES

1. Bolognia JL. Biopsy techniques for pigmented lesions. Dermatol Surg. 2000;26(1):89-90.
2. Mir M, Chan CS, Khan F, et al. The rate of melanoma transection with various biopsy techniques and the influence of tumor transection on patient survival. Am Acad Dermatol. 2013; 68(3):452-8.
3. Mendese GW. (2007). The Diagnostic and Therapeutic Utility of the Scoop-Shave for Pigmented Lesions of the Skin. University of Massachusetts Medical School. Senior Scholars Program: Office of Educational Affairs. Paper 46. [online] Available at http://escholarship.umassmed.edu/ssp/46. [Accessed March, 2017].
4. Buka RL, Ness RC. Surgical pearl: the pendulum or "scoop" biopsy. Clin Med Res. 2013;6(2):86-7.
5. Geisse JK. Biopsy techniques for pigmented lesions of the skin. Pathology (Phila). 1994 2(2): 181-93.
6. Nischal U, Nischal KC, Khopkar U. Techniques of skin biopsy and practical considerations. J Cutaneous Aesthetic Surg. 2008;1(2):107-11.
7. Zhang J, Rosen A, Orenstein L, et al. Factors associated with biopsy site identification, postponement of surgery and patient confidence in dermatologic surgery practice. J Am Acad Dermatol. 2016;74(6):1185-93.
8. Skarsvåg TI, Wågø KJ, Tangen LF, et al. Does adjusting the pH of lidocaine reduce pain during injection? J Plast Surg Hand Surg. 2015;19:1-3.
9. Lui S, Carpenter RL, Chiu AA, et al. Epinephrine prolongs duration of subcutaneous infiltration of local anesthesia in a dose related manner. Reg Anesth. 1995;20:378-84.
10. Arndt KA, Bowers KE, Alam M, et al. Manual of dermatologic therapeutics with essentials of diagnosis. Philadelphia: Lippincott Williams and Wilkins; 2002. p. 214.
11. Maize JC, Ackerman AB. Pigmented Lesions of the Skin. Philadelphia: Lea and Febiger; 1987. pp. 19-25.
12. Harvey DT, Fenske NA. The razor blade biopsy technique. Dermatol Surg. 1995;21:345-7.
13. Goldber LH, Segal RJ. Surgical Pearl: A flexible scalpel for shave excision of skin lesions. J Am Acad Dermatol. 1996;35:452-3.
14. Eton O, Legha SS, Balch CM. Cutaneous Melanoma. N Engl J Med. 1992;326(5):345-6.
15. Harris MN, Gumport SL. Biopsy technique for malignant melanoma. J Dermatol Surg Oncol. 1975;1(1):24-7.
16. Bowan PH, Mitchel P, Goldman MD. Surgical pearl: Scalpel dermabrasion complements shave excision. J Am Acad Dermatol. 2003;48:789-90.
17. Peterson AJ, Peterson SR, Jensen KJ. Surgical Pearl: The DermaBlade as a curett. J Am Acad Dermatol. 2006;54:518-9.
18. Camisa C, Roberts W. Monsel solution tattooing. J Am Acad Dermatol. 1983;8:753-4.
19. Larson PO. Topical hemostatic agents for dermatologic surgery. J Dermatol Surg Oncol. 1988;14: 623-32.
20. Smack DP, Harrington AC, Dunn C, et al. Infection and allergy incidence in ambulatory surgery patients using white petrolatum vs bacitracin ointment. A randomized controlled trial. JAMA. 1996;276(12):972-7.
21. Chen TM, Mellette JR. Surgical Pearl: Tomato—an alternative model for shave biopsy training. J Am Acad Dermatol. 2006;54:517-8.

22. Pariser RJ, Divers A, Nassar A. The relationship between biopsy technique and uncertainty in the histopathologic diagnosis of melanoma. Dermatol Online J. 1999;5(2):4.

23. Ho J, Brodell RT, Helms SE. Saucerization biopsy of pigmented lesions. Clin Dermatol. 2005;23(6): 631-5.

24. Charles CA, Yee VS, Dusza SW, et al. Variation in the diagnosis, treatment, and management of melanoma in situ: a survey of US dermatologists. Arch Dermatol. 2005;141(6):723-9.

25. Swanson NA, Lee KK, Gorman A, et al. Biopsy techniques. Diagnosis of melanoma. Dermatol Clin. 2002;20(4):677-80.

26. Cockerell CJ. Biopsy technique for pigmented lesions. Semin Cutan Med Surg. 1997;16(2): 108-12.

27. Sober AJ, Chuang TY, Duvic M, et al. Guidelines of care for primary cutaneous melanoma. J Am Acad Dermatol. 2001;45(4):579-86.

28. Stevens G, Cockerell CJ. Avoiding sampling error in the biopsy of pigmented lesions. Arch Dermatol. 1996;132(11):1380-2.

29. Gambichler T, Senger E, Rapp S, et al. Deep shave excision of macular melanocytic nevi with the razor blade biopsy technique. Dermatol Surg. 2000;26(7):662-6.

30. Witheiler DD, Cockerell CJ. Sensitivity of diagnosis of malignant melanoma: a clinicopathologic study with a critical assessment of biopsy techniques. Exp Dermatol. 1992;1(4):170-5.

31. Tran KT, Wright NA, Cockerell CJ. Biopsy of the pigmented lesion—when and how. J Am Acad Dermatol. 2008;59(5):852-71.

CHAPTER 6

Punch Biopsies and Other Uses for the Punch Tool

Michael T Cosulich, Anna Wile

HISTORY/OVERVIEW

The cutaneous punch instrument has been in use since 1879, when it was used to remove specks of burnt powder from a man's face following a firework accident.[1] Since then, the punch has become an essential skin biopsy tool. While there are many factors a clinician must consider when choosing a biopsy technique, punch biopsies are most commonly employed to evaluate the full thickness of the dermis. Larger punches (8–12 mm) can also be helpful in the evaluation of subcutaneous tissue. Currently, most clinicians prefer to use disposable instruments. The typical disposable punch tool consists of a cylindrical, sharp-edged metal blade attached to a plastic handle. The diameter of commercially available metal blades varies from 0.5 mm to 12 mm, although 3 mm and 4 mm instruments are the most commonly used.[2] Smaller punch sizes are most commonly used in cosmetically sensitive areas, but smaller punches can limit the diagnostic value of the biopsy specimens produced.

While a punch tool is most often used for diagnostic purposes, it is a versatile instrument with many therapeutic uses. It can often be used as an alternative to elliptical excision to quickly and effectively remove cysts, lipomas, and other benign neoplasms.

STANDARD PUNCH BIOPSY TECHNIQUE

The biopsy site is first cleaned, marked, and anesthetized with a local anesthetic agent. The instrument is pressed against the skin with downward force while simultaneously rotating the instrument along its long axis as the instrument pene-

trates the skin. The skin can be stretched with the index finger and thumb perpendicular to relaxed skin tension lines prior to insertion of the instrument. This will cause the resulting defect to be oval shaped rather than circular, which facilitates closure with minimal standing cone formation (Figs. 1A and B).

> Stretching the skin with the index finger and thumb perpendicular to the relaxed skin tension lines prior to insertion of the punch produces an oval defect that facilitates closure.

Typically, force is applied to the instrument until the junction of the blade and handle is flush with the skin. This is referred to as "hubbing" and maximizes the likelihood of reaching the subcutaneous fat and will allow for the greatest amount of tissue to be acquired for histological examination. In addition, larger punches (8 mm or larger) are often chosen when the intent is to include subcutaneous fat (see diagnosing suspected panniculitis below). However, depending on anatomical location and the expected depth of pathology, the clinician may choose to not "hub" the instrument. Particular care is taken on the face, neck and genitals to avoid damaging underlying nerves and vascular structures. The skin surrounding the biopsy site can also be squeezed to elevate the skin and subcutaneous fat away from deeper structures (Figs. 2A and B).

> To decrease the risk of damaging underlying structures, squeeze the surrounding area to elevate the skin and subcutaneous tissue.

Once the punch reaches the desired depth, the instrument is removed. The specimen can be

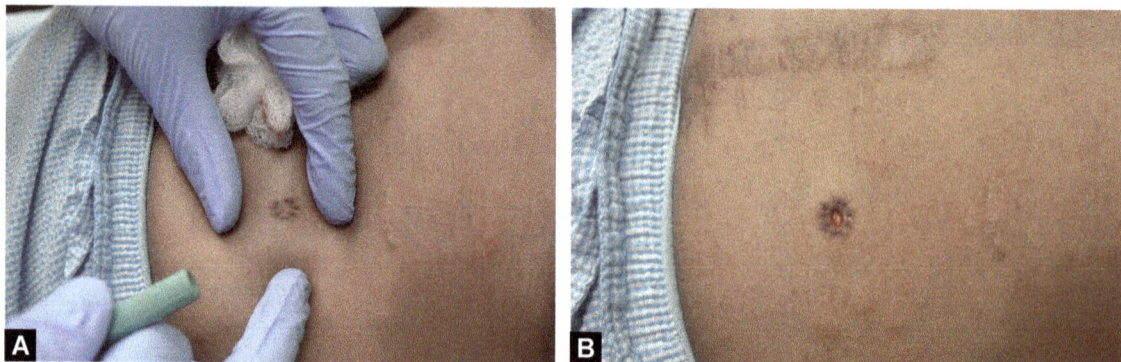

Figs. 1A and B: Creating an oval defect. (A) The skin is stretched in a perpendicular direction to relaxed skin tension lines. (B) The resulting oval-shaped defect.

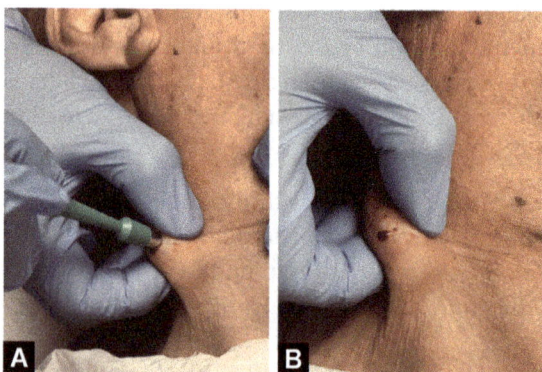

Figs. 2A and B: Avoiding neurovascular structures. (A) The skin can be squeezed together to avoid damaging underlying nerves and vascular structures. (B) The lesion after removal of punch tool.

gently extracted with forceps or a skin hook. Care should be taken not to crush the specimen which leads to histopathologic artifacts. Often the base of the specimen will need to be snipped with scissors to ensure that subcutaneous fat is removed with the epidermis and dermis. When the target to be sampled is in the epidermis or dermis, the specimen can often be retrieved by traction alone.

After the specimen is safely placed in a labeled specimen container, the clinician must determine the best method for closing the resulting wound. A number of methods that can be used effectively, and the clinician's choice is influenced by cost, efficiency, and desired cosmetic result.

Most often the wound is closed primarily with simple interrupted sutures. The choice of suture depends on the size of the punch tool used and the location of the body. For the standard 4 mm

punch on the trunk or extremities, a 4-0 nonabsorbable suture is appropriate. 5-0 or 6-0 sutures can be used on the face and areas with low tension at the wound edges. Absorbable sutures can be used for patients who are unable to return for suture removal. There was no significant difference detected in infection, dehiscence, scar hypertrophy, or patient's satisfaction when compared with nonabsorbable sutures in one study.[3] Punches 6 mm and greater can also be closed using an "X" suture which requires only one knot. This saves time in closing punches that would otherwise require two sutures[4] (Figs. 3A and B).

While suturing the defect, bleeding that obscures the physician's ability to see the wound clearly is a regular occurrence. Despite frequent blotting with gauze, the clinician's vision can still be affected. The need for frequent blotting also increases the risk of a needle stick accident. Greco and Cusack described a clever technique for controlling bleeding with minimal risk of needle stick accidents while promoting tissue eversion[5] (Fig. 4). Once the specimen is removed and the defect is ready to be closed, a sterile cotton-tipped applicator is inserted into the wound. Force is applied with the cotton-tipped applicator toward one side of the defect while gently pulling the skin upward. The suture needle is then placed into this everted wound edge and the cotton-tipped applicator is removed. The cotton-tipped applicator is then pressed down several millimeters from the opposite edge of the wound to create eversion. The suture needle is then inserted through this opposite edge to complete the simple interrupted stitch.

Figs. 3A and B: X-suture. To perform the closure, the needle is initially inserted as if placing a simple interrupted suture. After the needle exits on the opposite side of the wound, the suture is then pulled through the skin until only a small tail remains. Without cutting the suture, a second bite is taken parallel to the first. For both throws, the needle enters on the same side of the wound. (A) The configuration after both throws of the suture. (B) Final result after the knot has been tied.

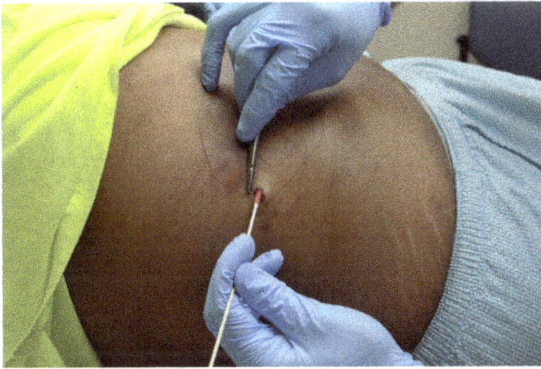

Fig. 4: Cotton-tipped applicator for hemostasis. A cotton-tipped applicator is used to aid in hemostasis during suture placement.

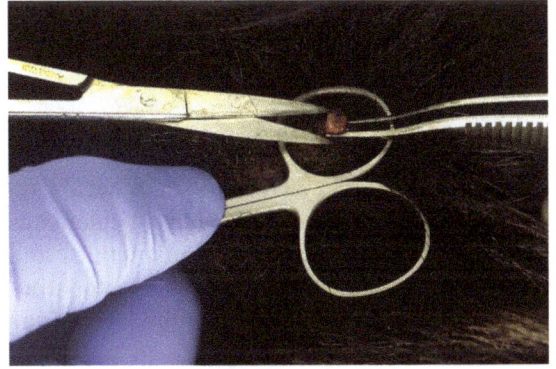

Fig. 5: Instrument tamponade. Pressure is applied to the area around a defect with the circular handle of an instrument.

> In patients with significant bleeding from a punch wound, a q-tip can be used to evert edges and minimize the chance of needle-stick injury.

Another tip for improved hemostasis was described by Whalen et al. as "instrument tamponade".[6] This is particularly useful for the scalp, an area notorious for excessive bleeding even when lidocaine with epinephrine is used to induce vasoconstriction 15 minutes before the procedure is begun. Just before the biopsy is performed, an assistant uses the circular handle of any instrument to apply firm pressure to the skin surface surrounding the biopsy site. The other steps of the punch biopsy are performed in the same manner described above. When performed properly, very little bleeding occurs during the procedure (Fig. 5).

> Firm pressure using a circular handle produces "instrument tamponade" at sites where excessive bleeding is common.

Although punch defects can be closed primarily, some clinicians favor healing by secondary intention. This produces good cosmetic results while maximizing efficiency and minimizing cost.[7] Several pieces of gel foam are packed in the wound to aid in hemostasis. The wound is then covered with petroleum jelly and a bandage (Fig. 6).

Fig. 6: Punch biopsy left to heal by secondary intention. The wound is packed with gel foam and covered with Vaseline before being bandaged.

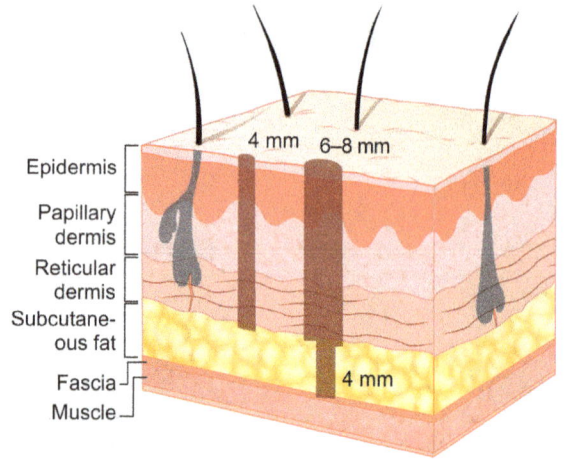

Fig. 7: Double-trephine punch technique for panniculitis. The double-trephine technique using a 6 or 8 mm punch tool followed by a 4 mm punch tool is able to sample deeper subcutaneous tissue than using a 4 mm punch tool in the standard fashion.

SPECIAL USES FOR A PUNCH

Diagnosing Suspected Panniculitis

The standard 4 mm punch biopsy does not always allow for the acquisition of enough subcutaneous tissue to properly diagnose panniculitides and other dermatoses where important histopathologic findings are present below the level of the dermis. In these cases, clinicians may elect to perform incisional biopsies or very large (10–12 mm) punch biopsies. However, such biopsies are associated with increased cost and time, as well as increased morbidity in the form of larger scars. Several techniques have been described that allow for the acquisition of adequate subcutaneous tissue for a proper diagnosis of panniculitis without the use of incisional biopsies or very large punch biopsies. Ha and Nousari developed one such method, termed as the "double-trephine punch".[8] In this method, an 8 mm punch tool is inserted with the traditional technique described above. After this initial tissue sample is removed, a 4 to 6 mm punch tool is then used to obtain additional subcutaneous tissue from the center portion of the previously created 8 mm defect. The defect is then closed in a normal fashion (Fig. 7).

> The "double trephine punch" method improves the sampling of subcutaneous fat.

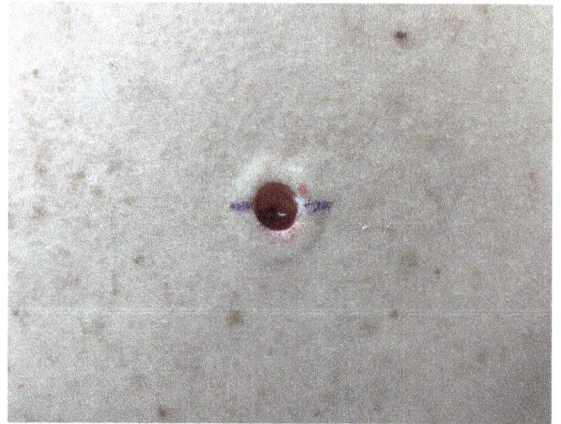

Fig. 8: Relaxing incisions for panniculitis. After the punch tool is removed, relaxing incisions are made along the marked lines. The same punch tool can be re-inserted deeper into the fat to sample deeper tissue.

Another variation on this technique was subsequently described by Ersoy-Evans.[9] In this method, a 4 mm instrument is inserted in the traditional fashion, but, at this point, the core is left in place. Two relaxation incisions, each 2 mm long, are then made using a #15 blade. These are placed perpendicular to the skin surface on opposite sides of the punch defect parallel to skin tension lines. The same 4 mm instrument is used with additional pressure into the previously punched area. The core is removed along with ample subcutaneous tissue (Fig. 8). Compared

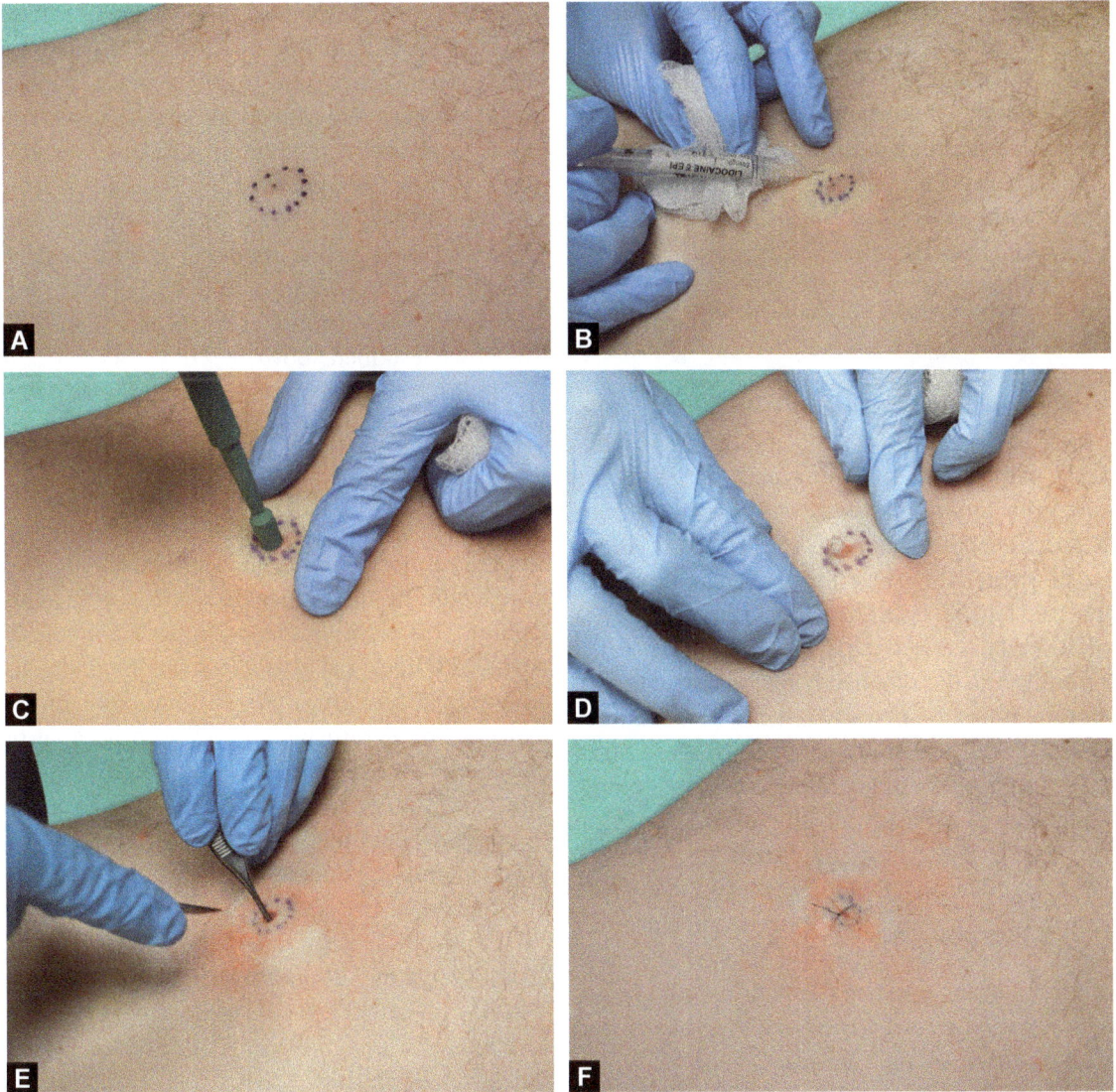

Figs. 9A to F: Punch excision of a cyst. (A) The borders of the cyst are marked prior to injection of anesthetic. (B) Anesthetic is injected into dermis surrounding cyst. (C) Punch instrument is inserted into center of lesion. (D) Firm pressure is applied to lesion. (E) Remaining cyst wall is removed. (F) Final result after suture placement.

to the "double-trephine punch", this technique has the benefits of being less expensive (only one punch tool required) and creating a smaller defect and scar. However, less subcutaneous tissue is usually obtained. For both of these methods, care must be taken to avoid damaging underlying nerves and vascular structures.

Excision of Cysts

While epidermal inclusion cysts and pilar cysts have traditionally been removed using ellip-

tical excision, the use of a punch tool is a quick and effective alternative that produces excellent results (Figs. 9A to F). A randomized prospective study demonstrated that, compared to elliptical excision, punch incision was quicker and cosmetically superior while having a similar recurrence rate.[10,11] It is important to remember that there is no special value in removing cysts intact. Even if the cyst wall is removed in pieces, the cyst will not recur so long as remnants of the cyst wall are not left in place. In addition, this technique is effective in removing infected, ruptured and inflamed cysts. Even though the cyst wall may be harder to visualize during the procedure, the recurrence rate is still low.[11] Also, just as draining an abscess is a critically important approach to effective treatment, draining a pocket of infection associated with a cyst is a positive intervention, not one that should be avoided until after pretreatment with systemic antibiotics.

> There is no special value to removing a cyst intact.

To perform the procedure, the area is prepared and anesthetized. It is important to manually palpate and mark the boundaries of the cyst prior to anesthetizing, as the infiltrate may obscure the border and make it difficult to visualize the center of the cyst. Lidocaine should not be injected into the cyst, but rather around the edges of the cyst to form a ring. A punch tool is inserted centrally into the skin overlying the cyst centered on the pore of the cyst when it can be visualized. Gentle lateral pressure is applied to the base of the cyst, resulting in expression of cyst contents and pieces of the cyst wall. The wound should be carefully evaluated for any remaining cyst wall. Residual cyst wall should be removed to prevent recurrence. Although use of larger punches may help to visualize the cyst wall after incision, generally a 4 to 6 mm punch is adequate even for larger cysts up to 4 cm. The wound can then be sutured with one or two simple interrupted sutures.

Excision of Lipomas

Like cysts, lipomas are frequently encountered by dermatologists and have traditionally been treated with elliptical excision (Figs. 10A to F). However, a number of studies describe an efficient technique for punch removal of lipomas that demonstrates a low recurrence rate.[12,13] First, the borders of the lipoma are marked and the overlying skin is anesthetized. A 6 to 8 mm punch tool is used to make a round incision into the skin above the center of the lipoma. Firm lateral pressure is applied to both sides of the lipoma with one or two hands to squeeze the lipoma out of the central incision. Often a significant amount of pressure is needed for removal of the lipoma. For large or fibrosed lipomas, blunt dissection may be required, and the lipoma can then be removed in a piecemeal fashion. In many cases, cutting the lipoma capsule with an iris scissor allows the lipoma to be delivered more easily. Once most of the tumor has been delivered, the adjacent subcutaneous space should be checked through the defect for any residual lipoma to decrease risk of recurrence. The wound is then closed with one or two simple interrupted sutures or a single "X" suture as described above.

In the authors' experience, lipomas of up to 6 cm can be removed using this technique. It is particularly useful in patients with multiple painful lipomas that are more easily expressed with lateral pressure than other lipomas. If for any reason the lipoma cannot be removed using this technique, conversion to an elliptical excision is always an option. This technique can be more difficult in areas with thicker skin and less skin pliability, as obtaining a firm grasp laterally and beneath the lipoma is more difficult. Furthermore, lipomas of the forehead may be closely associated with the frontalis muscle, making them difficult to remove using this technique.[14] Caution is recommended when attempting lipoma removal in this anatomical region.

> Multiple painful lipomas are more easily expressed with lateral pressure than other lipomas.

Excision of Large Oval Lesions with a Smaller Round Punch

Often dermatologists are asked to remove benign neoplasms such as benign melanocytic nevi or dermatofibromas for cosmetic purposes. Although an elliptical excision could be considered, a punch excision is usually faster and less costly. When a standard punch excision is performed, the size of the punch chosen is typically at least 0.2 mm larger than the widest diameter of the lesion that is to be excised. A modified punch technique has been described. A smaller-diameter punch is used to remove larger lesions, thereby decreasing the overall final scar length and improving cosmetic outcomes[15] (Figs. 11A to D). This technique is only applicable when the long axis of the lesion

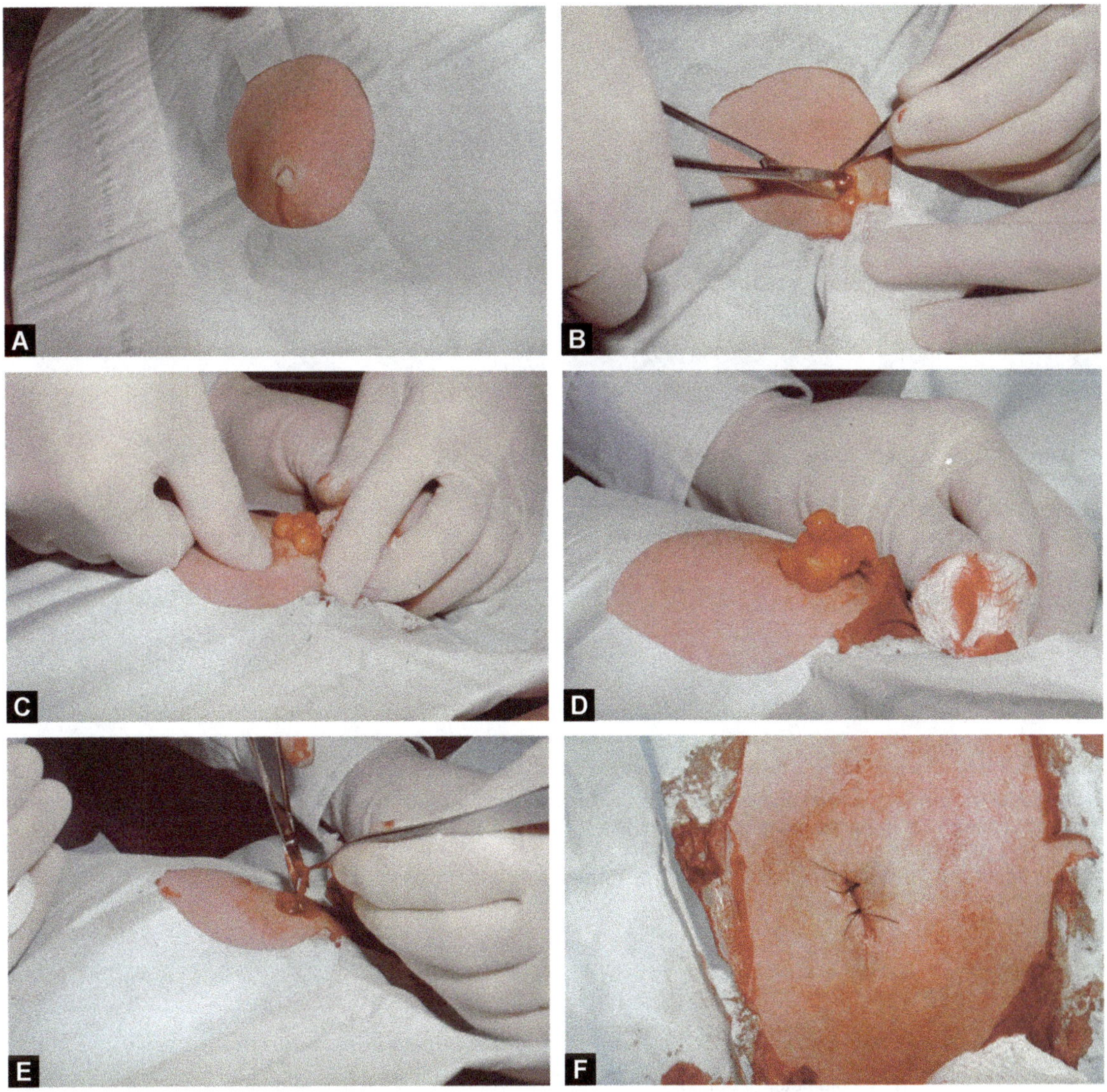

Figs. 10A to F: Punch excision of lipoma. (A) Punch incision has been made over center of lesion. (B) Dissection being performed to loosen fibrous tissue. (C) Firm pressure is applied to lesion. (D) The majority of the lesion has been extracted. (E) Any remaining lesion is removed. (F) Final result after suture placement.

is less than one-third larger than the diameter of the punch tool used (which will be ~1 mm larger than the short axis of the lesion). For example, if the short axis of a lesion is 5 mm and a 6 mm punch tool is selected, the long axis of the lesion should be less than 8 mm (Fig. 12).

The metal cutting edge of the punch is placed at one end of the lesion along the long axis at a 45° angle to the surface of the skin. The oval lesion can then be squeezed into the aperture of the punch as the handle is repositioned perpendicular to the skin, so that the cutting edge is level with the skin.

The lesion is essentially "stuffed" into the opening of the punch tool. The punch tool is rotated with downward pressure in the standard fashion and the instrument is removed, leaving an oval-shaped defect. The specimen is removed and the defect is sutured and closed.

It should be noted that if the long axis of the lesion is perpendicular to the skin tension lines, this technique will cause the suture line to be perpendicular to the direction that would normally produce the best cosmetic result. A clinician must use their best judgment to determine whether this

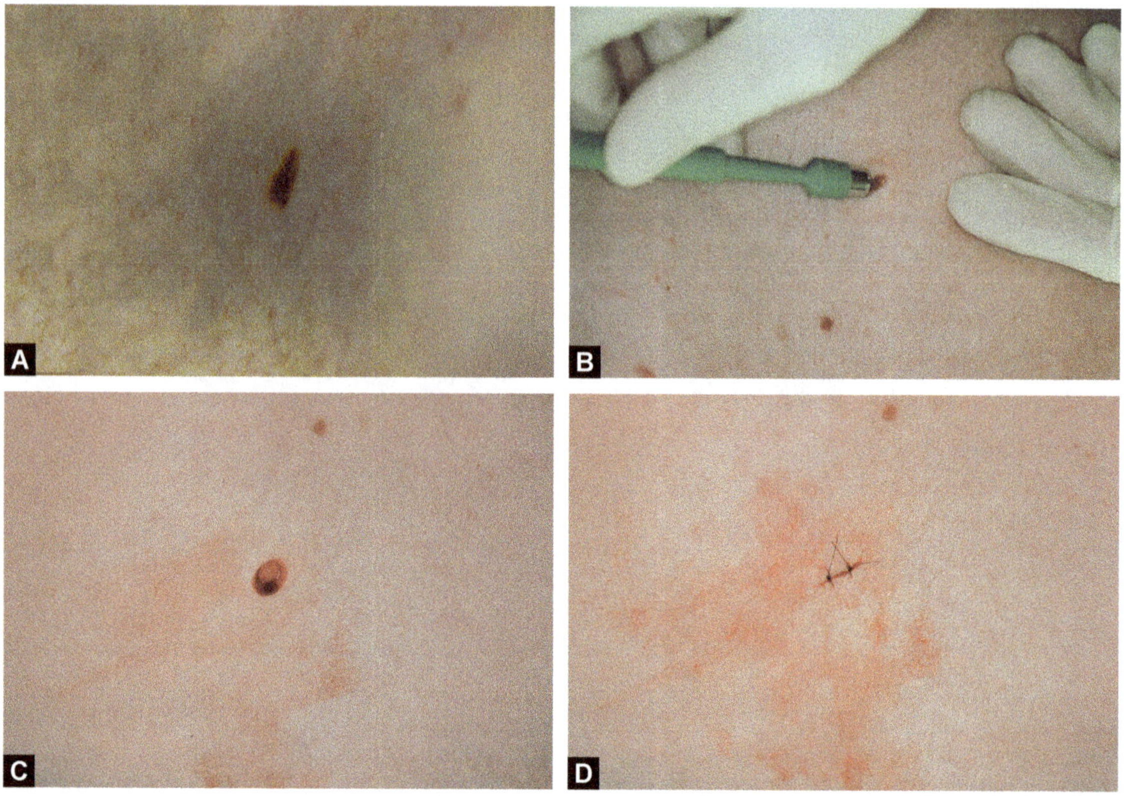

Figs. 11A to D: Removing a large oval lesion with a small round punch. (A) An ideal lesion. (B) The edge of the punch tool is placed at one end of the lesion along the long axis at a 45° angle. (C) The resulting oval-shaped defect. (D) The final result after suture placement.

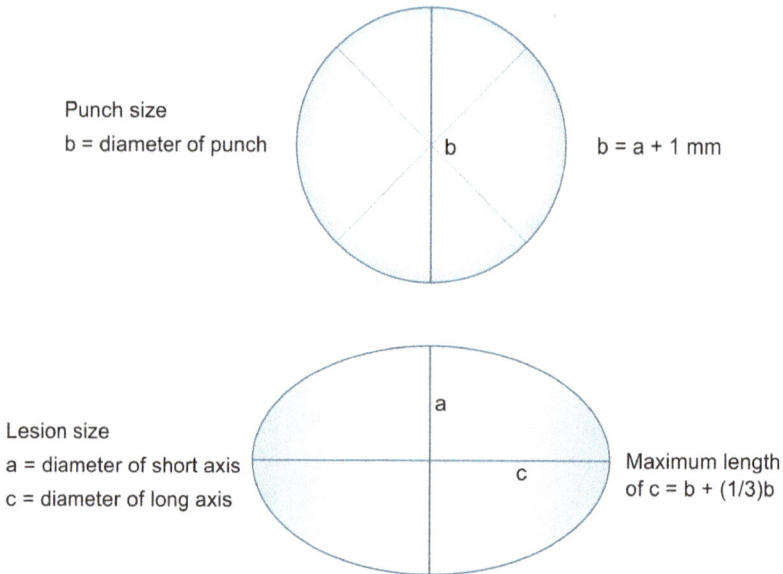

Punch size
b = diameter of punch

b

b = a + 1 mm

Lesion size
a = diameter of short axis
c = diameter of long axis

a

c

Maximum length
of c = b + (1/3)b

Fig. 12: Maximum size of an oval lesion that can be removed with a round punch. The size of the punch used should be 1 mm greater than the short axis of the lesion. The maximum length of the long axis is diameter of the punch plus one-third the diameter of the punch.

technique will still yield a favorable cosmetic outcome. Furthermore, potentially malignant lesions should be excised with proper margins to avoid incomplete excision. Finally, if this technique is used for lesions on areas where the dermis is very thick, there is significant beveling produced at each long end of the excision that can produce a suboptimal result.

Bisecting a Punch Biopsy Specimen at the Bedside

A common scenario that dermatologists encounter is a patient that requires two biopsy specimens from the same area. Examples of this include conditions with tense blisters that require a hematoxylin and eosin (H&E) specimen of the blister edge and direct immunofluorescence from perilesional skin, or a patient that needs an H&E specimen as well as a specimen for tissue culture. Instead of performing two separate punch biopsies, performing a single larger biopsy, that is then bisected at the bedside is a cost-effective alternative that produces equivalent specimens.[16,17] To maintain orientation when this technique is used on tense blisters, a line is drawn from the tense blister onto the adjacent normal skin centered on the site to be punch biopsied (Figs. 13A and B). This is classically performed by using a 15-blade in a sawing motion to bisect the specimen after it has been removed. One-half of the specimen is placed in formalin for H&E and one-half is placed in Michel's media for direct immunofluorescence. Both specimens will show adjacent skin and the take-off point of the blister. When immunoglobulin G (IgG) and complement are present, it can be localized to the roof or the floor of the blister producing "salt split skin-like information".

> Bisecting a punch biopsy specimen at the bedside after removal with a number 15 blade is a cost-effective alternative to obtaining two separate biopsy specimens.

This technique, however, requires some practice to perform this "grossing" technique without producing crush artifact. An alternate way to bisect the specimen without crushing tissue is to split the tissue before it has been removed from this skin.[18] The punch tool is introduced into the skin in the normal fashion, but only advanced into the papillary dermis and withdrawn as soon as bleeding is noted. An 11-blade is then inserted into the center of the specimen and advanced completely through the dermis to bisect the specimen. The punch tool is then reinserted and now extended to the subcutaneous fat before withdrawal. The specimen is then retrieved as two pieces.

> An alternative way to bisect a punch specimen without crushing the tissue is to split the tissue before it has been removed from the skin.

Benefits Compared to Alternatives

Compared to shave biopsies and "saucerization" approaches, the punch biopsy allows for visualization of the deep dermis and even subcutaneous tissue. This is critically important in the diagnosis of some dermatologic conditions. While traditional excision or excisional biopsy may also be utilized for evaluation of the deep dermis and subcutaneous fat, punch techniques are less time consuming, heal faster, and commonly result in smaller scars.

RISKS/LIMITATIONS

As this technique more deeply invades the skin and subcutaneous tissue when compared to shave and "saucerization" biopsies, punch biopsies can pose a risk to underlying structures, such as blood vessels and nerves in certain areas. This is particularly true when using the "double-trephine punch" technique. Sampling error is another concern when punch biopsies are performed to sample large lesions. The punch specimen may not be representative of the most significant pathology in this circumstance. Incisional biopsies or "saucerization" techniques may be preferred for large pigmented lesions, so that a broader portion of the dermoepidermal junction can be assessed.

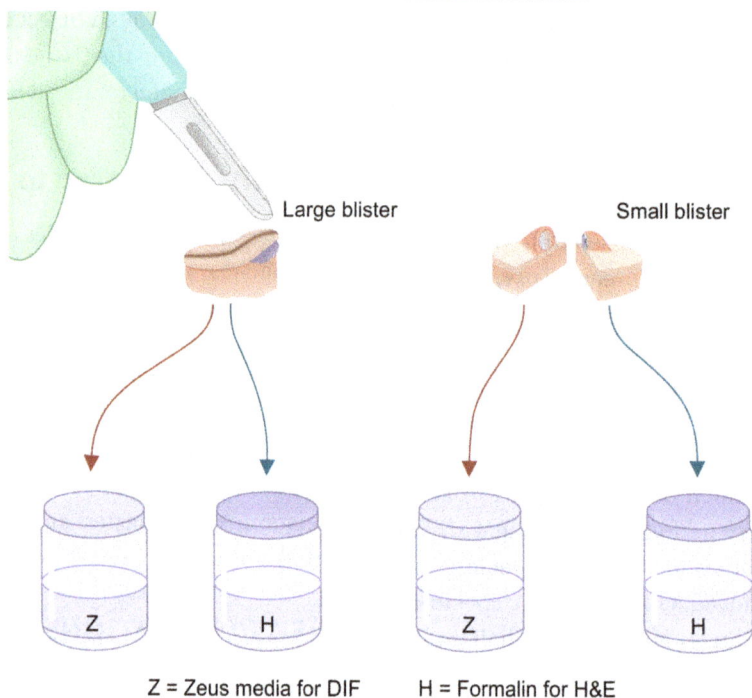

Figs. 13A and B: Biopsy technique for blisters. (A) For larger blisters, a line is drawn from the roof of the tense blister onto the surrounding perilesional skin. The biopsy should be obtained from the edge of the blister with roughly 75% of the sample representing perilesional skin. For smaller blisters, the entire blister should be excised along with perilesional skin. (B) Specimens from large blisters are bisected at the bedside with a 15-blade along the previously drawn line to ensure that both perilesional skin and the take-off point of the blister will be visible when the cut edge is properly embedded in the laboratory. Specimens of smaller blisters are bisected as well, but can be bisected at any orientation. Half of each specimen is placed in formalin for hematoxylin and eosin (H&E) processing, and the other half is placed in Zeus (or Michel's) medium for direct immunofluorescence.

REFERENCES

1. Keys EL. The cutaneous punch. J Cutan Genitourin Dis. 1887;5:98-101.
2. Fernandez EM, Helm T, Ioffreda M, et al. The vanishing biopsy: the trend toward smaller specimens. Cutis. 2005;76(5):335-9.
3. Gabel EA, Jimenez GP, Eaglstein WH, et al. Performance comparison of nylon and an absorbable suture material (Polyglactin 910) in the closure of punch biopsy sites. Dermatol Surg. 2000;26(8):750-2; discussion 752-3.
4. Reynolds MB, Ratz JL. Surgical pearl: Mini-running or "X" suture for closure of punch wounds. J Am Acad Dermatol. 2002;46(3):423-5.

5. Greco JF, Cusack CA. Surgical pearl: The use of a cotton-tipped applicator for tissue eversion during punch biopsy. J Am Acad Dermatol. 2005;53(2):329-30.

6. Whalen JG, Gehris RP, Kress DW, et al. Surgical pearl: Instrument tamponade for punch biopsy of the scalp. J Am Acad Dermatol. 2005;52(2):347-8.

7. Christenson LJ, Phillips PK, Weaver AL, et al. Primary closure vs second-intention treatment of skin punch biopsy sites: a randomized trial. Arch Dermatol. 2005;141(9):1093-9.

8. Ha CT, Nousari HC. Surgical pearl: double-trephine punch biopsy technique for sampling subcutaneous tissue. J Am Acad Dermatol. 2003;48(4):609-10.

9. Ersoy-Evans S. Surgical pearl: A novel punch biopsy technique for diagnosing panniculitis. J Am Acad Dermatol. 2015;72(6):e161-2.

10. Lee HE, Yang CH, Chen CH, et al. Comparison of the surgical outcomes of punch incision and elliptical excision in treating epidermal inclusion cysts: a prospective, randomized study. Dermatol Surg. 2006;32(4):520-5.

11. Mehrabi D, Leonhardt JM, Brodell RT. Removal of keratinous and pilar cysts with the punch incision technique: analysis of surgical outcomes. Dermatol Surg. 2002;28(8):673-7.

12. Rao SS, Davison SP. Gone in 30 seconds: a quick and simple technique for subcutaneous lipoma removal. Plast Reconstr Surg. 2012;130(1):236e-8e.

13. Christenson L, Patterson J, Davis D. Surgical pearl: Use of the cutaneous punch for the removal of lipomas. J Am Acad Dermatol. 2000;42(4):675-6.

14. Salasche SJ, McCollough ML, Angeloni VL, et al. Frontalis-associated lipoma of the forehead. J Am Acad Dermatol. 1989;20(3):462-8.

15. Warino LA, Brodell RT. Surgical pearl: Removal of large oval lesions with a smaller round punch. J Am Acad Dermatol. 2006;55(3):509-10.

16. Braswell MA, McCowan NK, Schulmeier JS, et al. High-yield biopsy technique for subepidermal blisters. Cutis. 2015;95(4):237-40.

17. Loh E, Armstrong AW, Fung MA. Pre-bisection of a single skin biopsy does not produce technically inadequate specimens for direct immunofluorescence: a review of 3450 specimens. J Cut Pathol. 2014;41(11):890-2.

18. Inman VD, Pariser RJ. Biopsy technique pearl: Obtaining an optimal split punch-biopsy specimen. J Am Acad Dermatol. 2003;48(2):273-4.

CHAPTER 7

Curettage

Jess (Logan) Rush, Lauren M Craig

HISTORY

Curettage is a basic in-office procedure in which a sharp curette is used to treat superficial skin lesions. Curettage is often combined with electrosurgery in a technique known as "electrodesiccation and curettage" (ED&C). ED&C represent a relatively safe, effective, and inexpensive treatment for selected nonmelanoma skin cancers and certain benign lesions.

The history of dermal curettage dates back to the late 19th century. The earliest dermal curette, a variant of the uterine curette, was a cup-shaped tool developed by Volkmann in 1870.[1] Originally used to treat lupus vulgaris, Wigglesworth expanded the role of the dermal curette to treat a variety of skin lesions, including psoriasis and syphilitic condylomas.[2] GH Fox improved on the engineering of the dermal curette in 1902 with the introduction of the Fox curette—the most popular style used today.[3]

The use of electrodesiccation on skin lesions was first documented by William Clark in 1911, who dried or desiccated skin lesions with the application of high voltage, low current using a monoterminal electrode.[4] He reported successful treatment of a number of skin lesions, including basal cell carcinoma, utilizing this method. As the availability of curettes and instruments for electrodesiccation grew during the 20th century, the method of curettage with electrodesiccation became increasingly popular (Table 1).

PROCEDURES

Periprocedural care involves cleaning the surgical area with alcohol wipes or other cleansing agents,

Table 1: Skin lesions commonly treated by curettage ± electrodesiccation.*	
Benign	*Malignant or premalignant*
Acrochordons	Actinic keratosis
Dermatosis papulosa Nigra	Well-differentiated squamous cell carcinoma, squamous cell carcinoma in-situ
Molluscum contagiosum	Nodular basal cell carcinoma
Pyogenic granuloma	Superficial basal cell carcinoma
Seborrheic keratosis	
Verrucae vulgaris	

*This list is representative of conditions commonly treated, but not comprehensive.

such as chlorhexidine gluconate (Hibiclens®) or povidone-iodine (Betadine®). Once dry, the visible borders of macular or barely elevated lesions should be marked with a surgical pen. It is important to ensure the surgical area is dry of any antiseptic agents prior to electrodesiccation, as many are flammable.

> Borders should be marked with a surgical pen.

Anesthesia is usually achieved using an injection of 1% lidocaine with or without epinephrine. If the lesion is cancerous, it is wise to avoid injecting directly into the lesion to avoid the theoretical possibility of transplanting cancerous tissue into healthy tissue.[5] It is important to delineate the lesion with a marker prior to injection of the anesthetic. The vasoconstrictive effects of epinephrine and the wheal from the injection can obscure the clinical borders of the lesion. This increases the

Figs. 1A and B: (A) Lesion prior to injection with lidocaine with epinephrine; (B) Wheal visualized after injection with lidocaine with epinephrine.

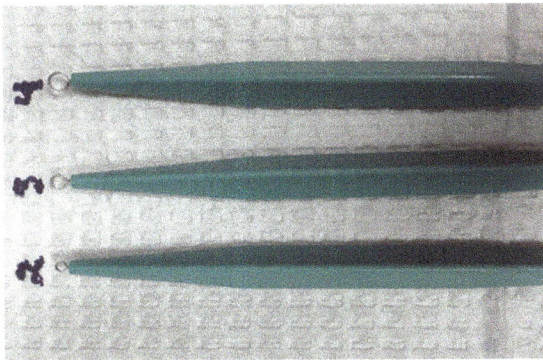

Fig. 2: Various sizes of disposable curettes.

potential of incomplete treatment or unnecessary treatment to healthy tissue (Figs. 1A and B).

Selecting the proper curette is an important aspect of the procedure. The type and size of curette and the choice of reusable or disposable curettes is largely based on personal preference. There are a variety of curette types available, but most clinicians use either a standard round curette or the oval head Fox curette.

Curettes range in size from 0 to 8 mm in diameter (Fig. 2). There is an art to choosing the proper curette. Small curettes can cause fragmentation of the specimen. Curettes which are too large for the specimen may cause unnecessary damage to the surrounding tissue. Smaller curettes are often preferred for lesions on the face. Some clinicians prefer using a larger curette initially and switching to a smaller curette to finish deeper and peripheral areas within the lesion for finer control.[6]

Reusable curettes have certain disadvantages that make them less preferable. Reusable curettes require meticulous cleaning to remove any tissue that may remain on the curette prior to autoclaving. Reusable curettes also tend to become dull after repetitive use, while disposable curettes are always sharp. Because so many physicians have moved away from reusable instruments, it can be hard to find a professional to sharpen these instruments.

> Disposable curettes are generally favored over reusable ones.

Although the focus of this chapter is more on curettage than electrosurgery, an understanding of electrosurgical modalities is important for performing an ED&C. *Electrodesiccation* is the high-voltage, low-amperage use of a monoterminal electrode used for superficial destruction. This is the modality that is commonly used in conjunc-

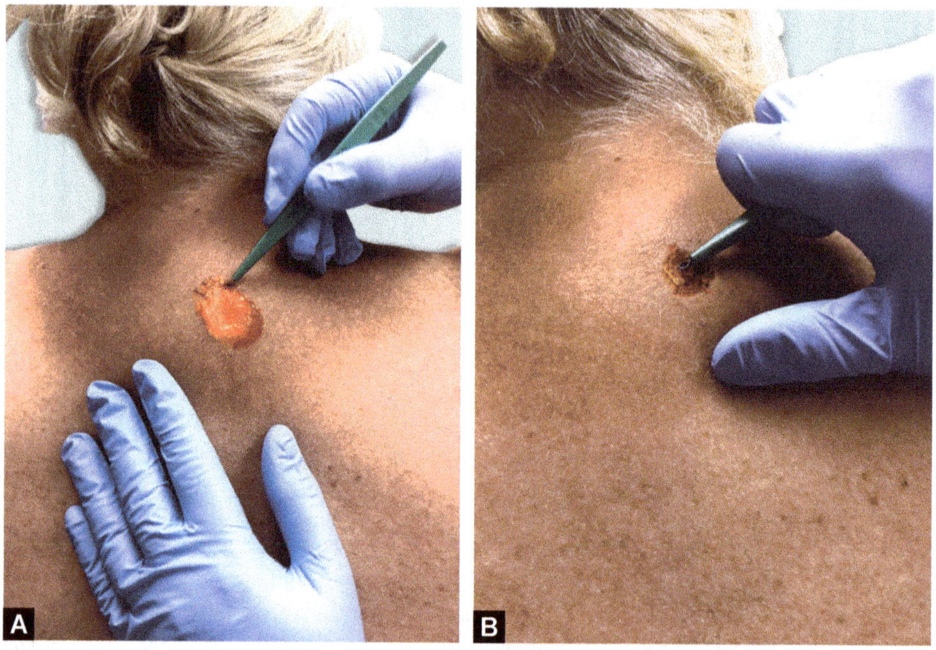

Figs. 3A and B: (A) Curettage using "pencil" technique; (B) Curettage using "potato peeler" technique.

tion with curettage. *Electrofulguration* is also the high-voltage, low-amperage use of a monoterminal electrode, although in this case, the spark is applied without actually touching the tip of the instrument to tissue. *Electrocautery*, in contrast, is the low-voltage, high-amperage use of a biterminal electrode. This tends to be more deeply destructive than the former two modalities.

> Electrodesiccation is the modality used with curettage for superficial tissue destruction.

Curettage ± Electrodesiccation of Malignant Lesions

After the lesion is appropriately anesthetized, raised lesions are shaved flush with the skin using a No. 10 scalpel blade or a Dermablade® prior to curetting. If there is no previous pathologic confirmation of the diagnosis, tissue may be submitted in formalin for pathologic examination prior to curettage. This produces an optimal pathologic specimen, which is submitted to the laboratory in formaldehyde.

> If cancer is suspected, tissue can be submitted for pathologic examination prior to curettage.

Two curettage techniques are commonly utilized: The pencil technique and the potato peeler technique (Figs. 3A and B).[7] In the pencil technique, the curette is held like a pencil. The base of the palm can be rested on the skin for stability. The natural cleavage plane between the lesion and surrounding skin should be identified. The free hand should be used to hold the skin taut. In the potato peeler technique, which is used for larger lesions, the curette is held in the distal interdigital fold of the index finger and other bent fingers. The thumb is used to counter skin traction exerted by the thumb and index fingers of the free hand. The curette tip is firmly pressed at the farthest point of the lesion and pressed toward the nearest point of the lesion, as if peeling a potato.

The base is scraped until the gritty sensation of the underlying dermis is identified. A softer, gelatinous feel of the tissue is appreciated when curetting the mass of squamous cell or basal cell carcinomas. The ability to appreciate the differences in feel between healthy and cancerous tissue promotes removal of the tumor and insures that subsequent stages of electrodesiccation will produce an adequate margin beneath the tumor.

> Cancerous tissue will have a softer, gelatinous feel compared to healthy tissue.

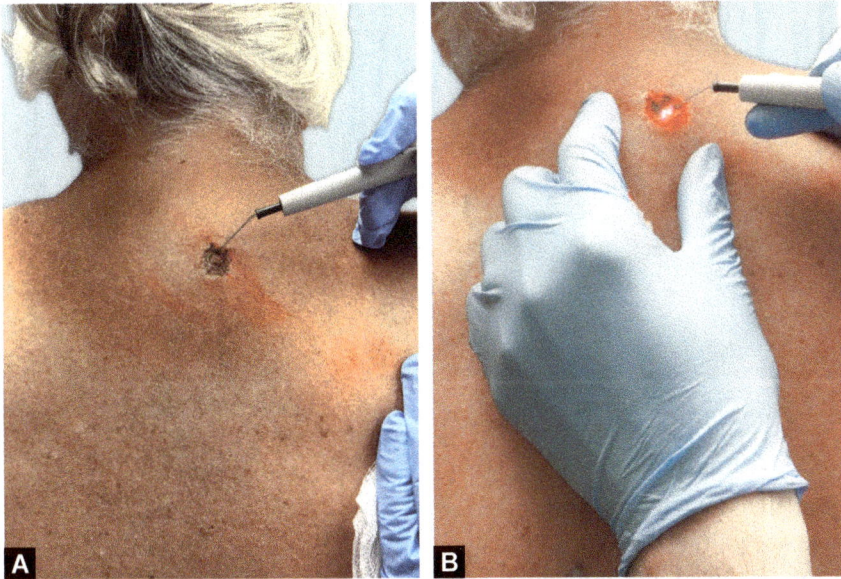

Figs. 4A and B: (A) Electrodesiccation with denatured skin char; (B) Electrodesiccation providing homeostasis.

The rest of the lesion should be scraped in multiple directions to insure that any residual strands of tumor are removed. It has been demonstrated for a basal cell carcinoma less than 2 cm, a 4 mm margin was necessary to eliminate the entire tumor in 98% of cases.[8] If the curette breaks through to subcutaneous tissue, it is wise to convert to an excisional procedure to prevent tumor seeding of the subcutaneous fat.[6]

The bleeding associated with curetting is wiped with gauze, followed by achievement of hemostasis with 25% aluminum chloride solution or Monsel's solution. Electrodesiccation may also be used to control local bleeding. Application of the cautery tip in a backward and forward motion on a dry lesion not only achieves coagulation, but also denatures the cancerous tissue (Figs. 4A and B). The curettage following each pass of electrodesiccation removes the denatured tissue.

There is some debate on the optimum number of ED&C cycles to effectively treat skin cancers. The evidence is not clear whether one, two, or three cycles of ED&C is the most effective, although there is sufficient evidence of higher rates tumor clearance with increased number of cycles.[7,9] For this reason, we recommended more than one cycle.

Postoperative care of the wound involves gentle washing of the affected area, which is usually covered with a light bandage. Many dermatologists prefer the application of petroleum jelly to the wound, such as Vaseline®, as opposed to an antibacterial ointment such as Neosporin®, due to the risk of contact sensitivity reactions to those products. The wound heals by secondary intention over 2–4 weeks. Descriptive documentation or photographing the lesion before and after the procedure can assist with identifying the site to monitor for any signs of reoccurrence.

> Photographing the lesion aids in identifying recurrence.

Curettage ± Electrodesiccation of Benign Lesions

Molluscum Contagiosum

The core of molluscum contagiosum (which contains the intracytoplasmic inclusion bodies known as *Henderson-Paterson bodies*) is quickly and easily curetted and most lesions require only one treatment (Fig. 5). One randomized trial of 124 children found curettage of molluscum contagiosum to be the most efficacious treatment option.[10] EMLA cream (2.5% lidocaine and 2.5% prilocaine) applied under occlusive tape (Blenderm®) 1 hour before treatment and reapplied

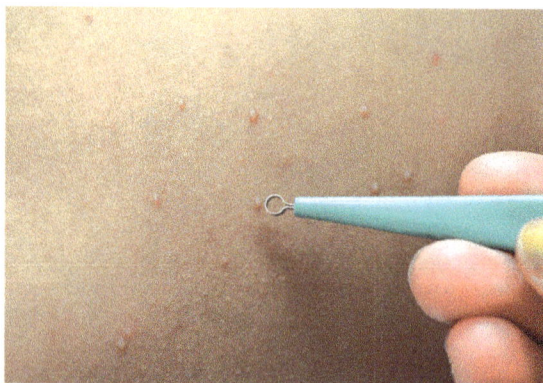
Fig. 5: Curettage of molluscum contagiosum.

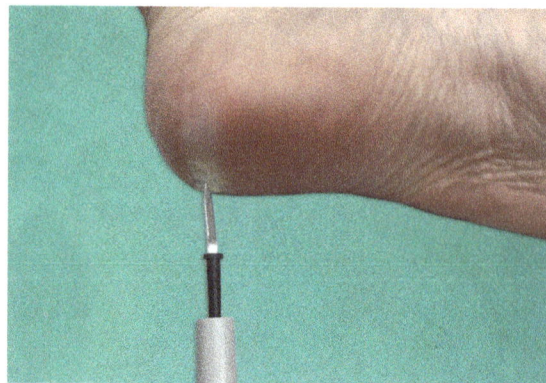
Fig. 6: Light electrodesiccation of a wart prior to removal with curettage.

30 minutes before treatment is frequently used for local anesthesia. The pain associated with curetting is significantly reduced, but not eliminated. A follow-up visit in 3–4 weeks is suggested to ensure that any lesions too small to identify or missed are promptly curetted. Once clear, the parents or patients are instructed to return with any sign of recurrence before the molluscum spreads.

Verrucae

Warts (verrucae) are benign lesions that can be treated with electrodesiccation and curettage. Although no single treatment has been found uniformly to be the most effective, chemical destruction (i.e. salicylic acid) and local destruction (cryotherapy) are more commonly recommended as first-line treatment because of the increased risk of scarring potential associated with ED&C.[11]

Anesthesia is usually achieved with local injection of 1% lidocaine with epinephrine. Once anesthetized, the wart is lightly electrodessicated so that it can be more easily scraped away with a lateral motion of the curette (Fig. 6). Further electrodesiccation may be necessary to achieve hemostasis. Warts are epidermal lesions. So, it is important to avoid deep electrodesiccation into the dermis to lessen the chance of scarring. Since human papillomavirus (HPV) DNA is present in the plume of smoke from electrodesiccation, a mask and a smoke evacuator should be used to prevent transmission of HPV to the operator's nose, throat or vocal cords.[12]

> A mask and smoker evacuator should be used when electrodesiccation is used on any wart.

Seborrheic Keratoses

Although cryotherapy remains the most common treatment of seborrheic keratoses, curettage (±electrodesiccation) is a viable treatment option. Curettage allows for immediate healing of the lesion and avoids the necrosis caused by cryotherapy.[6] Following anesthesia via injection of lidocaine plus epinephrine, the seborrheic keratoses are peeled off the dermis quite easily with smooth strokes of the curette. Special care must be taken to avoid curetting the mid and deeper dermal layers or breaking through to the subcutaneous fat. Larger curettes may be used to remove the bulk of the lesion, followed by treatment with a smaller size curette for finer control (Fig. 7).

Dermatosis Papulosa Nigra

Dermatosis papulosa nigra (DPN) are dark, tag-like benign skin lesions seen primarily in adult African-Americans. DPN can be quickly and easily treated with curettage. One study comparing curettage, pulsed dye laser, and electrodesiccation for the treatment of DPN found curettage to have the highest lesion clearance rate (96%).[13] Although the cosmetic outcome is typically very good, hypopigmentation of the treatment site is a possibility with any of the treatment options (Fig. 8).

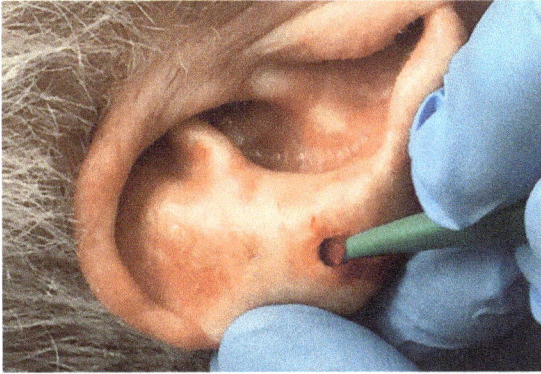

Fig. 7: Curettage of a seborrheic keratosis.

Fig. 8: Curettage of dermatosis papulosa nigra.

Postoperative care of the wound involves gentle washing of the affected area and application of petroleum jelly. The wound can be left exposed to air or covered with a light bandage. Healing occurs via secondary intention over 2–4 weeks. The scar result for most of these benign lesions is typically minimal.

Benefits Compared to Alternative Procedures

Curettage, with or without electrodesiccation, is a simple, inexpensive, and time-efficient procedure to perform. No sutures are required as healing occurs via secondary intention. There is usually a good cosmetic result with minimal complications. Curettage has the advantage of not only producing a specimen that will be analyzed to confirm the diagnosis (via biopsy prior to curettage), but treatment is also performed in the same visit. As long as the pathology does not demonstrate an aggressive form of tumor (e.g. morpheaform or sclerotic basal cell carcinoma) and the tumor does not recur with careful clinical follow-up, then additional treatment is not required.

The cost-effectiveness of curettage ± electrodesiccation makes it a popular option for many clinicians and dermatologic surgeons. Mohs micrographic surgery is widely recognized as the gold standard for treatment of nonmelanoma skin cancers. However, due to the expense and time involved in this procedure, it is indicated only with aggressive tumors and cases where disfigurement or functional impairment is a risk.[14]

One study that evaluated the cost comparison of treatment modalities for nonmelanoma skin cancer found ED&C to be, by far, the most cost-effective treatment option.[15]

Cure rates for curettage and electrodesiccation of nonmelanoma skin cancer are largely user dependent and depend on the type and location of lesion. There have been many studies reporting cure rates of ED&C. A review of studies reporting cure rates of basal cell carcinoma reported an average 5-year reoccurrence rate of 7.7%.[16] Although a number of studies support the efficacy of ED&C, the cure rate of nonmelanoma skin cancers remains a topic of debate.[17,18] In a study by Spiller et al., the cure rate for basal cell carcinoma with ED&C was 97% after 5 years. While this percentage seems high, the clinician needs to select the lesion to be treated appropriately. For example, superficial lesions as well as lesions in areas of decreased hair density are more successfully treated with ED&C.[19]

> Cure rates for superficial and nodular basal cell carcinomas are often reported to be greater than 90%.

The practice of using curettage alone is gaining traction as several studies have showed it can lead to similar cure rates and better cosmetic outcomes as ED&C for treating superficial and nodular basal cell carcinomas.[20] However, many practitioners believe the char from the electrodesiccation improves cure rate by damaging cancerous tissue, but the evidence supporting this assertion is unclear.[7]

Fig. 9: The "H" zone of the face.

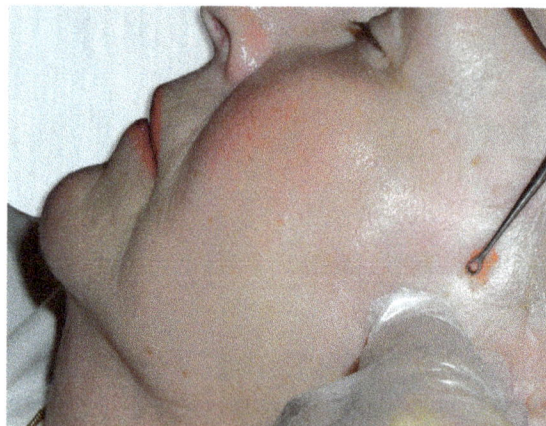

Fig. 10: Feathering of a biopsy with curettage.

RISKS AND LIMITATIONS

Anesthesia

Injections of 1% lidocaine with epinephrine are generally avoided in distal extremities, such as the tips of digits or distal penis, to prevent distal necrosis. In patients allergic to lidocaine, injecting diphenhydramine (25 mg/dL) diluted in 1–5 mL of sterile normal saline is effective for small lesions.[21]

EMLA cream toxicity has also been reported. Most reactions are local skin reactions, but more serious conditions, such as methemoglobinemia, central nervous system toxicity, and cardiotoxicity have occurred.[22] Factors that have led to these toxicities include excessive amount of EMLA application, prolonged application time, and application to diseased or inflamed skin.

Surgical Side Effects

Complications of the procedure include hypertrophic scarring or keloid formation, lesion recurrence, hypopigmentation, infection, and bleeding. Excessive electrodesiccation can result in delayed healing or hypertrophic scarring. Electrodesiccation also has the potential to interfere with implanted cardiac devices.[23]

Curettage is not indicated in the treatment of recurrent tumors, melanomas, tumors larger than 2 cm, tumors extending into subcutaneous tissue, or lesions with ill-defined borders.[6] Curettage should not be used for morpheaform and micro-nodular types of basal cell carcinomas and poorly differentiated, infiltrative squamous cell carcinomas. It is also contraindicated in perigenital areas and the "H" zone of the face, which includes the periauricular areas, periorbital areas, nasal alar, and nasolabial folds (Fig. 9). Recurrence may occur in scars, which might result in the recurrence being overlooked for years. As mentioned previously, cure rates for curettage ± electrodesiccation have been widely debated.

OTHER USES FOR CURETTES

There are a number of other miscellaneous uses for a dermal curette. Curettes have been used to "feather" the edges of a lesion following a shave biopsy. A 2–3 mm curette is used to lightly blend the edge of the shave-so-the demarcation between the lesion and the surrounding skin is less sharp. This has no treatment value, but has great utility as it enhances the cosmetic outcome (Fig. 10).

Curettes can also aid in scabies preparations. The curette is used to scrape the burrows of mites. After scraping, the wooden end of a cotton tip applicator can be placed through the ring of the curette to push the material onto the mineral oil on a slide for examination (Fig. 11).[24]

Author attribution: Logan Rush performed library research on this subject and wrote the first draft of this manuscript. Lauren Craig reviewed, edited the manuscript and approved the content of the

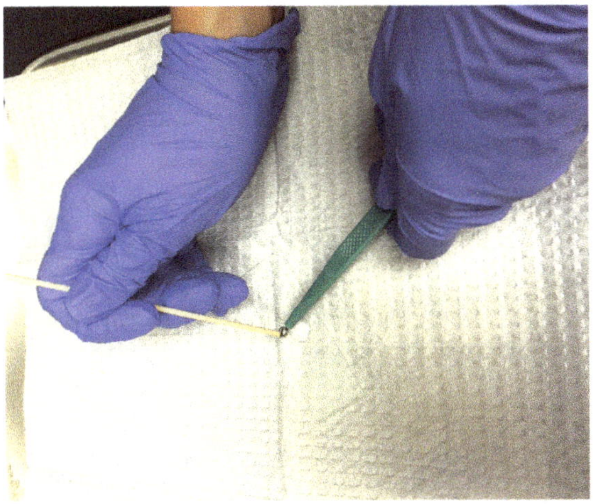

Fig. 11: Use of curette to obtain sample for mineral oil preparation in scabies. A cotton tip application is used to push contents onto the glass slide.

final draft. This article has not been previously published in the literature.

Conflict of Interest

Jess (Logan) Rush and Lauren Craig have no conflicts of interest. There was no financial support for the preparation of this manuscript.

REFERENCES

1. Pifford HG. Histological contribution. Am J Syph Dermatol. 1870;1:217.
2. Wigglesworth, E. The curette in dermal therapeutics. Boston Med Surg J. 1876;94:143.
3. Fox GH. Photographic atlas of the disease of the skin in four volumes, Philadelphia: JB Lippincott; 1905.
4. Clark WL. Oscillatory desiccation in the treatment of accessible malignant growths and minor surgical conditions: new electrical effect. J Adv Therap. 1911;29:169-83.
5. Chrissey JT. Curettage and electrodessication as a method of treatment for epitheliomas of the skin. J Surg Oncol. 1971;3:287-90.
6. Goldman G. The current status of curettage and electrodesiccation. Dermatol Clin. 2002;20(3):569-78.
7. Sheridan AT, Dawber RP. Curettage, electrosurgery, and skin cancer. Australas J Dermatol. 2000; 41(1):19-30.
8. Wolf DJ, Zitelli JA. Surgical margins for basal cell carcinoma. Arch Dermatol. 1987;123:340-4.
9. Edens BL, Bartlow GA, Haghighi P, et al. Effectiveness of curettage and electrodesiccation in the removal of basal cell carcinoma. J Am Acad Dermatol. 1983;9:383-8.
10. Hanna D, Hatami A, Powell J, et al. A prospective randomized trial comparing the efficacy and adverse effects of four recognized treatments of molluscum contagiosum in children. Pediatr Dermatol. 2006;23(6):574-9.
11. Sterling JC, Gibbs S, Hussain H, et al. British Association of Dermatologists' guidelines for the management of cutaneous warts 2014. Br J Dermatol. 2014;171(4):696-712.
12. Lewin JM, Brauer JA, Ostad A. Surgical smoke and the dermatologist. J Am Acad Dermatol. 2011;65 (3):636-41.
13. Garcia MS, Azari R, Eisen DB. Treatment of dermatosis papulosa nigra in 10 patients: a comparison trial of electrodesiccation, pulsed dye laser, and curettage. Dermatol Surg. 2010;36(12):1968-72.
14. Neville JA, Welch E, Leffell DJ. Management of nonmelanoma skin cancer in dermatology in 2007. Nat Clin Pract Oncol. 2007;4(8):462-9.
15. Rogers HW, Coldiron BM. A relative value united-based cost comparison of treatment modalities for nonmelanoma skin cancer: effect of the loss of the Mohs multiple surgery reduction exemption. J Am Acad Dermatol. 2009;61(1):96-103.
16. Rowe DE, Carroll RJ, Day CL Jr. Long-term recurrence rates in previously untreated (primary) basal cell carcinoma: implications for patient follow up. J Dermatol Surg Oncol. 1989;15(3):315-28.
17. Werlinger KD, Upton G, Moore AY. Recurrence rates of primary nonmelanoma skin cancers treated by surgical excision compared to electrodesiccation-curettage in a private dermatological practice. Dermatol Surg. 2002;28(12)1138-42.
18. Reschly MJ, Shenefelt PD. Controversies in skin surgery: electrodessication and curettage versus excision for low-risk, small, well-differentiated squamous cell carcinomas. J Drugs Dermatol. 2010;9(7):773-6.
19. Spiller WF, Spiller RF. Treatment of basal cell epithelioma by curettage and electrodesiccation. J Am Acad Dermatol. 1984;11(5 Pt 1):808-14.
20. Barlow JO, Zalla MJ, Kyle A, et al. Treatment of basal cell carcinoma with curettage alone. J Am Acad Dermatol. 2006;54(6):1039-45.
21. Pavlidakey P, Brodell E, Helms SE. Diphenhydramine as an alternative local anesthetic agent. J Clin Aesthet Dermatol. 2009;2(10):37-40.
22. Tran AN, Koo JY. Risk of systemic toxicity with topical lidocaine/prilocaine: a review. J Drugs Dermatol. 2014;13(9):1118-22.
23. Snow JS, Kalenderian D, Colasacco JA, et al. Implanted devices and electromagnetic interference: case presentations and review. J Invasive Cardiol. 1995;7(2):25-32.
24. Jacks SK, Lewis E, Witman PM. The curette prep: a modification of the traditional scabies preparation. Pediatr Dermatol. 2012;29(4):544-5.

CHAPTER 8

Suturing

Jeremy R Etzkorn, Ilya Lim, Thuzar M Shin

HISTORY/OVERVIEW

Visible scarring alters the gaze patterns of observers, stigmatizes patients, and impairs psychosocial functioning.[1-3] Patients with altered physical appearance, particularly with asymmetries such as poorly camouflaged scars, will go to great lengths to prevent or correct these changes.[1,4] Patients value timely restoration of their physical appearance after surgery, and wound closure via suturing aims to expedite wound healing and create a resultant scar that is minimally apparent to the casual observer. The earliest use of suturing for wound closure appears to date back to 50,000 to 30,000 BC when suture needles were made from bone, and sutures were fashioned from hemp, bark fibers, and hair.[5] Since then, a variety of technical and material innovations related to suturing have evolved. The characteristics of appropriately sutured wounds, however, remain the same (Box 1).

SELECTION OF SUTURING MATERIALS

Suture Instruments

Needle Driver

The needle driver jaw size should be appropriately matched to the suture needle size (Fig. 1). Needle driver jaw width should be no greater than 30–50% of the radius of the needle.[6] A needle driver with jaws that are too large bends and straightens out the curvature of the needle. A needle driver with jaws that is too small allows the needle to move (by allowing rotation around the long axis of the

> **Box 1:** Characteristics of appropriately sutured wounds.
> - Elimination of dead space
> - Tension-free approximation of wound edges
> - Opposing faces of the sutured wound aligned at the same height

needle) and may damage the ability of the needle driver jaws to come into apposition in the future.

> Failure to match the needle driver jaw size with the suture needle size will damage the suture needle or the needle driver.

Each jaw of the needle driver can be smooth or serrated (Figs. 2A and B). Serrations can damage smaller needles, but provide additional grip security that is useful when handling larger needles or when closing wounds under high tension. However, serrated jaws may tear the suture thread when pulling on the thread. As a general rule, larger, serrated needle holder jaws should be used with larger needles and thicker suture thread, while smaller, nonserrated smooth jaws should be used with smaller needles and thinner suture thread.

> Larger, serrated needle holder jaws should be used with larger needles and thicker suture thread, while smaller, nonserrated jaws should be used with smaller needles and thinner suture thread.

Forceps

Forceps may be smooth, serrated, or toothed. For dermatologic surgery, toothed forceps (particularly 1v2 Adson forceps) are most commonly used

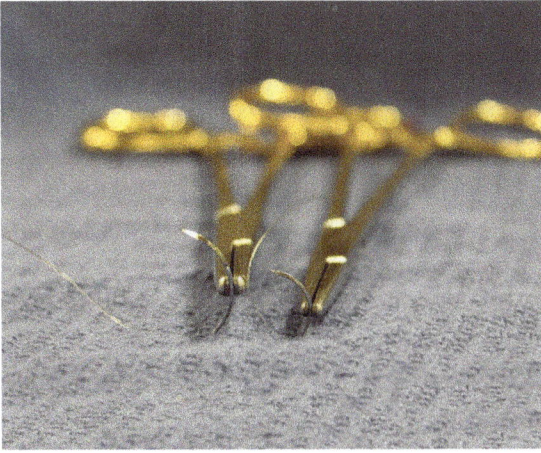

Fig. 1: Needle driver size. The size of the needle driver should match the needle size.

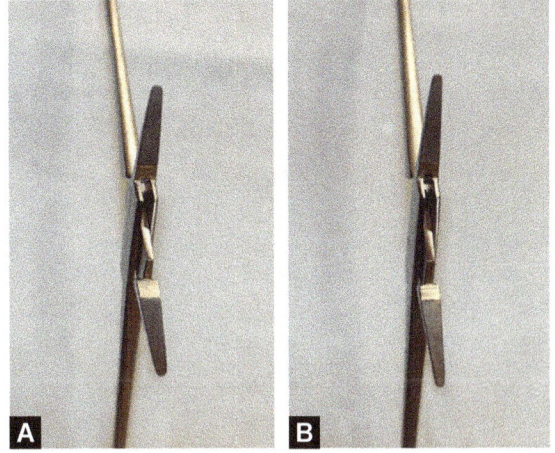

Figs. 2A and B: Needle driver jaws. (A) Serrated jaws. (B) Smooth jaws.

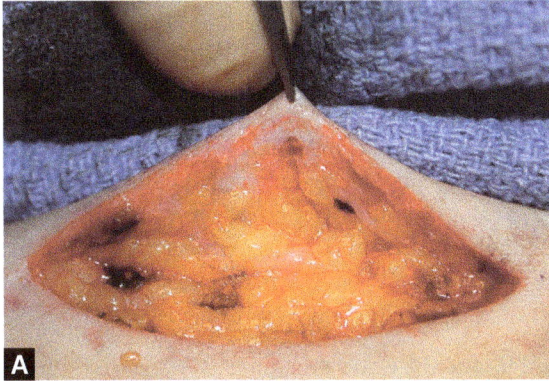

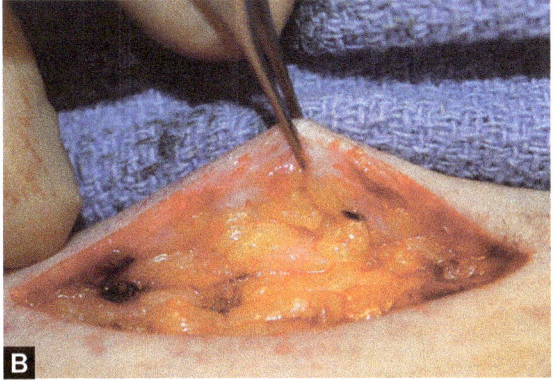

Figs. 3A and B: Retraction with forceps. (A) Appropriate retraction via grasping the papillary dermis exposes a large dermal target for suturing. (B) Retracting too deeply compresses the dermis and makes the target for suturing smaller.

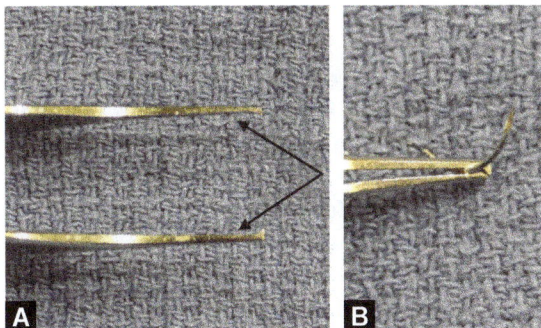

Figs. 4A and B: Utilizing the suture platform to grasp the needle. (A) 1v2 Adson forceps with suture platform (black arrows). (B) Suture grasped with platform, not suture teeth.

delicate forceps (such as the Bishop Harmon forceps). Forceps may have a platform immediately proximal to the teeth that permits grasping of the suture needle; utilizing this platform allows for more efficient needle grasping than attempting to grab the needle with the teeth of the forceps (Figs. 4A and B).

Skin Hooks

As an alternative to forceps, many surgeons choose to use a skin hook for retraction when placing deep sutures (Figs. 5A and B). This ensures atraumatic retraction close to the epidermis, but has the down side of requiring manipulation of a sharp instrument.[7] Skin hooks also facilitate retrieval of suture needles in tight or deep spaces

since their opposing teeth ensure a good grip and gentle tissue handling (Figs. 3A and B). For thin skin, such as the eyelid, use lighter weight,

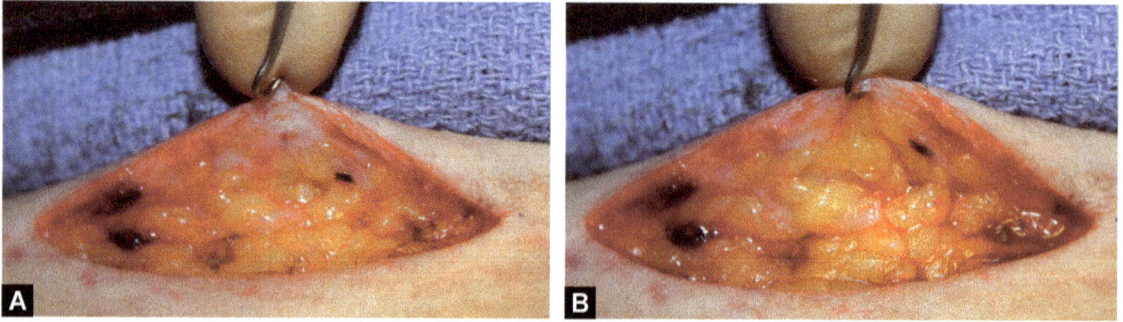

Figs. 5A and B: Retracting with a skin hook. (A) Retracting with the skin hook applied to the more superficial aspect of the dermis exposes a large dermal target. (B) Retracting too deeply compresses the dermis and collapses the target for suturing.

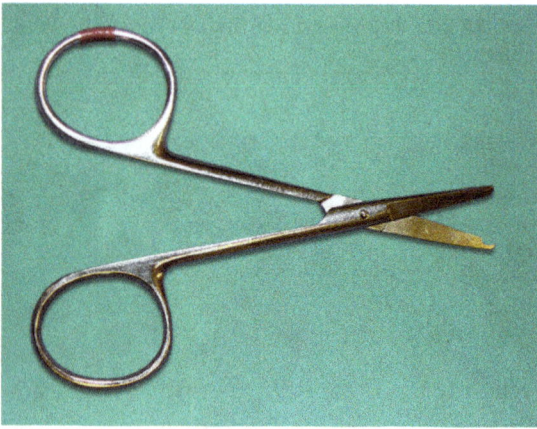

Fig. 6: Spencer suture scissors.

with less risk of bending the suture needle compared to forceps.

Suture Scissors

Suture scissors come in a variety of shapes and sizes. The authors prefer to use Spencer stitch scissors (Fig. 6). These suture scissors have a small curved tip that allows the surgical assistant to easily maneuver the scissor tip into the wound in order to reach the knot.

Wound Closure Materials

The choice of wound closure material should be tailored to the thickness of the skin, the tension of the wound, anatomic location, and patient preference.

Suture

Suture thread: Suture thread can be absorbable or nonabsorbable, synthetic or biological, and

monofilament or braided. Absorbable sutures (Table 1) are generally used to close the dermis and deeper tissue layers. These sutures are not removed because they degrade via hydrolysis or enzymatic degradation. Additionally, certain rapidly absorbing sutures, such as fast-absorbing surgical gut can also be used as a cuticular surface stitch. Nonabsorbable sutures (Table 2) are often used for cuticular surface closure and are removed 4–14 days after skin surgery, depending on the anatomic location and tension on the wound. As a general rule, the smallest suture thread caliber that will provide adequate tensile strength for the indicated repair should be utilized.

> The smallest suture caliber that will provide adequate tensile strength for the indicated repair should be utilized.

In addition to the initial tensile strength of the suture, an important consideration when choosing which deep absorbable suture to use is the breaking strength retention (BSR) curve of the suture. The BSR curve is a representation of how quickly the initial tensile strength of the suture diminishes over time. For example, poliglecaprone 25 (Monocryl®) has a higher initial tensile strength than polydioxanone (PDS II®) or polytrimethylene carbonate (Maxon®) for the same cross sectional diameter, however, its tensile strength diminishes more rapidly over time. After 2 weeks, poliglecaprone (Monocryl®) retains only 30% of its initial tensile strength, while at the same time polytrimethylene carbonate (Maxon®) and polydioxanone (PDS II®) retain 80% and 70% of the initial tensile strength at 2 weeks, respectively.[8] For this reason, polytrimethylene carbonate (Maxon®) and polydioxanone (PDS II®) are fre-

Table 1: Absorbable sutures.

Generic name	Trade name	Multifilament or monofilament	Duration of tensile strength	Time to complete absorption	Tissue reactivity	Knot security	Author notes
Plain surgical gut	N/A	Multifilament twisted	Lost in 7–10 days	70 days	High	Poor	
Fast-absorbing gut	N/A	Multifilament twisted	Lost in 3–7 days	21–42 days	High	Poor	• For fine epidermal approximation of skin grafts • For patients who cannot return to the office for suture removal • 6-0 fast gut mostly broken apart within 7 days; 5-0 fast gut often lasts 1–2 weeks prior to breaking apart
Chromic surgical gut	N/A	Multifilament twisted	Lost in 10–21 days	90 days	Moderate to high	Fair	• May persist beyond desired duration so consider delayed follow-up for suture removal • May be used for mucosal wound for prolonged support, although suture stiffness may bother patients
Poliglecaprone 25	Monocryl (Ethicon)	Monofilament	1 week: 50% 2 week: 20–30%	90–120 days	Very low	Very good	• Easy to handle • Great for running subcuticular stitch • Can be used for the deep dermal as well as superficial stitches • Highly elastic, will stretch to accommodate tissue swelling and return to original size without compromising approximation
Polydioxanone	PDS II (Ethicon)	Monofilament	2 weeks: 70–80% 4 weeks: 50% 6 weeks: 25%	180–210 days	Low	Poor	• Used for high-tension wounds that requires prolonged support. • Delayed spitting sutures may occur (up to 6 months)
Polyglactin 910	Vicryl (Ethicon)	Multifilament braided	2 weeks: 65% 3 weeks: 40% 4 weeks: 8%	56–70 days	Low to intermediate	Good	Increased risk of inflammatory spitting suture at 3–4 weeks when placed too superficially.
Polyglycolic acid	Dexon II (Covidien)	Multifilament braided	1 week: 65% 2 weeks: 35% 4 weeks: 5%	90–120 days	Low to intermediate	Good	
Polytrimethylene carbonate	Maxon (Covidien)	Monofilament	2 weeks: 75–80% 4 weeks: 50% 6 weeks: 25%	60–180 days	Very low	Very good	• Used for high tension wounds that require prolonged support • Better handling than PDS • Delayed spitting suture may occur (up to 6 months)
Lactomer	Polysorb (Covidien)	Multifilament braided	2 weeks: 80% 3 weeks: 30%	56–70 days	Low to intermediate	Good	

Table 2: Nonabsorbable sutures.

Generic name	Trade name	Multifilament or monofilament	Tissue reactivity	Knot security	Author notes
Silk	Sofsilk (Covidien) Perma-Hand (Ethicon)	Multifilament braided	High	Excellent	Soft, ideal for sensitive mucosal and intertriginous areas
Nylon	Monosof (Covidien) Dermalon (Covidien) Ethilon (Ethicon)	Monofilament	Low	Poor	
Nylon	Nurolon (Ethicon) Surgilon (Covidien)	Multifilament	Low	Fair	
Polypropylene	Prolene (Ethicon) Surgipro (Covidien)	Monofilament	Low	Poor	Most commonly used non-absorbable suture by the authors
Polyester, uncoated	Dacron (Covidien) Mersilene (Ethicon)	Multifilament braided	Very good	Moderate	
Polyester, coated	Ti-Cron (Covidien)	Multifilament braided Silicon coated	Moderate	Good	
Polyester, coated	Ethibond Excel (Ethicon)	Multifilament braided Polybutulane coated	Moderate	Good	
Polybutester	Novafil (Covidien)	Monofilament	Low	Good	

quently chosen for high tension wounds that require prolonged support.

> When choosing deep absorbable suture, poly-trimethylene carbonate (Maxon®) and polydioxanone (PDS II®) are frequently chosen for high tension wounds that require prolonged support.

Suture needle: The surgical needle consists of three parts: point, body, and shank (Fig. 7). The body of the needle is the middle portion between the shank and the point of the needle. This is the strongest part of the needle and is the only part of the needle that should be grasped by the needle holder. Grasping the needle body avoids crushing/bending of the weaker swaged shank of the needle, and prevents damage to the delicate sharp point. The ideal position to grasp the needle with the needle holder jaw is the area approximately one-third to one-half of the distance from the swaged end to the point (Figs. 8A and B). The needle should be grasped at the very tip of the needle driver jaws to maximize dexterity and to prevent the needle driver jaws from interfering with suture placement (Figs. 9A and B). Reverse cutting needles are the most frequently used needles in dermatologic surgery.

> The needle should be grasped 1/3–1/2 the distance from the swaged end to the point with the tip of the needle driver jaws.

The curvature of the needle is designated by the fraction of a circle it approximates. Needle curvature preference depends on the location and depth of the defect. The most commonly used needle arc in cutaneous surgery is the 3/8 circle. Use of the 3/8 circle better facilitates needle passage through the dermis, as it requires less pronation of the forearm and wrist as compared to the 1/2 circle needle. The 1/2 circle needle arc is sometimes used when working in deep confined spaces (such as on the scalp) or for suturing small flaps.

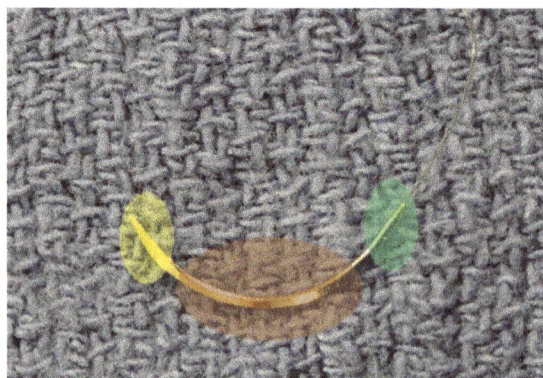

Fig. 7: Parts of the needle—tip (yellow), body (orange), shank (green).

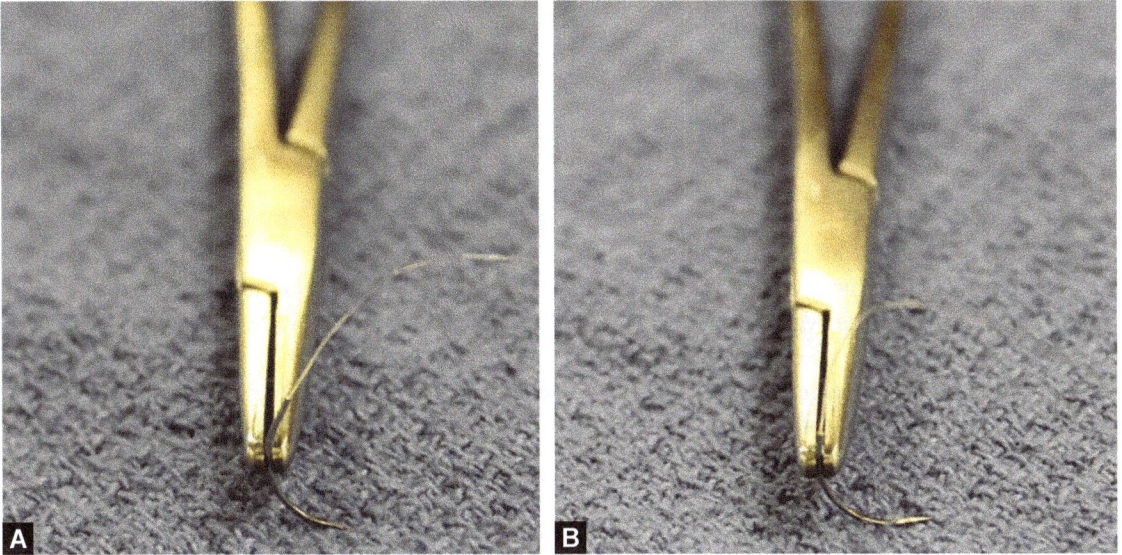

Figs. 8A and B: Grasping the needle. (A) Appropriately grasping the needle between 1/3 and 1/2 the distance from the shank to the tip. (B) Grasping the needle too far back (toward the shank).

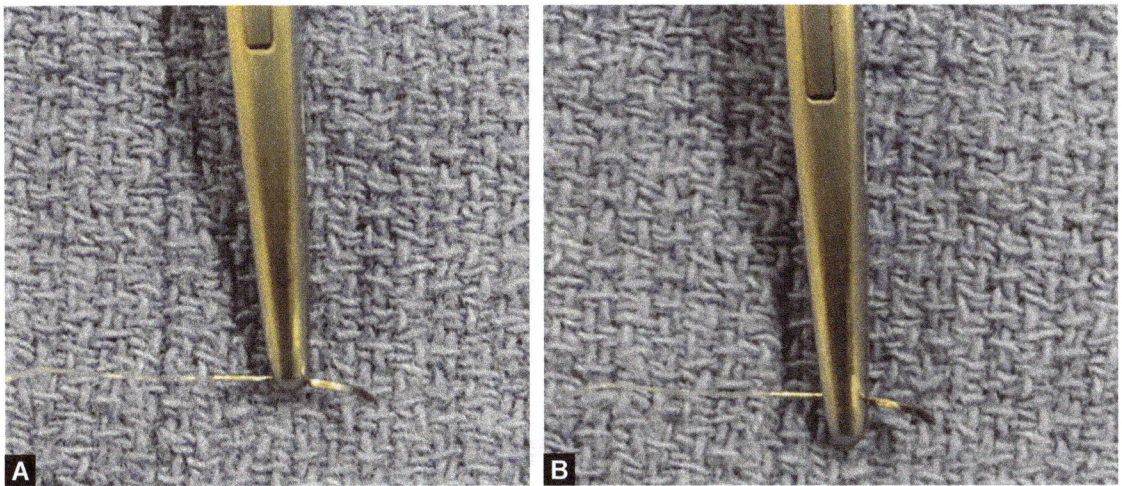

Figs. 9A and B: Grasping the needle at the tip of the jaws. (A) Appropriately grasping the needle with the tip of the jaws maximizes dexterity for suture placement. (B) Needle grasped too far back.

The 3/8 circle needle is most commonly used because it facilitates needle passage through the dermis by requiring less pronation and supination of the wrist.

The 1/2 circle needle is useful for defects on the scalp and for suturing small flaps.

The ideal needle size for placing deep dermal sutures allows for easy passage of the needle through the dermis with sufficient needle body available after the exit point for grasping by the needle holder. Most commonly used needle curvature lengths in dermatologic surgery range from 11 mm to 19 mm.[9]

Tissue Adhesives

Tissue adhesives are an excellent option for closing the epidermal surface and have the advantage of speed, lack of skin puncture holes that could lead to track marks or wound infection, and elimination of the need for bandage changes by the patient. Tissue adhesives should be used judiciously for well-selected, well-approximated wounds, as this modality lacks the ability to evert wound edges or correct height discrepancies. These products are particularly useful for wounds that are located in difficult to bandage locations, such as the back and the scalp, in young patients where the risk for track marks is elevated, or in patients who may have difficulty with daily wound care. Tissue adhesives may also be used adjunctively with absorbable sutures, especially in atrophic skin, to prevent epidermal sutures from tearing through the wound edges.

> Tissue adhesives may be used adjunctively with absorbable sutures in atrophic skin to prevent the epidermal sutures from tearing through the wound edges.

Octyl cyanoacrylate (Dermabond®, Ethicon) is a common tissue adhesive used in dermatologic surgery. After polymerization, which takes about 2.5 minutes, octyl cyanoacrylate provides wound strength equivalent to 5-0 nylon suture.[10] The aesthetic outcome of epidermal closure with octyl cyanoacrylate versus suturing has been found to be noninferior.[11-13] Octyl cyanoacrylate should be applied to clean, dry, and well-approximated wound edges. It is important not to get any of the adhesive into the wound itself, as this can result in delayed wound healing as well as foreign body granuloma reaction. Although the authors only apply one layer of surgical glue, the process may be repeated two more times after the preceding application has dried completely. The polymerization process results in the generation of heat, which may cause minor discomfort to some patients (although this is virtually never noted by patients who are anesthetized with local anesthesia).[14] Of note, tissue adhesives are typically more expensive than suture, but the cost is partially offset by the increased speed of wound closure (especially for larger incision lines) and decreased staff utilization (easier and quicker postoperative patient counseling and wound care instructions, no need for a postoperative visit to remove sutures).

Staples

Surgical stapling is a quick and effective wound closure modality. When used on properly selected wounds, staples have equivalent aesthetic outcomes when compared to sutures.[15] Stapling in dermatologic surgery should generally be reserved for relatively flat surfaces on the trunk and scalp, as well as large full thickness or split thickness skin grafts. Staples should not be used over bony prominences in the intertriginous areas, or on delicate skin (e.g. eyelids). In these areas, they result in significant patient pain and discomfort.[8] Since tissue approximation with staples lacks precision, the two edges of the wound should not have major height discrepancies, as major step off anomalies cannot be corrected.[6] Finally, staples are typically more expensive than suture so their use is typically reserved for larger incisions that would require multiple suture packets and/or significant time for wound closure.

SUTURING TECHNIQUE

Deep Sutures

Appropriate placement of deep sutures redistributes closure tension away from the surface of the wound, approximates the epidermal wound edges, and eliminates dead space. Prior to placement of the deep sutures, undermining or loosening of the adjacent subcutaneous tissue is often performed. The amount of undermining will depend on the location and intrinsic elasticity of the skin, as excessive undermining can increase risk of bleeding and threaten the vascularity of the wound edges.

Buried Vertical Mattress Suture

The buried vertical mattress suture is the most commonly used deep suture in dermatologic surgery.[16] When correctly placed, the path of vertical mattress suture resembles a heart-shaped loop. On each side of the wound, the suture path peaks in the deep papillary or mid dermis. In the middle of the wound, the suture path is lower than these peaks at the sites of suture entry and exit from the wound edges. The knot is below the suture path (Fig. 10).

> When correctly placed, the path of vertical mattress suture resembles a heart shaped loop.

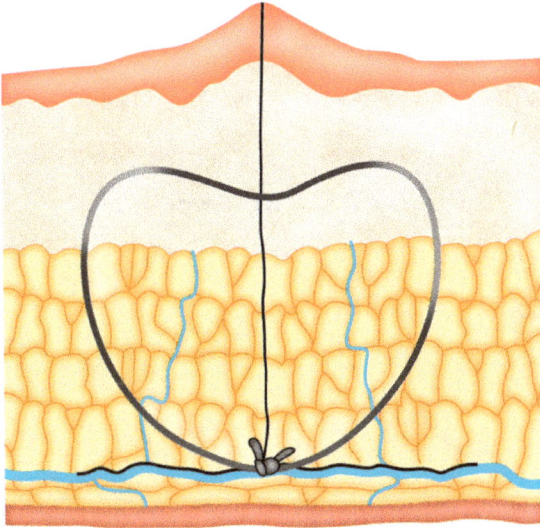

Fig. 10: Buried vertical mattress. The ideal path of the buried vertical mattress creates a heart shaped loop.

Prior to initiating the stitch, the wound edge should be retracted tautly with the forceps or skin hook (*see* Figs. 4 and 5); presenting tissue to the suture needle in an everted position eases and almost guarantees creation of a heart-shaped loop and eversion of the wound edges. If the depth difference between the peak and the exit point is adequate, after the retracting instrument is released, the epidermis and papillary dermis should snap back toward the center of the wound.[7] The suture is tied, and the knot secured with the ends pulled in the direction parallel to the wound to prevent dead space around the knot, and to allow the wound edges to come together.

Eversion refers to the upward sloping wound edges that meet precisely at the crest without inward sloping or plateau. Eversion counters the contractile forces during wound healing and prevents inversion or depression of the scar. Additionally, eversion is a marker that the wound tension has been correctly transferred to the reticular dermis, leaving the papillary dermis and epidermis to heal with minimal tension. The degree of eversion should be tailored to the magnitude of wound tension and the anatomic location with more eversion on areas of the body under high tension (such as the back, chest, and shoulders). Lower tension areas and anatomic regions with natural creases (such as the nasolabial fold and glabella) benefit from less eversion in the authors' experience.

While wound eversion has traditionally been the standard in wound closure,[17-20] not all dermatologic surgeons agree that it is necessary.[21] A randomized, comparative, split-scar intervention study of everted wounds compared to planar ones failed to reveal any differences in aesthetics, pain, or complications at 3 and 6 months postoperatively, as judged by blinded observer and patient assessment.[21] This study was limited by arbitrary selection of everting technique, widespread distribution of anatomic sites, and small study size. Further investigation of eversion is warranted.

Sequence of Suturing

The proper suturing sequence can greatly facilitate the efficiency and execution of the closure. For high-tension wounds, the authors will usually place the initial deep suture in the area of greatest tension and then move on to the areas of sequentially lower tension. For low-tension wounds, starting at one end of the wound and progressing to the other end may be easier and provide equivalent results.

Tying the Knot

An instrument tie is used to create the knot and ensure adequate approximation of the wound edges. With the exception of the key tarsal suture during a wedge repair of the eyelid, the knot is typically buried at the depth of the undermining plane. Prior to initiating the throw, it is critical that each end of the suture lies on the same side of the loop of the buried vertical mattress suture. The number of throws made by the surgeon will be guided by the knot security of the suture and the tension on the wound.[7]

> With the exception of the key tarsal suture during a wedge repair of the eyelid, the knot is buried at the depth of the undermining plane.

The authors typically use a slipknot for the initial throws and then lock the knot in place with a square knot. Throwing a slipknot may be accomplished by following the steps outlined below:

- Form a V that points to the center of the wound with the suture ends (Fig. 11).
- Place the needle holder between both arms of the V during knot tying (Fig. 12).

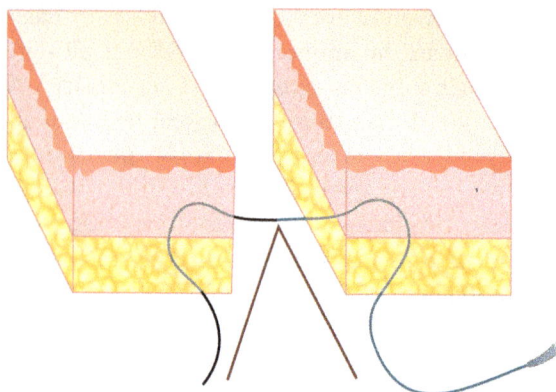

Fig. 11: Form a V that points to the center of the wound with the suture ends.

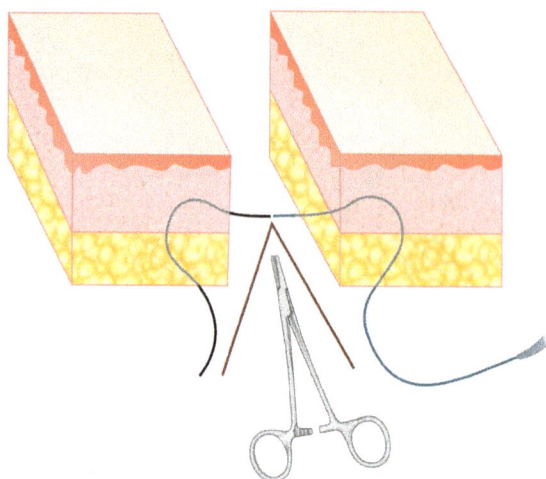

Fig. 12: Place needle driver within the imaginary V formed by the suture strands.

Fig. 13: Wrap the suture thread connect to the needle around the needle driver.

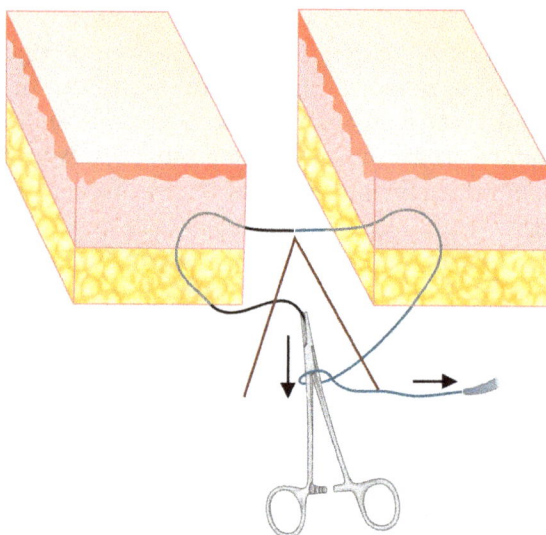

Fig. 14: Grasp the trailing end of the suture and pull it parallel to the long axis of the wound and toward the same side (red arrow) that it originally positioned.

- With the nondominant hand, wrap the needle end of the suture once around the needle holder toward the opposite side of the wound (Fig. 13).
- Grasp the trailing end of the suture with the needle holder and pull it parallel to the long axis of the wound toward the same side that the suture ends initially lay relative to the loop of the buried vertical mattress suture (Fig. 14).
- Bring the needle holder back to center (Fig. 15).
- Throw another loop around the needle holder and pull the suture in the same direction as the first throw. Cinch this throw with the dominant hand pulling rapidly and confidently

along the long axis of the wound (Fig. 16). The final configuration of the slipknot is shown in Figure 17.

Selected Variants: Pulley Suture

The buried pulley suture facilitates approximation of wound edges under tension.[22] The dermal buried pulley suture is essentially comprised of two (or more) adjacent buried dermal sutures. Multiple passes of the suture thread through the dermis

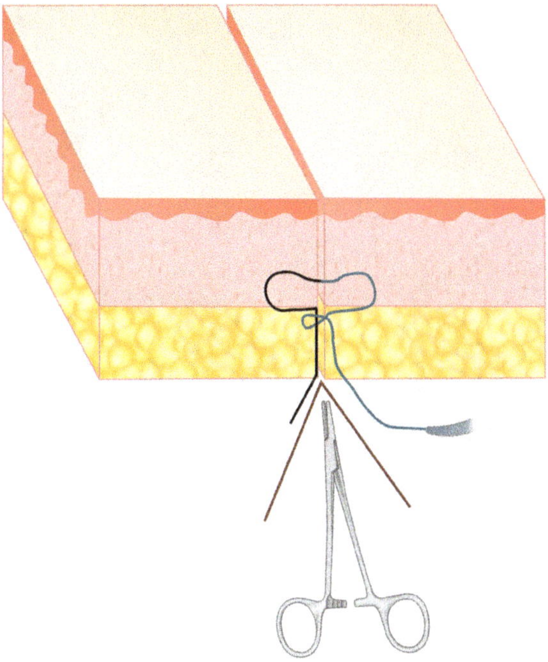

Fig. 15: Return the needle driver to the middle of the V. Note that the relationship of the ends of the suture thread is the same as prior to the first knot throw.

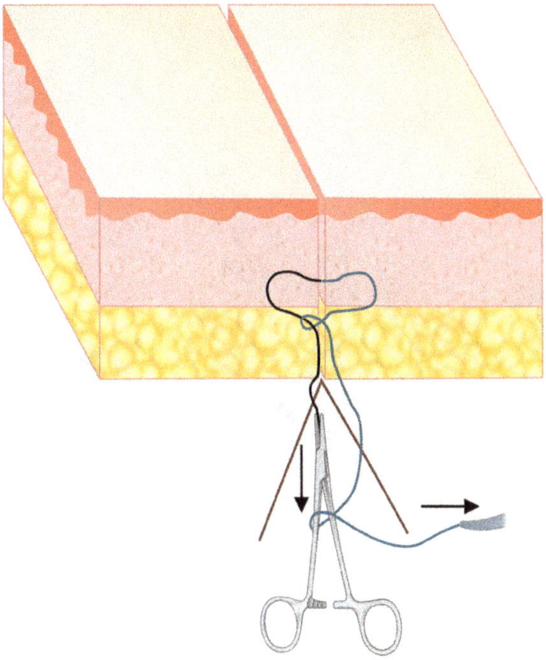

Fig. 16: Another loop is placed around the needle holder in the same fashion as the first loop. Then pull the suture in the same direction as the first throw. Cinch this throw with the dominant hand (grasping the needle driver) pulling rapidly and confidently along the long axis of the wound.

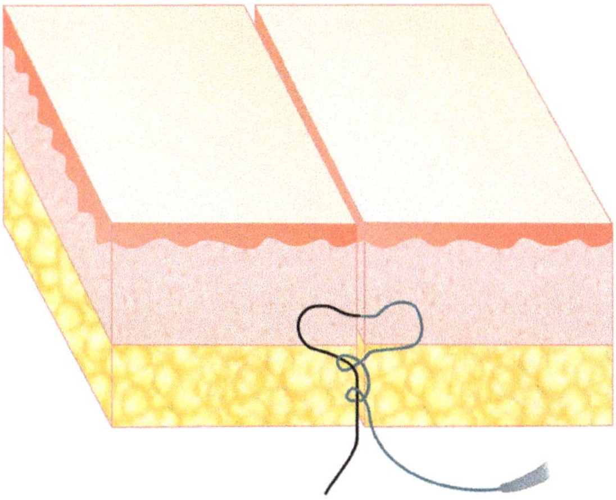

Fig. 17: Slip knot completed.

create increased resistance to sliding movement. Due to this resistance, the suture does not slide after it is pulled to approximate the edges and released to tie the second knot, maintaining the approximation of the wound edges (Figs. 18A to C).

Superficial Sutures

Superficial sutures correct minor height differences between the wound edges that remain after placement of the buried sutures, and should have minimal to no tension. Correction of minor height discrepancies is usually best approached by placing the first bite of the top suture through the high side. A useful guideline to correct height discrepancies with top sutures is: "Bite high on the high side, and bite low on the low side".[7] Approach the high side with a shallow bite of the suture needle that exits the wound edge superficially (i.e. in the papillary dermis). Show the tip of the needle between the wound edges and then depress the wound edge of the "high side" until it matches the height of the "low side". Then pass the needle with a deeper and wider bite through the "low side", at which point the wound edges should be precisely approximated. Placement of superficial sutures in a running or continuous stitch without interruption by knots is faster when compared to interrupted stitches and is commonly used in dermatologic surgery.

> When correcting wound edge height discrepancies, a useful guideline is to "bite high on the high side, and bite low on the low side."

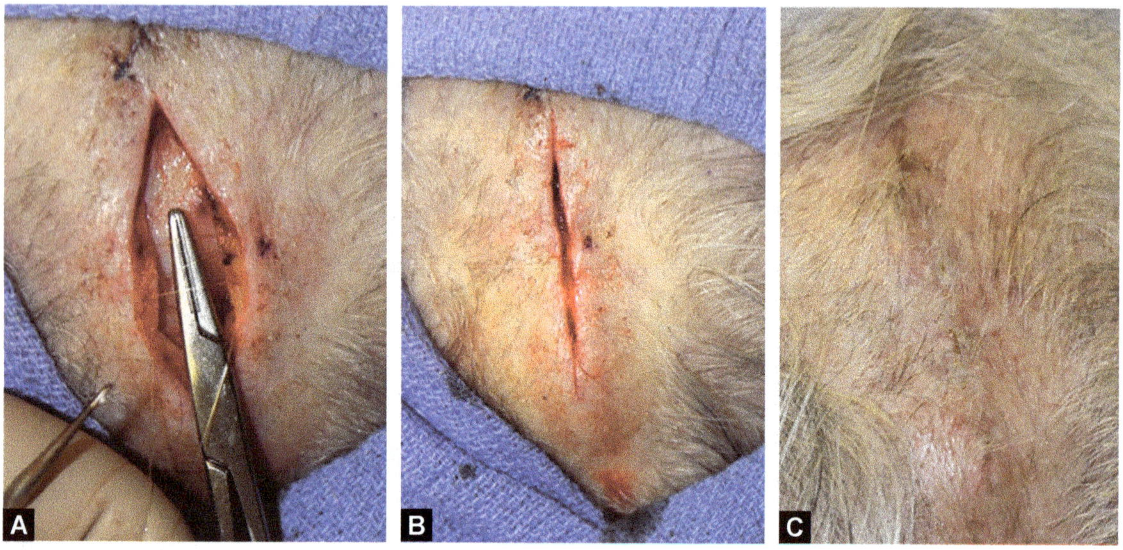

Figs. 18A to C: Pulley suture for closure of a high-tension wound on the scalp. Note that the galea, not the dermis, is the tissue target for the pulley suture in this example. (A) Two adjacent passes of suture shown prior to tying the knot. (B) Wound apposition after a single galeal pulley suture. (C) Wound at 2-week follow-up.

Running Subcuticular Suture

The major advantage of the running subcuticular suture is the lack of epidermal punctures and avoiding visible suture marks. To initiate the suture, place a deep dermal stitch and then run it by taking horizontal loops at the same dermal plane on each side of the wound. Upon reaching the end of the defect, the suture is then tied off on itself beneath the skin surface. Alternatively, the two ends of the suture can be left out and taped down with a tape strip and subsequently removed at a follow-up visit. If utilizing the latter technique, a central epidermal release loop on the skin surface can be placed for easier removal. A suture with a low coefficient of friction is usually used such as poliglecaprone if the suture is to be left in place to dissolve on its own; or polypropylene if the suture is to be removed (Fig. 19).

Vertical Mattress Suture

The vertical mattress suture can help to decrease the tension on the wound edges as well as achieve closure of dead space and wound eversion. The suture is placed with the far-far-near-near sequence. In wounds under high tension, bolsters made of cotton, cardboard, or rubber can be placed between the exposed loops of the suture and the epidermis to prevent the suture from

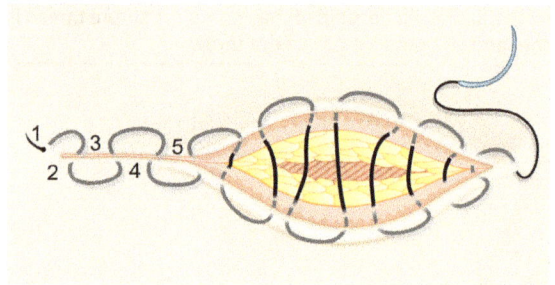

Fig. 19: Running subcuticular suture.

cutting into and injuring the skin in the setting of postoperative edema (Figs. 20A to C).

Horizontal Mattress Suture

The horizontal mattress suture can be used to redistribute wound tension and maximize wound edge eversion. It is started as a simple interrupted stitch by taking a bite with the needle from one wound edge to the next. Then the needle direction is reversed, and it is reentered into the skin 3–5 mm lateral to the last point of exit, taking a second bite of the skin before being tied off with an instrument knot. Moody et al. noted improvement in physician assessed aesthetic outcomes for facial Mohs surgery defects closed with a running horizontal mattress suture in a split scar study (Figs. 21A and B).[23]

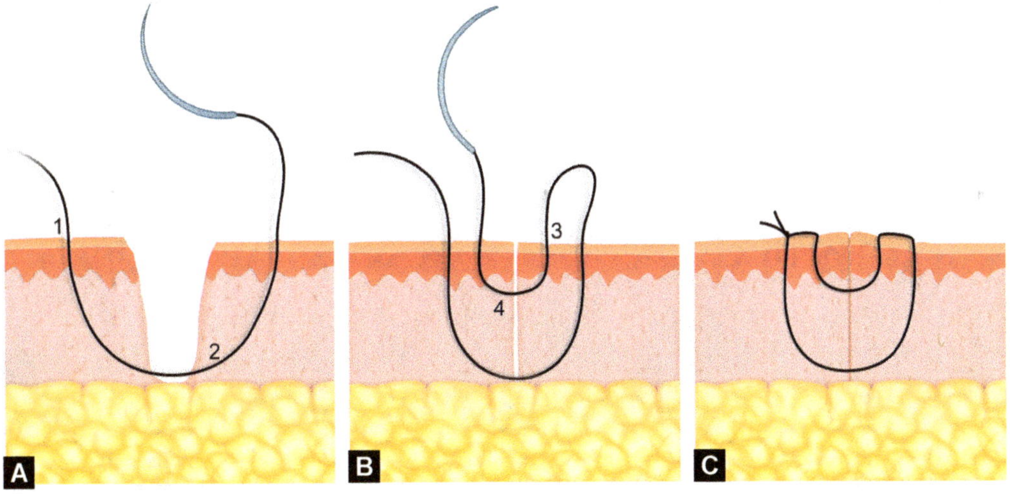

Figs. 20A to C: Vertical mattress suture.

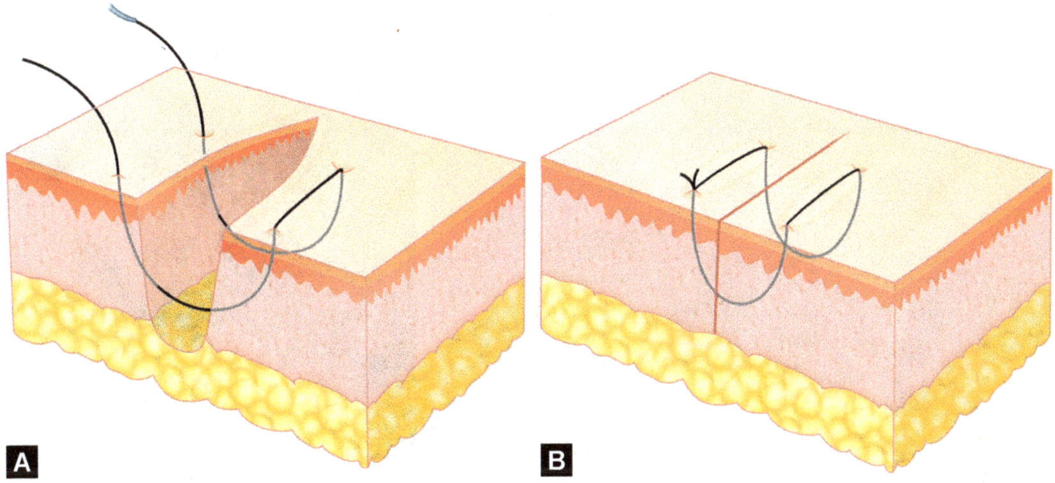

Figs. 21A and B: Horizontal mattress suture.

TROUBLESHOOTING HIGH-TENSION WOUNDS

Several techniques can alleviate frustration when closing high-tension wounds.

Positioning

Back Squeeze (Figs. 22A to D)

Prior to excisions on the back, ask the patient to sit up straight and squeeze their scapulae (shoulder blades) together with their arms by their sides. Tell the patient to visualize squeezing a quarter between the shoulder blades. The resting skin tension lines will become very prominent and can facilitate the excisional design. Asking the patient to repeat the "back squeeze" movement during placement of deep sutures can wound edge approximation.

> Ask the patient to "squeeze your shoulder blades together" to decrease wound closure tension when placing deep sutures for wounds on the back.

Shoulder Flexion (Figs. 23A to F)

Asking the patient to flex the shoulder can help to relieve tension on shoulder wounds, which facilitates placement of deep sutures and wound edge

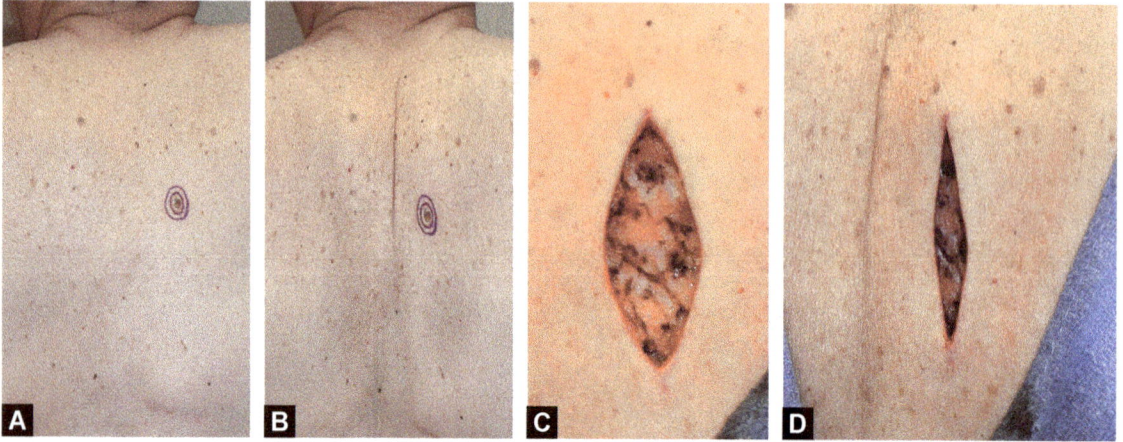

Figs. 22A to D: Back squeeze maneuver. (A) Basal cell carcinoma outlined with 4 mm margins. (B) "Back squeeze maneuver" performed to facilitate design of the orientation for excision. (C) Defect after excision prior to placement of sutures. (D) "Back squeeze maneuver" nearly results in wound edge apposition prior to placement of any sutures.

Figs. 23A to F: Shoulder flexion maneuver. (A) Broad wound on shoulder after excision. (B) Diameter of wound reduced with shoulder flexion. (C) Difficulty apposing wound edges with first dermal suture. (D) Wound edges easily appose when shoulder flexion is performed. (E) Key central sutures placed with shoulder in flexion. (F) Tension-free wound edge approximation after placement of deep sutures.

approximation. For some shoulder wounds, having the patient abduct the shoulder is equally or more effective in reducing tension during wound closure.

Knee Bend

The skin of the pretibial area can be especially challenging to close due to high tension. Asking the patient to bend their knee, so that the calf is suspended off the table allows access to the skin reservoir of the posterior lower leg and facilitates wound closure.

> For pretibial wounds, having the patient bend their knee while keeping their heel on the operating table assists wound closure.

Use of Fascial Structures

Closure of or plication of deeper fascial layers allows the surgeon to offset tension from the dermis and epidermis; this can be useful for facial defects, large defects on the trunk and on the scalp.[24] The galea aponeurotica is the tough fibrous fascial band connecting the frontalis muscle anteriorly to the occiput posteriorly. Scalp dermis often lacks sufficient strength to allow closure of large defects, likely because a portion of the dermis is replaced by follicular structures. Placement of deep sutures that grasp the galea often permits direct closure of defects that might otherwise not be amenable to linear closure (Figs. 24A to E).

> Use the galea to help close high tension wounds on the scalp that might otherwise not be amenable to linear closure.

BENEFITS COMPARED TO ALTERNATIVES

The principal alternative to suturing a wound is second intention healing during which a wound is left to heal on its own. A detailed discussion of when to utilize second intention healing versus when to suture is beyond the scope of this chapter; the principal advantage of suturing a wound is more expedient wound healing with modest wound care requirements and decreased postoperative bleeding. As discussed previously, tissue adhesives and staples can be used in place of percutaneous sutures. However, suturing is still typically necessary to close deeper tissue layers, and epidermal closure with sutures may allow more precise tissue approximation when compared to these modalities.

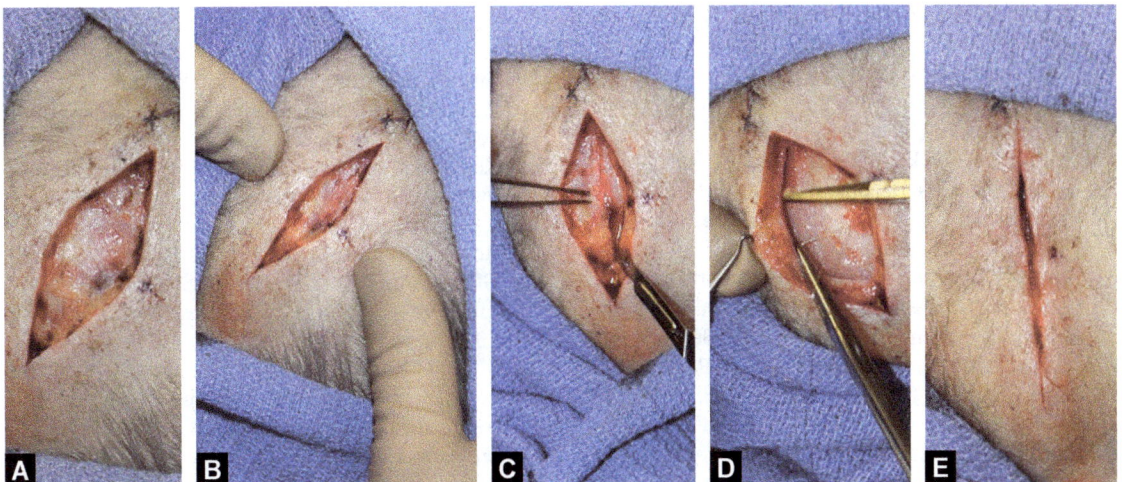

Figs. 24A to E: Closure of scalp wound utilizing galea to displace tension. (A) Scalp defect after removal of standing cones. (B) Manual pressure applied demonstrating high tension and difficulty approximating wound edges. (C) Incision through galea to permit removal of galea from center of wound. (D) Suture placed through galea. (E) Wound appearance immediately after placement of a single pulley suture through the galea.

RISKS/LIMITATIONS

There are several predictable complications that may arise in sutured wounds. Failure to properly close the dead space of deeper wounds or to adequately stop bleeding can result in the formation of seromas or hematomas, respectively. Buried sutures may give rise to spitting sutures and suture granulomas. In the authors' experience, these complications from buried sutures are minimized by using monofilament buried sutures and with appropriate knot cutting technique. Failure to cut the suture thread flush with the knot may increase the risk for spitting sutures. Occasionally, scars may spread or track marks may result from suturing. Meticulous suturing technique with wound tension entirely offset to the buried sutures usually prevents scar spread and track marks. Additionally, timely removal of the superficial sutures (i.e. in 5–7 days on the face) may help avoid track marks. In younger patients, the authors' preference is to use skin adhesives in place of percutaneous sutures to obviate the possibility of track marks, especially on the trunk and extremities.

REFERENCES

1. Sobanko JF. Optimizing design and execution of linear reconstructions on the face. Dermatol Surg. 2015;41 Suppl 10:S216-28.
2. Sobanko JF, Sarwer DB, Zvargulis Z, et al. Importance of physical appearance in patients with skin cancer. Dermatol Surg. 2015;41(2):183-8.
3. Rankin M, Borah GL. Perceived functional impact of abnormal facial appearance. Plast Reconstr Surg. 2003;111(7):2140-6.
4. Borah GL, Rankin MK. Appearance is a function of the face. Plast Reconstr Surg. 2010;125(3):873-8.
5. Mackenzie D. The history of sutures. Med Hist. 1973;17(2):158-68.
6. Baker SR. Local Flaps in facial reconstruction, 2nd edition. Philadelphia, PA: Elsevier; 2007. pp 58
7. Miller CJ, Antunes MB, Sobanko JF. Surgical technique for optimal outcomes: Part II. Repairing tissue: Suturing. J Am Acad Dermatol. 2015;72(3): 389-402.
8. Robinson JK, Hanke CW, Siegel DM, et al. Surgery of the Skin: Procedural Dermatology, 3rd edition. London, England: Elsevier/Saunders; 2015. pp 196-7.
9. Leffell DJ, Brown MD. Manual of Skin Surgery: A Practical Guide to Dermatologic Procedures, 2nd edition. Shelton, Connecticut, USA: People's Medical Publishing House; 2011.pp 96-8.
10. Shapiro AJ, Dinsmore RC, North JH Jr. Tensile strength of wound closure with cyanoacrylate glue. Am Surg. 2001;67(11):1113-5.
11. Toriumi DM, O'Grady K, Desai D, et al. Use of octyl-2-cyanoacrylate for skin closure in facial plastic surgery. Plast Reconstr Surg. 1998;102(6): 2209-19.
12. Sniezek PJ, Walling HW, DeBloom JR 3rd, et al. A randomized controlled trial of high-viscosity 2-octyl cyanoacrylate tissue adhesive versus sutures in repairing facial wounds following Mohs micrographic surgery. Dermatol Surg. 2007;33 (8): 966-71.
13. Kim J, Singh Maan H, Cool AJ, et al. Fast absorbing gut suture versus cyanoacrylate tissue adhesive in the epidermal closure of linear repairs following Mohs micrographic surgery. J Clin Aesthet Dermatol. 2015;8(2):24-9.
14. Ammirati CT. Advances in wound closure materials. Adv Dermatol. 2002;18:313-38.
15. Edlich RF, Becker DG, Thacker JG, et al. Scientific basis for selecting staple and tape skin closures. Clin Plast Surg. 1990;17(3):571-8.
16. Adams B, Levy R, Rademaker AE, et al. Frequency of use of suturing and repair techniques preferred by dermatologic surgeons. Dermatol Surg. 2006; 32(5):682-9.
17. Moy RL, Waldman B, Hein DW. A review of sutures and suturing techniques. J Dermatol Surg Oncol. 1992;18(9):785-95.
18. Alam M, Goldberg LH. Utility of fully buried horizontal mattress sutures. J Am Acad Dermatol. 2004;50(1):73-6.
19. Zide MF. Scar revision with hypereversion. J Oral Maxillofac Surg. 1996;54(9):1061-7.
20. Krunic AL, Weitzul S, Taylor RS. Running combined simple and vertical mattress suture: A rapid skin-everting stitch. Dermatol Surg. 2005;31(10): 1325-9.
21. Kappel S, Kleinerman R, King TH, et al. Does wound eversion improve cosmetic outcome?: Results of a randomized, split-scar, comparative trial. J Am Acad Dermatol. 2015;72(4):668-73.
22. Giandoni MB, Grabski WJ. Surgical pearl: The dermal buried pulley suture. J Am Acad Dermatol. 1994;30(6):1012-3.
23. Moody BR, McCarthy JE, Linder J, et al. Enhanced cosmetic outcome with running horizontal mattress sutures. Dermatol Surg. 2005;31(10):1313-6.
24. Dzubow LM. The use of fascial plication to facilitate wound closure following microscopically controlled surgery. J Dermatol Surg Oncol. 1989; 15(10):1063-6.

PART 2

Tips and Tricks: Chemical Destruction of Skin Lesions

—Robert T Brodell

CHAPTER 9

Dichloroacetic Acid in Dermatology

Jacqueline Graham, Elaine Kunzler, Kristen N Ramey, Robert T Brodell

> *"To a man with a hammer, a lot of things look like nails that need pounding"*
>
> —Abraham Maslow, 1966
>
> *"And, sometimes that's not a bad thing"*
>
> —Robert T Brodell

HISTORY

Dichloroacetic acid (DCA) is an efficacious and cost-effective chemical used to treat a variety of superficial lesions, especially those composed of sebaceous glands and cholesterol deposits. Some healthcare workers may be more familiar with the name bichloroacetic acid (BCA), the historic trade name for this chemical. The official scientific name for this compound, according to the International Union of Pure and Applied Chemistry (IUPAC) rules of nomenclature, is 2,2-dichloroacetic acid. The name simplification accepted by IUPAC is DCA, which is the name most commonly used when ordering this agent.[1]

Dichloroacetic acid may be purchased at a standard strength of 100%. One ounce costs less than $30 and two ounces cost $45 in 2016, making DCA an accessible and inexpensive treatment (*see* Appendix 1). It is generally safe in pregnant women and children, currently being listed as US Food and Drug Administration (FDA) pregnancy category N, or not classified.

> The accepted name for the chemical commonly called bichloroacetic acid in the past is now dichloroacetic acid (DCA).[1]

Until recently, monochloroacetic acid (MCA) was available as a crystal or solution for the treatment of warts. Trichloroacetic acid (TCA) is a crystalline solid at room temperature used in varying strengths diluted to different concentrations depending on the lesion being treated. We are unaware of any direct comparisons between TCA and DCA for the treatment of the lesions covered in this chapter.

DESCRIPTION OF PROCEDURE

Dichloroacetic acid treatment has a broad range of indications including xanthelasma, sebaceous hyperplasia, verrucae, corns, seborrheic keratoses, ingrown nails, cysts, and benign erosions of the cervix. The evidence supporting the use of DCA is largely in the form of case reports and case series, while retrospective and prospective studies support the use of TCA for chemical peels. The authors are unaware of any randomized controlled trials comparing BCA and cryotherapy, laser, or electrosurgical options. However, evidence suggests similar efficacy between BCA and cryotherapy for warts.[2]

During the Procedure

This simple technique consists of carefully applying standard full-strength 100% DCA in its natural liquid state with a pointed toothpick to each lesion. The concentration of TCA must be diluted according to the lesion being treated. Although the volume of acid applied cannot be adequately quantified, BCA is applied sparingly with less than 0.01 mL used in any treatment. It is recommended that only a few lesions be treated initially as a test to ensure that the patient will be satisfied with the final cosmetic result before initiating treatment of a large number of lesions.[1]

> Full-strength 100% DCA in its natural liquid state is applied with a toothpick to each lesion.

> Only a few lesions should be treated initially to ensure that the patient will be satisfied with the final cosmetic result.[1]

Care must be taken to avoid contact with normal skin, and it is important to be cautious around the ocular region.[3] Asking the patient to keep their eyes closed during the entire procedure while treating lesions on the face is a safe practice. A frosted white coating appears as the DCA and TCA air-dries within seconds of the acid application and the treatment is associated with a transient burning or stinging sensation. The acids do not need to be neutralized or washed off, unless accidentally applied on an area of normal skin. In the case of larger lesions like xanthelasma, petroleum ointment may be applied around the lesion to avoid irritation of the adjacent skin. The application of DCA and TCA in total will take approximately 5–10 minutes.[4]

Postprocedure

A superficial erosion develops at the site of treatment within 24 hours. Tenderness resolves and complete re-epithelialization occurs in 4–5 days, with healing usually complete by a few weeks postprocedure. If DCA is spilled or mistakenly applied to adjacent normal skin, or if excessive pain is produced, it can be neutralized with soap and water or sodium bicarbonate. Sodium bicarbonate, found in the common household baking soda, may be mixed with just enough water to make a paste and applied to the affected area. In the vast majority of cases, the stinging sensation is transient and pain medication is not required. Skin irritation is the most common complaint during the healing phase. This can be ameliorated by applying mupirocin 2% ointment, bacitracin-polymyxin ointment, or petroleum jelly twice daily until healing is complete.[1] The latter approach avoids the potential for development of allergic contact dermatitis and petroleum jelly has been shown to promote healing without increased risk of infection for a variety of clean wounds.[5] It is not necessary to apply an adhesive bandage though this is permissible if the patient wishes to cover the treated area.

> Petroleum jelly has been shown to promote healing without increased risk of infection for a variety of clean wounds.

Follow-up visits are arranged for patients within 4 weeks to ensure that the final cosmetic result is acceptable and to treat additional lesions. In the case of xanthelasma, or large sebaceous hyperplasia, retreatment of a persistent lesion is performed at the follow-up visit.[6] Patients with xanthelasma may have recurrences that can be treated as necessary years after the first treatment.[6] Thus, DCA is efficacious in dramatically reducing number of visible lesions, improving cosmetic appearance, and achieving patient satisfaction.

Mechanism

Dichloroacetic acid applied topically penetrates and destroys targeted areas by coagulating proteins and dissolving lipids in the manner of a nonspecific chemical cauterant.[7] The ideal lesion is composed primarily of lipid with small amounts of protein in cell walls and fibrous septae (e.g. sebaceous hyperplasia or xanthelasma). After the DCA quickly dissolves any lipid component of the lesion, the process stops when the acid comes in contact with the underlying dense collagen protein. A thin layer of denser, denatured dermal protein prevents further destruction.[1]

This explains why DCA effectively and uniformly destroys sebaceous hyperplasia and xanthelasma with minimal scar formation.

> After DCA dissolves the lipid component of the lesion, the process stops when the acid comes in contact with the underlying dense collagen protein.

While there is very little evidence comparing the effects of chlorinated acetic acids on skin, it is well established that all three acids, MCA, DCA and TCA, are effective tissue cauterants when used in high concentrations.[6] Of the chloroacetic acids, MCA is considered to be the most deeply destructive of the tissues due to its greater ability to penetrate membranes. The acid strength of these agents decreases with each additional chlorine atom [MCA is stronger than DCA (previously called BCA because it has two chlorine atoms) which is stronger than TCA]. It appears, however, that the degree of tissue destruction in practice likely varies more proportionately with the concentration of acid used rather than with the choice of acid.[6]

> The strength of these agents decreases with each additional chlorine atom [MCA is stronger than DCA (formerly BCA) which is stronger than TCA].

Xanthelasma Palpebrarum

Xanthelasma palpebrarum (XP) is the most common cutaneous xanthoma with a prevalence of 1.1% in women and 0.3% in men.[6] Clinically, XP consists of soft-to-calcareous yellow plaques near the inner canthus of the eyelid found more often on the upper than lower lid. The lesions have a tendency to progress, coalesce, and become permanent.[6] Treatment options include surgical and nonsurgical modalities. XP is a difficult condition to manage and has a strong history of recurrence, regardless of treatment modality used.[8] Although eruptive xanthomas may improve with diet and lipid-lowering agents, xanthelasma seldom resolve entirely with diet or pharmacologic therapy.[6]

Dichloroacetic acid use in XP has been demonstrated in several case reports and case series. In one study, 11/13 (85%) of patients treated with a single uniform application of topical DCA to the entire plaque of xanthelasma responded with complete clearing.[6] Lesions immediately frosted, became eroded within 24 hours, and healed within 2 weeks. At 1-month follow-up, all lesions crusted and healed with only mild residual erythema that faded progressively over several weeks. Of those who responded, less than one-third had a recurrence within 15 months. Patients with incomplete resolution or recurrence were treated until the lesions resolved to the patient's satisfaction. At follow-up 6.5 years later, 100% of recurrent lesions responded to a second treatment and did not require a third treatment. None of the patients experienced infections, scars, or serious complications.[6] Figures 1A to C and 2A to D illustrate the progression of two additional cases of xanthelasma treated in a similar fashion using DCA and producing excellent cosmetic results. Adverse effects from treatment include dyspigmentation, inflammation, scarring, and accidental application to nonaffected areas.[8]

> Xanthelasma treated with DCA immediately frosts, becomes eroded within 24 hours and heals within 2 weeks.

Although literature on treatment of xanthelasma with DCA is mostly limited to patient case reports, other prospective and retrospective studies have evaluated the effect of TCA on xanthelasma. Concentration of TCA used depends on the type of lesion, as an evaluation of the three strengths of TCA on xanthelasma showed that 100% TCA gives the best results in papulonodular lesions, 100% or 70% TCA gives similar results in flat plaque xanthelasma; in macular lesions, 50% is sufficient.[9] A prospective study of 24 patients assessed the results of treatment of eyelid xanthelasma with 70% TCA with regard to efficacy, cosmetic appearance, patient's satisfaction, and recurrence rate.[4] The average number of treatments was 1.5. One hundred percent of patients expressed satisfaction with treatment results, and a recurrence of the xanthelasma lesions was only seen in 25% of patients.[4] Furthermore, a retrospective review measured outcomes of TCA treat-

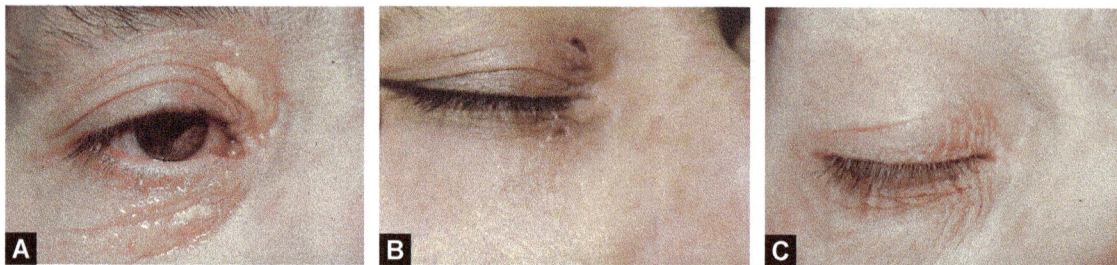

Figs. 1A to C: (A) A 47-year-old male with a 10-year history of a 19 mm × 9 mm yellowish plaque on the right medial upper eyelid and a 3-year history of a smaller 8 mm × 3 mm plaque on the right medial lower eyelid. Petroleum jelly was applied to the surrounding skin producing a reflection seen in this image. Dichloroacetic acid (DCA) 100% was applied with a toothpick until the lesions frosted. The patient was instructed to apply petroleum jelly four times daily at home. (B) Erosion persisting 1 week after treatment with DCA. (C) Excellent final cosmetic result seen at 6 weeks after healing is complete.

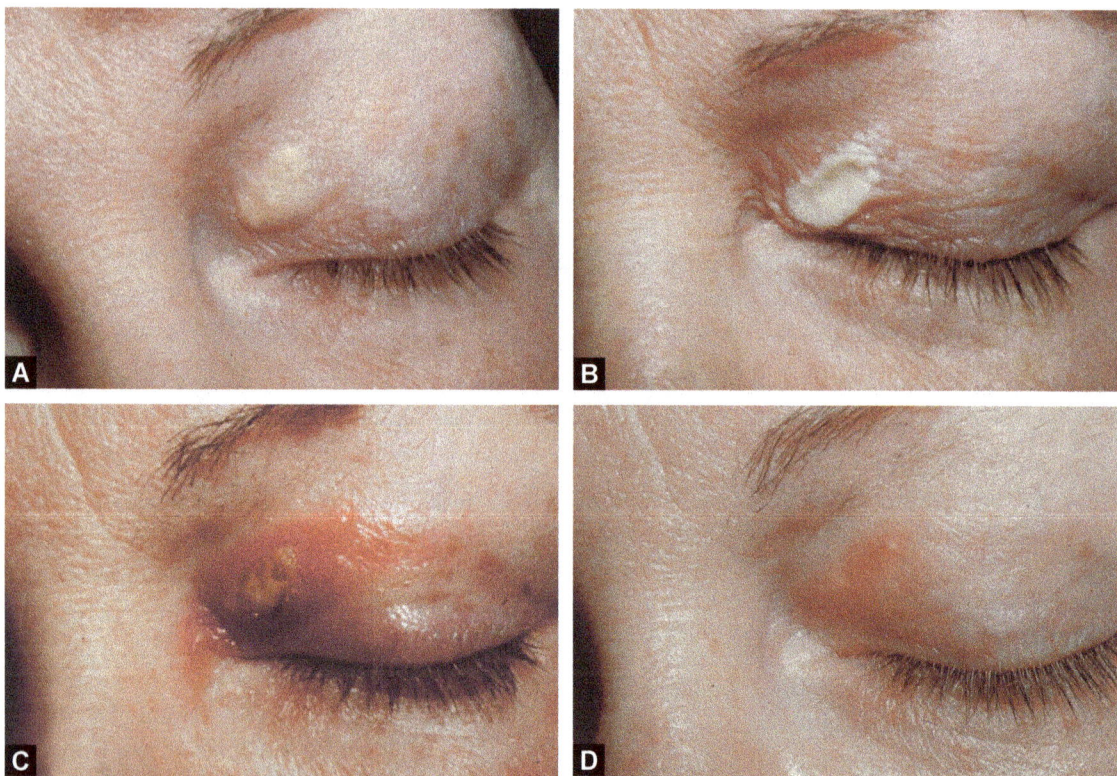

Figs. 2A to D: (A) A 45-year-old female presented with a 12 mm × 10 mm yellow plaque on the left medial upper eyelid. The patient had normal lipoproteins. A diagnosis of xanthelasma was made. (B) 10 seconds after the lesion was treated with dichloroacetic acid (DCA) using a toothpick, the plaque became frosted. (C) The patient returned in 24 hours for a wound check. Erythema and edema are noted, typical of the inflammatory response of DCA on the eyelids. (D) After 3 weeks the wound is healed with post-inflammatory erythema. A milia cyst is noted reflecting the fact that some scarring occurs as a result of this treatment, even recognizing the excellent cosmetic result.

ment for XP and the results presented seemed to show a favorable outcome with TCA treatment.[8] At a mean follow-up of 31.8 months, the overall success rate, determined by a combination of recurrence rate as well as patient's satisfaction with TCA treatment, was 61%.[8] Despite a high recurrence rate of 66%, patient's satisfaction with the procedure was high and many patients whose lesions recurred did not seek further treatment as they were satisfied with their results.[8]

Sebaceous Glands

Ectopic sebaceous glands are common and occur in more than 70% of the adult population. First described by Fordyce in 1896, these glands appear as light yellow, milia-like papules with well-demarcated borders.[1] Ectopic sebaceous glands have been reported to occur on the lips, penis (Tyson's glands), vaginal mucosa, labia majora, and clitoris, as well as on the mucosa of the esophagus, the epibulbar area after a buccal mucous membrane graft, and on the tongue, palate, and gingiva.[1] Papules are frequently distributed bilaterally and occasionally coalesce into plaques. Ectopic sebaceous glands function by holocrine secretion and represent a variation of normal sebaceous glands.[1] The glands rarely occur in children, and hormonal activity at the onset of puberty appears to play a role in their development.

Fordyce Spots

Fordyce spots are enlarged sebaceous glands commonly found on the vermilion zone of the lips and the buccal mucosa. They appear as multiple 0.1–1.0 mm yellow-white papules often occurring bilaterally and occasionally forming plaques. They are similar to sebaceous glands found in the skin except that they lack an association with hair follicles and have ducts that open directly onto the skin's surface. Hormonal changes with puberty can stimulate enlargement of normal sebaceous glands that are present at birth.[7] Although they can have a troubling cosmetic appearance, they are asymptomatic.

> Fordyce spots have been shown to respond well to DCA treatment.

Fordyce spots have been shown to respond well to DCA treatment. A 32-year-old male presented with Fordyce spots that were previously treated with predictable lack of success after treatment with valacyclovir (Fig. 3A). The 100% DCA preparation was applied with a toothpick to Fordyce spots in a central test area. Just as occurs in the DCA treatment of xanthelasma, a frosty white appearance is noted within seconds of the application (Fig. 3B) associated with a stinging sensation. After 1 month, the central test area showed excellent cosmetic results (Fig. 3C) and the remainder of the upper lip was treated with equally excellent results (Fig. 3D).[7] In each treated area, superficial erosions develop at the site within 24 hours and healed completely in 5 days. The patient was instructed to keep the area moist with 2% mupirocin ointment applied twice daily until healing was complete. The lesions had not recurred on any portion of the treated area 3 months post-treatment.[7]

Montgomery Tubercles

Montgomery tubercles are another form of ectopic sebaceous glands that open directly to the skin surface on areola of the breast. Mild epithelial trauma may incite these lesions in specific locations after introduction of a stimulatory hormonal milieu. The treatment of ectopic sebaceous glands is purely for cosmetic purposes.

In one case report, cosmetically distressing Montgomery tubercles on the areola were successfully treated with a single application of DCA in a 15-year-old girl.[1] A 4 mm punch biopsy confirmed the diagnosis prior to DCA treatment (Fig. 4A). 6 weeks after successful treatment of a test area (Fig. 4B), 2 dozen lesions were treated (Fig. 4C). The treatment was associated with a minor burning sensation that resolved after 24 hours, and bacitracin-polymyxin ointment was applied twice daily during the healing phase under a nonstick pad. Initial post-inflammatory erythema faded slowly and the patient and physician were satisfied with the cosmetic result at 6 weeks (Fig. 4D).[1]

> Montgomery tubercles on the areola were successfully treated with a single application of DCA.

Sebaceous Hyperplasia

Sebaceous hyperplasia is a benign skin lesion that most commonly occurs on the cheeks, nose, and forehead of individuals greater than 50 years of age. These lesions are usually 2–6 mm umbilicated

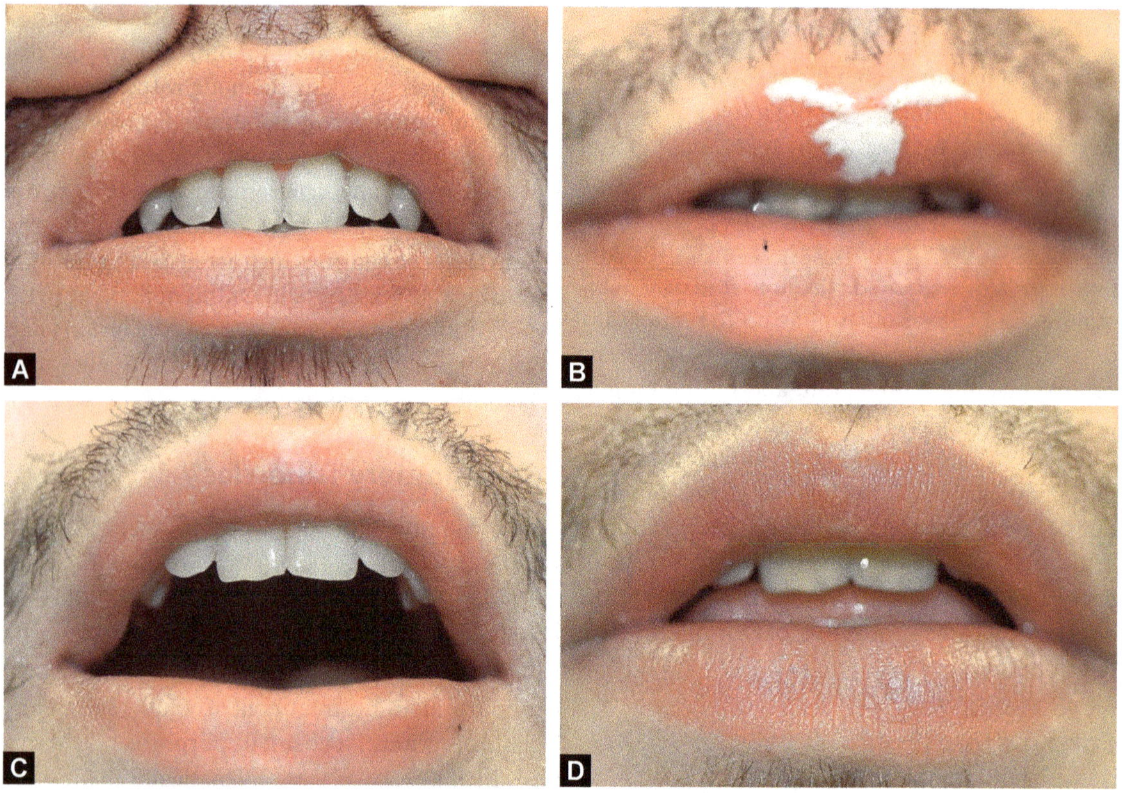

Figs. 3A to D: (A) A 32-year-old male presented with hundreds of 0.5–1.0 mm yellowish papules on the upper lip typical of Fordyce spots. (B) A test area was treated with bichloroacetic acid (BCA) 100% and the frosty white appearance is seen within seconds of contact with the acid. (C) After 4 weeks, the test area had marked reduction in the number of Fordyce spots without significant scarring. (D) Final photo taken 4 weeks post-treatment of left and right upper lip areas, demonstrating 80–90% improvement without any significant scarring.
Source: Reprinted from reference 7, with permission from Wolters Kluwer Health, Inc.

papules that are soft, yellow-to-tan in appearance. The application of BCA is a safe, quick, and effective method for treatment of sebaceous hyperplasia. Topical application of 100% DCA to areas of sebaceous hyperplasia can significantly reduce, if not totally eliminate, these lesions with minimum scarring. In one study, 63 facial lesions of sebaceous hyperplasia in 20 patients were treated with DCA.[10] All lesions treated with a single application of DCA, except one, resolved with good or excellent results as judged by both the patients and their physicians.[10]

> In one study, 62 out of 63 sebaceous hyperplasia lesions responded to one treatment with DCA with good-to-excellent results.[10]

The one lesion that did not resolve responded to a second treatment with an excellent cosmetic result. The treated areas typically form a crust and heal with only mild residual erythema at 1 month that continued to fade over time. Close examination revealed a slight depression and/or shininess of the treated areas in some patients, clinically suggestive of a mild atrophic scar. Hypertrophic scarring was not a problem in any case.[10] Figures 5A to C and 6A to C illustrate the progression of two additional cases of benign sebaceous hyperplasia treated in a similar fashion using DCA and producing excellent cosmetic results.

Sebaceous hyperplasia may also present in a linear fashion as described in an 8-year-old African-American male who presented with an asymptomatic birthmark in the right retroauricular area. Physical examination revealed a 4 mm × 6 cm linear lesion composed of minute yellow papules without even a hint of verrucous change. The posterior pole of the lesion was associated with an 8 mm × 8 mm tan-brown plaque. The

Figs. 4A to D: (A) A 15-year-old female presented with a patch of yellow papules on her left breast. A 4 mm punch biopsy revealed a morphologically normal sebaceous gland in the superficial dermis that drained to the surface through a dilated infundibulum. (B) Scattered 0.5–0.75 mm yellowish papules (Montgomery tubercles) present on the upper medial quadrant of the right areola. Post-inflammatory erythema present 6 weeks after treatment of three 0.75 mm papules with dichloro-acetic acid (DCA) 100%, with the largest area of erythema (directly above the nipple) from the punch biopsy done 9 weeks earlier. (C) Frosty white appearance of Montgomery tubercles seen seconds after DCA 100% application. (D) Resolution of lesions with some persistent post-inflammatory erythema seen 6 weeks post-treatment.
Source: Reprinted from reference 1, with permission from Wolters Kluwer Health, Inc.

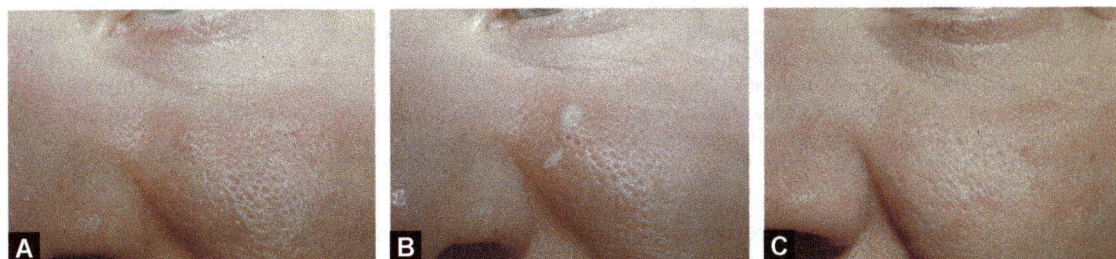

Figs. 5A to C: (A) A 55-year-old male presented with a 4 mm × 4 mm yellowish plaque with a central umbilication on the left medial cheek. (B) 10 seconds after application of dichloroacetic acid 100%, the lesion is frosted and an area of normal skin inferior to the lesion also became frosted after the acid inadvertently touched this area. A surrounding flare of erythema which was associated with a stinging sensation is also noted. This is seen in many patients treated by this modality. (C) After 4 weeks, the patient was quite satisfied with this excellent cosmetic result.

overall appearance was that of the Nike™ swish (Fig. 7A). A 3 mm punch biopsy was performed to include a portion of the brown plaque and adjacent yellow papules. The pathology revealed superficially placed ectopic sebaceous glands emptying directly to the surface without draining

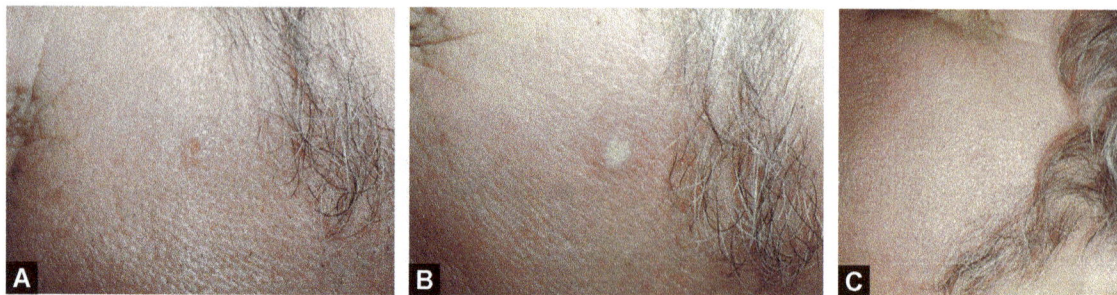

Figs. 6A to C: (A) A 68-year-old male presented with a 5 mm × 5 mm yellowish plaque with a central umbilication on the left pre-auricular area. A diagnosis of sebaceous hyperplasia was made and the dichloroacetic acid 100% was applied with a toothpick. (B) The lesion frosted white within 10 seconds after the application. (C) An excellent cosmetic result is noted at 6 weeks.

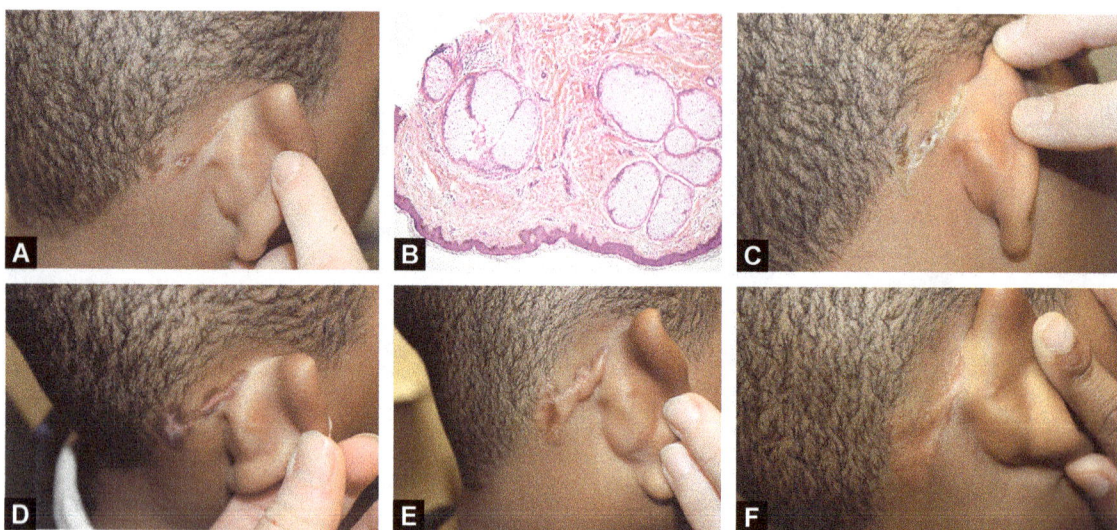

Figs. 7A to F: (A) An 8-year-old African-American male presented with a 4 mm × 6 cm linear lesion composed of minute yellow papules with an 8 mm × 8 mm tan-brown plaque in the posterior pole, giving the overall appearance of a Nike™ swish located in the right retroauricular area. (B) A 3 mm punch biopsy revealed superficially placed ectopic sebaceous glands emptying directly to the surface without draining into hair follicles. The hyperpigmented pole of the lesion demonstrated lentiginous melanocytic hyperplasia without melanocyte atypia or nesting. (C) One week after the dichloroacetic acid treatment, the wound is not completely healed. (D) 2 weeks after the dichloroacetic acid treatment, the wound is healed with some post-inflammatory hypopigmentation at the center and hyperpigmentation in a rim around the treatment site. (E) Three months post-treatment, the patient returned for evaluation of a hypertrophic scar in the footprint of the original lesion treated with DCA. 1 cc of triamcinolone 10 mg/cc was injected into this scar. (F) One month after intralesional triamcinolone injection, the scar flattened and no further treatment was required.

into hair follicles (Fig. 7B). There was no acanthosis, papillomatosis, or heterotopic apocrine glands. The hyperpigmented pole of the lesion demonstrated lentiginous melanocytic hyperplasia without melanocyte atypia or nesting. The lesion was treated with DCA 100% and mupirocin ointment three times daily was recommended for home care. One week after the DCA treatment, the wound was not completely healed (Fig. 7C). Two weeks after the DCA treatment the wound healed with some post-inflammatory hypopigmentation at the center and hyperpigmentation in a rim around the treatment site (Fig. 7D). Three months post-treatment, the patient returned for evaluation of a hypertrophic scar in the footprint of the original lesion treated with DCA (Fig. 7E). One cubic centimeter of triamcinolone 10 mg/cc was injected into this scar. One month after intralesional triamcinolone injection, the scar flattened and no further treatment was required (Fig. 7F).

Warts and Molluscum Contagiosum

Both TCA and DCA have been used in the treatment of warts. The mechanism of action of these acids appears to be related to physical destruction of lesions through its action as a cauterant inducing local inflammation that may lead to memory T-cell production specific to attack the infectious particles causing these lesions. Clearance rates for external genital warts range from 64% to 88%, with a recurrence rate of 36%, similar to the efficacy of cryotherapy.[2] Because DCA and TCA are potent chemicals, they should not be provided for home treatment.[11] Before applying the chemical, it may be helpful in the case of warts to pare away the callous and soak the lesions in warm water.[11] Hydrating the keratin allows better penetration of the liquid or agent that is being applied.[11] Clinicians apply a thin layer of DCA to warts using a toothpick. The lesions frost in seconds signifying that the acid is effectively denaturing proteins and destroying cellular tissues. Treatments are applied by the clinician up to three times per week until the lesion has resolved, with an estimated total cost of $986.[2] Care must be taken to avoid treatment of uninvolved adjacent skin since the solutions of TCA and DCA have a thin consistency and will quickly spread from the application site.[2] It appears that the best results are achieved when small, moist warts are treated.[12]

> Clearance rates for warts range from 64% to 88% with a recurrence rate of 36%, similar to the efficacy of cryotherapy.[2]

Molluscum lesions are treated in a similar manner without the need for paring or hydration. TCA has been successfully used to treat pediatric patients with facial molluscum without resulting in any significant irritation or pigment alteration.[13] Although the lesions of molluscum are typically self-limited, experts recommend treating genital molluscum to decrease risk of transmission.

BENEFITS COMPARED TO ALTERNATIVE APPROACHES

The treatment of DCA offers the advantage of simplicity; the procedure can be performed quickly, easily and requires no special technical skills. In addition, DCA has been used safely for years in the treatment of a variety of skin lesions. Surgical modalities (shave or elliptical excision, electrodesiccation, and curettage) have been described to treat each of the skin lesions described above, but many of these approaches require local or topical anesthesia and no single technique has emerged as a preferred method. Furthermore, the skill of the operator is critically important and significant scarring can occur. Surgical methods can be particularly painful and traumatic in pediatric patients.[13] Cryotherapy with cryospray or cryoprobe [Refer to Chapter 14 (Cryotherapy of Warts, Actinic Keratoses)] can also be used for many of the lesions described, but again the skill of the operator is critical to avoid post-inflammatory hyperpigmentation and hypopigmentation and scarring.

In the case of warts and XP, carbon dioxide (CO_2) superpulsed laser therapy is another treatment modality that has the advantage of enhancing hemostasis with an essentially bloodless field, has better visualization, does not require suturing, results in less postoperative pain, and is a faster speed in comparison to surgery.[6] Disadvantages of CO_2 therapy include lack of availability in all offices, the expense of this technology, and the potential for scarring and pigmentary changes, especially if treatment extends deeper than involved tissue.[7] A prospective study comparing the ultrapulse CO_2 laser and 30% TCA in treatment of XP showed that the CO_2 laser was more effective in severe lesions as there was a significant difference in cure rate, improvement in appearance, number of treatments needed, and recurrence rates.[14] On the other hand, there was no significant difference in any of these categories between TCA and CO_2 laser in treatment of clinically mild lesions and TCA resulted in significantly less pigmentary change. The authors concluded that both 30% TCA and ultrapulse CO_2 laser are safe options with low risk of serious side effects such as visible scarring and ectropion.[14] Another study examined the clinical efficacy of different concentrations of topical TCA versus the CO_2 laser in XP treatment.[15] There was statistically significant clinical improvement with usage of 70% TCA and CO_2 laser compared to patients treated with 35% and 50% TCA, but the difference in clinical efficacy between patients treated with TCA 70% and patients with CO_2 laser was insignificant.[15] Although lasers are an effective treatment, DCA and TCA treatments are certainly more cost-effective than laser and cold steel options.

Xanthelasma lesions can be treated by erbium: YAG (yttrium aluminum garnet) laser. A prospective study found that there was no significant difference in efficacy or complications of xanthelasma lesions treated with 70% TCA versus YAG laser.[16] YAG has the disadvantage of high cost and maintenance of the apparatus and specialized training equipment for its use. Since both have similar effectiveness and complication rates, the treatment of XP with TCA is advantageous because it is more cost-effective and easier to use.

The 5-aminolevulinic acid photodynamic therapy has been reported to treat Fordyce spots.[7] After several sessions with the therapy, only mild clinical improvement has been shown, rendering 5-aminolevulinic acid-photodynamic therapy minimally effective in treating patients with ectopic sebaceous glands.[1,7] It is associated with significant adverse effects, such as painful swelling, vesiculation, and post-inflammatory hyperpigmentation.

Other treatments have been used to treat sebaceous lesions. In the 1980s, researchers found that isotretinoin could help transiently clear lesions of sebaceous hyperplasia within 2–6 weeks, but lesions recurred once the therapy was discontinued.[1,3] Isotretinoin is less ideal as risks of long-term systemic therapy are significant and recurrence is anticipated when therapy is discontinued.[7]

In the case of xanthelasma, surgical excision is a widely utilized technique. Surgery has the advantage of providing a pathologic specimen to confirm diagnosis. The surgical approach may be especially appropriate for smaller bulging lesions.[6] Despite this evidence, surgical excision is time-consuming and expensive when compared to DCA.[6] Removal of larger areas risks eyelid retraction, upper eyelid fold asymmetry, ectropion, scarring, or the need for more complicated coverage with grafts or other reconstructive procedures. Surgery has been shown to cause higher recurrence rates, as high as 40% after the primary

excision and 60% after the second.[17] DCA or TCA is a simpler technique than surgery that does not require high levels of surgical skill to obtain excellent results.

RISKS AND LIMITATIONS

Sufficiently powered, prospective double-blind, controlled studies are needed to determine the risks and benefits of DCA application. Reported side effects have included post-inflammatory erythema or hyperpigmentation that can take approximately 6–12 weeks to resolve. Post-inflammatory hypopigmentation may occur, more predominantly in patients with darker skin tones.[1] Physicians must take great care in application to avoid dripping or splashing the acid into the eyes producing a potentially catastrophic ocular injury. Patients should certainly be instructed to keep their eyes closed at all times. Other possible side effects include bacterial infection and scarring. However, previously reported cases with Fordyce spots, xanthelasma, and sebaceous hyperplasia suggest that the risk of significant scarring is small.[1] Lastly, patients should be informed that regardless of modality employed, recurrence is possible.

> Physicians must take great care in application to avoid dripping or splashing the acid into the eyes producing a potentially catastrophic ocular injury.

More important issues with this procedure can arise if a treated lesion is misdiagnosed as benign sebaceous hyperplasia when it is actually a basal cell carcinoma (BCC) or another type of invasive malignant tumor.[10] BCC and sebaceous hyperplasia share many clinical features, both being pearly, papular lesions, and the central erosion in a BCC can mimic the dimple in the center of sebaceous hyperplasia. There is no evidence in the literature that DCA would be curative for BCC, and would therefore delay appropriate treatment. Thus, should any question about diagnosis arise, a shave biopsy would be indicated. In order to reduce the risks of side effects, it is recommended to apply petroleum jelly or topical antibiotic ointments post-treatment to keep the wound bed moist until healing has occured.[7] Performing the first DCA treatment on a small test area or a few lesions before treating a large number of lesions may also help ensure that the patient will tolerate the treatment and be satisfied with the result.[1] Overall, it is expected that the side effects of DCA would be less pronounced than with tangential excision, CO_2 laser vaporization, or electrodesiccation, where the destructive effect of treatment is not as focused on the sebaceous glands.[1] Thus, DCA should be considered as a quick, effective, and safe treatment plan for a variety of common skin lesions.

REFERENCES

1. Tulbert B, Brodell RT. A simple and effective treatment for ectopic sebaceous glands on the areola. Dermatol Surg. 2010;36(8):1332-5.
2. Karnes JB, Usatine RP. Management of external genital warts. Am Fam Physician. 2014;90(5):312-8.
3. Richey DF. Aminolevulinic acid photodynamic therapy for sebaceous gland hyperplasia. Dermatol Clin. 2007;25(1):59-65.
4. Nahas TR, Marques JC, Nicoletti A, et al. Treatment of eyelid xanthelasma with 70% trichloroacetic acid. Ophthal Plast Reconstr Surg. 2009;25(4):280-3.
5. Trookman NS, Rizer RL, Weber T. Treatment of minor wounds from dermatologic procedures: a comparison of three topical wound care ointments using a laser wound model. J Am Acad Dermatol. 2011;64(3 Suppl):S8-15.
6. Haygood LJ, Bennett JD, Brodell RT. Treatment of xanthelasma palpebrarum with bichloroacetic acid. Dermatol Surg. 1998;24(9):1027-31.
7. Plotner AN, Brodell RT. Treatment of Fordyce spots with bichloroacetic acid. Dermatol Surg. 2008;34(3):397-9.
8. Cannon PS, Ajit R, Leatherbarrow B. Efficacy of trichloroacetic acid (95%) in the management of xanthelasma palpebrarum. Clin Exp Dermatol. 2010;35(8):845-8.
9. Haque MU, Ramesh V. Evaluation of three different strengths of trichloroacetic acid in xanthelasma palpebrarum. J Dermatolog Treat. 2006;17(1):48-50.
10. Rosian R, Goslen JB, Brodell RT. The treatment of benign sebaceous hyperplasia with the topical application of bichloroacetic acid. J Dermatol Surg Oncol. 1991;17(11):876-9.
11. Tuggy ML, Garcia J, Oswald L, et al. (2009). Procedures Consult: Wart Treatment (Family Medicine). [online] Available from www.clinicalkey.com/#!/content/medical_procedure/19-s2.0-mp_FM-007. [Accessed March, 2017].
12. Rivera A, Tyring SK. Therapy of cutaneous human Papillomavirus infections. Dermatol Ther. 2004;17(6):441-8.
13. Bard S, Shiman MI, Bellman B, et al. Treatment of facial molluscum contagiosum with trichloroacetic acid. Pediatr Dermatol. 2009;26(4):425-6.
14. Goel K, Sardana K, Garg VK. A prospective study comparing ultrapulse CO_2 laser and trichloroacetic acid in treatment of xanthelasma palpebrarum. J Cosmet Dermatol. 2014;14(2):130-9.
15. Mourad B, Elgarhy LH, Ellakkawy HA, et al. Assessment of efficacy and tolerability of different concentrations of trichloroacetic acid vs. carbon dioxide laser in treatment of xanthelasma palpebrarum. J Cosmet Dermatol. 2015;14(3):209-15.
16. Güngör S, Canat D, Gökdemir G. Erbium: YAG laser ablation versus 70% trichloroacetic acid application in the treatment of xanthelasma palpebrarum. J Dermatolog Treat. 2014;25(4):290-3.
17. Mendelson BC, Masson JK. Xanthelasma: follow-up on results after surgical excision. Plast Reconstr Surg. 1976;58(5):535-8.

APPENDIX 1

- Delasco website for convenient purchase of dichloroacetic acid: https://www.delasco.com/pcat/1/sds.php.
- The authors have no financial interest in the Delasco Company and we are certain that there are other sources available.

PART 3

Tips and Tricks: Complex Surgical Procedures

—*Ashish C Bhatia*

"There is no condition so bad that a surgeon can't make it worse"

—Volksweisheit

CHAPTER 10

Mohs Surgery

Brittany L Vieira, Lara E Rosenbaum, Ashish C Bhatia

HISTORY

Dr Frederic E Mohs originally pioneered Mohs micrographic surgery (MMS) at the University of Wisconsin-Madison in the 1930s, when he began using zinc chloride paste for in vivo fixation of tumors in rats. Zinc chloride paste consisted of zinc chloride, granulated stibnite, and extract of blood root (*Sanguinaria canadensis*), and had been used since the 1800s as an escharotic agent. In his preliminary experiments, Dr Mohs observed that intralesional injection of the 20% zinc chloride paste not only caused tumor necrosis, but also preserved histology so that the tumor could be microscopically examined upon removal. In 1936, Dr Mohs began using his technique on humans and in 1941, he first published a description of his technique.[1]

Unfortunately, the zinc chloride paste could be quite uncomfortable and sometimes required several days of application to clear the tumor. In the 1950s, Dr Mohs began performing excisions of the eyelid and other small discrete tumors using a fresh tissue technique. This technique gained popularity in the 1970s when Dr Tromovitch and Stegman published a detailed paper delineating this fresh-frozen tissue technique.[2] This fresh-frozen technique allowed for same-day resection and immediate reconstruction, a significant advantage compared to the use of zinc chloride.

In 1967, the American College of Micrographic Surgery and Cutaneous Oncology was established, followed closely thereafter with the first fellowship in 1970. The technique has continued to be refined over the decades. It is now estimated that one in every four skin cancers is treated with MMS.[3] In recent years, use of Mohs surgery has expanded beyond basal cell carcinoma and squamous cell carcinoma and may be utilized for more unusual cutaneous malignancies.

DESCRIPTION OF PROCEDURE HIGHLIGHTING TIPS AND TRICKS

Preoperative Evaluation

To ensure optimal outcomes, a detailed medical history and focused skin examination should be performed at the time of consultation. Specific preoperative considerations include patient allergies (drugs, latex, iodine, and anesthetics), current medications (including herbal supplements and over-the-counter agents), and implants that may affect use of a hemostatic device (cardiac pacemakers/defibrillators or deep brain stimulators). Special attention should be paid to the use of anticoagulants or other substances that may increase the risk of perioperative bleeding: ginko, garlic, ginseng, ginger, and vitamin E. Some Mohs surgeons may discontinue all supplements and over-the-counter drugs that are not medically necessary.[4]

Prophylactic antibiotics may be used to prevent surgical site infections, and reduce the risk of endocarditis or seeding of prosthetic devices in high-risk patients. For optimal prophylaxis, a single dose should be given 30–60 minutes prior to surgery. Recommendations for indications, selection, and timing of antibiotics in cutaneous surgery are usually based on the most recent American Heart Association guidelines[5] and should be reviewed prior to initiation.[6-8]

Given the temporal latency and hand-offs that typically occur between initial biopsy and MMS, it is important to confirm correct site in all patients.[9] Some surgeons also employ additional quality-assurance practices, such as the utilization of their own dermatopathologists to review biopsy slides of all referred patients. Indeed, one study reviewed 3,345 referred cases and found that 2.2% of preoperative diagnoses were incorrect, resulting in a revision of the management plan in the majority (61%) of those cases.[10]

Additional considerations include evaluating the need for preoperative imaging or establishing a multidisciplinary team for the patient. Consultation with other specialties, such as oculoplastics or otolaryngology may be indicated when a complex repair is anticipated. The day of surgery, patients can eat a light meal in the morning and continue all regular medications, and should also be encouraged to bring a friend or relative with them on the day of the procedure.

Technique of the Procedure

Though individual surgeons may use small variations, the technique of MMS employs a sequence of fundamental steps. In brief, the malignancy and a small perimeter of benign tissue are excised. The layer is flattened such that epidermis, dermis and subcutaneous tissue or adipose are now aligned in a single plane. This tissue is then frozen, cut with a cryostat, mounted on a slide and stained for examination by the surgeon such that 100% of the margin is visualized microscopically. Positive margins are indicated on the map, and additional malignant tissue is precisely excised.

These three steps: (1) surgical excision, (2) histopathologic assessment and (3) precise mapping, are repeated until all malignant tissue has been excised from the defect and after that wound management can begin.

Surgical Excision

To prepare the site for excision, the area should be thoroughly cleansed with a surgical scrub (Betadine, chlorhexidine, or povidone-iodine). Visually examine tumor and carefully mark the clinical margins and important cosmetic lines using gentian violet or a surgical pen. Once the area is delineated, inject local anesthetic (typically lidocaine with epinephrine).

Tip: To minimize the discomfort of acidic lidocaine injection, consider buffering with 1 part sodium bicarbonate to nine parts lidocaine, slow injection, pinching adjacent skin, application of ice, vibration, or needle insertion through a pore (particularly helpful on the nose). Allow 5–10 minutes for vasoconstrictive action of the epinephrine to take effect.

Some surgeons debulk the clinically evident tumor with a scalpel or curette prior to excising the first layer. The purpose of a debulking step is to remove and discard gross pathologic tissue to help delineate tumor extension and facilitate removal of a specimen of uniform thickness from the base of the debulked region.

Next, the initial Mohs layer is excised. A single smooth incision is made with a scalpel to excise the area of clinically apparent malignancy and a small border of normal-appearing tissue (1–4 mm, depending on histologic subtype, likelihood of tumor extension or recurrence, and importance of tissue sparing). The incisions used are most often beveled at 30–60°, which allows the sides and bottom of the layer to be flattened during tissue processing. Some Mohs surgeons no longer bevel their incisions, opting for perpendicular incisions; however, a conventional bevel of the scalpel is most common (Fig. 1).[11]

Before removing the tissue, marks are created to help orient the Mohs layer relative to the defect.

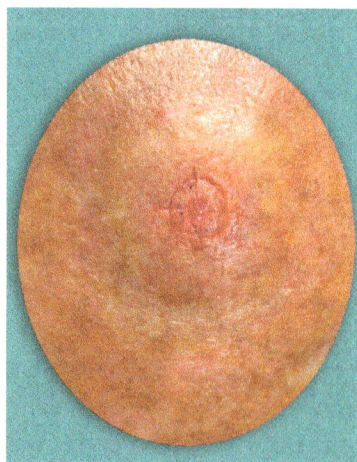

Fig. 1: The initial Mohs layer is excised with a small clinical margin. Nicks are made to help orient the Mohs layer relative to the defect.

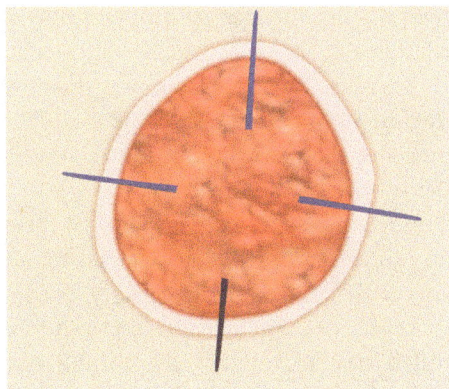

Fig. 2: Shallow nicks, bridging from the specimen to the adjacent skin, are typically placed at the 12, 3, 6 and/or 9 o'clock positions.

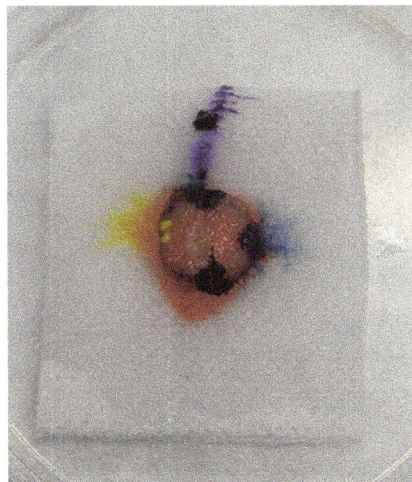

Fig. 3: The Mohs layer is placed on gauze and colored ink is applied to each nick for orientation and microscopic mapping.

These marks are typically created with a scalpel using shallow nicks, bridging from the specimen to the adjacent skin at 12, 3, 6 or 9 o'clock positions. This helps provide clear direction when correlating microscopic findings of positive margins later in the process (Fig. 2).

> *Tip:* Do not create symmetric marks in the specimen to decrease the risk of the specimen losing its proper orientation during transport from the patient to the tissue processing area.

Use a scalpel or tissue scissors to transect the base of the layer parallel to surface of the skin. Remove the layer and lay tissue on transfer card or marked gauze, ensuring correct orientation relative to the defect. Utilize electrocoagulation or thermocautery as indicated for hemostasis. The wound is temporarily dressed with a pressure bandage and the patient is discharged to the waiting room for 1–2 hours while the tissue is being processed and analyzed.

Precise Mapping

A "Mohs map" is carefully created to indicate tumor location relative to anatomic landmarks. Transfer information regarding shape, size, and orientation of markings, with corresponding ink colors to the specimen map (Fig. 3). Once the surgeon completes the histopathological assessment, areas of positive margins should be indicated on the specimen map, so residual tumor foci can be precisely excised.

Histopathologic Assessment

Next, the histotechnician processes the excised tissue layer. The histotechnician performs many precise steps prior to tissue assessment by the Mohs surgeon. Each processing step has the potential to introduce error and affect overall cure rate without careful recognition, correction and quality control measures.

Correct tissue processing is achieved by flattening the three-dimensional layer completely into a two-dimensional shape, so that the epidermis lies in the same plane as the dermis and deep margin. The tissue is then mounted in embedding medium and frozen using a cryostat. Frozen sections are cut using a microtome. The sections are set onto glass slides and stained with hematoxylin and eosin (H&E) or toluidine blue stain.

If tissue preparation is effective, the surgeon can microscopically assess of 100% of the excised surgical margin. Each section is carefully evaluated to confirm that 100% of the epidermis is present (Fig. 4). Epidermal or dermal tissue dropout may occur due to incorrect flattening or separation with microtome use, and may cause an incorrect interpretation of margin clearance.[12-14] Once 100% of the epidermis, continuous inked edges and deep margin is confirmed visually, the histology bordering these edges is evaluated. If positive margins are seen, the areas of residual tumor foci can be located and marked on the specimen map

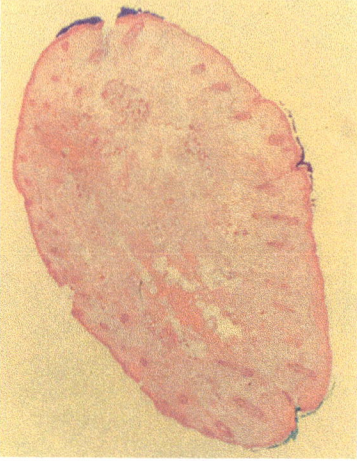

Fig. 4: The en face Mohs section allows for 100% margin assessment.

using orienting inked nicks. Directed by this map, the surgeon can precisely remove additional tissue until all margins are free of malignant tissue.

Wound Management

A multifaceted decision must be made whether to allow the tumor-free defect to heal by second intention or surgically repair the wound using a primary closure, delayed closure, local skin flaps or skin grafts. Important considerations in this wound management strategy include local tissue movement, need for adjacent anatomic and functional preservation, patient comorbidities, cosmesis, and likelihood of future surgery.

Allowing the wound to heal by second intention can result in excellent cosmetic results in the appropriate clinical setting, particularly with superficial wounds in concave areas (such as the medial canthus and conchal bowl), lip mucosa or in patients with limited cosmetic concerns.

The Mohs surgeon usually performs a surgical repair of the postoperative defect; however, involvement of other surgical specialties may be appropriate.[15,16] Linear closures are discussed in Chapter 11, while cutaneous reconstruction with graft and flaps is addressed in Chapter 13.

Postoperative Care

Postoperative wound care regimens are typically simple and restrictions are minimal. Wounds healing by second intention must be cleansed daily over a healing period of 4–8 weeks while those surgically repaired usually require care for only 1–2 weeks. If adherence to a proper wound care regimen is a concern, such as in debilitated patients, some surgeons will add oral antibiotics to the postoperative regimen.

Significant postoperative pain is rare following Mohs surgery. The typical postoperative discomfort is managed adequately with non-opioid analgesics. Specifically, one randomized controlled trial found that the combination of 1,000 mg acetaminophen with 400 mg ibuprofen offered significantly superior pain relief to both acetaminophen alone, and acetaminophen in combination with 30 mg codeine following Mohs surgery.[17] Evaluation of the need for narcotic analgesics occurs on a case-by-case basis, and may be appropriate in complex reconstructions, wide defects, or in areas of high tension.

Follow-up and ongoing dermatologic examination is typically recommended every 6 months for all patients.

BENEFITS COMPARED TO ALTERNATIVE APPROACHES

The most distinct advantages of Mohs surgery include: highest evidence-based initial cure rate and lowest recurrence rates of cutaneous neoplasms, immediate histological confirmation of 100% clear margins, maximal functional and cosmetic preservation, immediate reconstruction, safe outpatient procedure with increased patient convenience, and cost-effectiveness.

Mohs surgery offers the highest 5-year cure rates for both basal cell carcinoma (BCC) (primary 99%, recurrent 94.4%) and squamous cell carcinoma (SCC) (primary 96.9%, recurrent 90%).[18-20] The exceptional cure rate obtained by Mohs surgery can be attributed to the meticulous microscopic examination of 100% of excised tissue margins. This unique attribute facilitates precise excision of cancerous tissue, which allows for a smaller postoperative defect without forfeiting overall cure rates. The technique preserves benign tissue and inherently optimizes both aesthetic outcome and functional capacity of adjacent anatomic structures. The importance of the tissue-sparing benefits of Mohs surgery cannot be overstated given that 65% of non-melanoma skin cancer (NMSC) affects facial sites.

Moreover, in cases with aggressive, recurrent or invasive tumors, the microscopic assessment uniquely guides and informs the surgeon throughout the procedure. The unique position of the Mohs surgeon (as pathologist, clinician, surgeon) to facilitate curative therapy has been validated by data demonstrating a greater rate of incomplete excision of facial BCC performed by otolaryngologists (p < 0.02) and plastic surgeons (p < 0.008).[21] Additionally, for some patients with significant comorbid conditions or those of advanced age, Mohs surgery performed under local anesthesia may provide enhanced safety compared with more extensive anesthesia in the operating room. Indeed, the proven safety of MMS has been sustained even in patients greater than 90 years of age.[22] Wide excisions and complex reconstructions have been associated with increased postoperative complications in elderly patients undergoing cutaneous surgery, which

may have implications for the use of Mohs surgery to minimize these contributing factors.[23]

Amplified sensitivity to financial pressures and declining reimbursement rates has fueled a discussion of the cost-effectiveness of Mohs surgery. Mohs surgery was once thought to be more expensive and labor-intensive than other modalities;[24] however, several recent published analyses have validated its cost-effectiveness, particularly when compared to standard surgical excision, when used within appropriate indications (Box 1).[25,26]

A core cost consideration in favor of Mohs surgery regards its proven highest initial cure rates and lowest recurrence rates. The technique obviates the need for and cost of re-excisions. One study found that 29–32% of standard surgical excisions required at least one additional procedure to achieve clear margins.[27,28] Additional considerations to include in the cost of re-excision with standard surgical excision include the price of further reconstructive work, pathology

---

Box 1: Indications for Mohs surgery.

Appropriate Use Criteria Recommendations[3]
Basal cell carcinoma and cutaneous squamous cell carcinoma:
- High-risk anatomic locations of functional or cosmetic importance
  - Facial tumors ("Mask areas", eyes, ears, nose, lips)
  - Genital, anal, hand, foot and nail beds
- Recurrent tumors
- Large tumors (>0.5 cm on face; >2.0 cm on trunk or extremities)
- Tumors with poorly defined margins
  - Deeply infiltrating tumors with difficulty estimating depth
- Tumors of aggressive histologic subtypes
  - Perineural or perivascular invasion on biopsy
- Tumors in immunocompromised patients
- Tumors in patients at greater genetic risk of malignancy (e.g. basal cell nevus syndrome or xeroderma pigmentosa)
- Tumors in previously irradiated skin, scar or wound
- Tumors with positive margins on recent excision

Less common skin cancers that may benefit from treatment by Mohs surgery:[3]
- Adenocystic carcinoma
- Adnexal carcinoma
- Apocrine/eccrine carcinoma
- Atypical fibroxanthoma[44]
- Dermatofibrosarcoma protuberans[45]
- Extra-mammary Paget's disease[46]
- Leiomyosarcoma
- Malignant fibrous histiocytoma/undifferentiated pleomorphic sarcoma
- Merkel cell carcinoma (especially those on the head and neck)[47] (along with sentinel lymph node biopsy)
- Microcystic adenexal carcinoma[48]
- Mucinous carcinoma
- Sebaceous carcinomas[49]

Note: Mohs surgery is also being utilized in certain clinical scenarios for the treatment of melanoma (particularly lentigo maligna subtype) in conjunction with immunohistochemistry. This has shown very low recurrence rates in the current literature.[50]

charges and facility fees. If the costs of preventing both immediate re-excision and tumor recurrence with Mohs surgery are accounted for, this increases the cost-effectiveness of Mohs surgery compared to standard surgical excision. Overall, Mohs surgery has been shown to cost 12% less than frozen section office-based excisions, and 27% less than frozen section excisions in ambulatory surgical centers.[29]

Advancements in technique will only further aid in cost-savings, such as surgical curettage,[30] and use of confocal microscopy or adjuvant imiquimod,[31] which have all been shown to result in improved precision and fewer number of required Mohs stages.

Tip: Following the Mohs appropriate use criteria (Box 1) ensures that Mohs surgery is utilized in a cost-effective manner. If a tumor does not fall into these categories, it may be more appropriate and just as effective to use an alternate treatment option.

RISKS AND LIMITATIONS

With appropriate preoperative preparation and technique, Mohs surgery and repair of the associated defect can be very safely performed in the outpatient office-based setting. Expected postoperative events include scarring, bruising, swelling, and tenderness in the region of tumor extirpation. Additionally, like all surgical procedures, Mohs surgery carries a risk of adverse events, though the rate of unexpected complications is extremely low. In a prospective study of 1,358 outpatient cases, the complication rate was 1.64% and no complications were significant enough to require assistance of another specialist or patient hospitalization.[32] Rare complications include allergic reactions, cutaneous or motor nerve damage, hemorrhage, hematoma, seroma, surgical site infection, dehiscence, or necrosis.

Anecdotal concern for excessive bleeding in anticoagulated patients undergoing cutaneous surgery has prompted a recent surge of literature on the topic.[33-36] A consensus of these investigations shows that the risk of bleeding in patients who continue blood thinners perioperatively is significantly less than the risk of catastrophic thrombotic complications in patients who discontinue medically necessary anticoagulation.[37-39]

Additionally, the risk of postoperative infection in cutaneous surgery is low; however, published reports do vary widely from 0.7% to 8.7%.[40-42] Judicious use of prophylactic antibiotics should be practiced in cutaneous surgery, as should other interventions aimed to reduce infection. Alcohol-based hand rubs[43] have been associated with lower rates of surgical site infections, as has diligent hemostasis, as excessive bleeding and hematoma formation increase the likelihood of infection.[41] In addition to indications for antibiotic prophylaxis, antibiotics may be given 6 hours postoperatively in an unexpectedly extensive surgery or in those locations of high bacterial colonization such as sebaceous noses, nares, mouth, or distal lower extremities.[42] Postoperative prophylaxis of wound infection may be less effective than preoperative, as antibiotics are not incorporated into the coagulum of the wound.[6]

Finally, local recurrences after Mohs surgery are extremely rare. When recurrences do occur, they can often be attributed to errors in histological interpretation or tumor mapping, the presence of dense inflammation or tissue dropout on histology, or correlation with aggressive tumor subtype.[13,14] Recurrence rates have been reported to be about 1% after Mohs surgery.[13,26]

REFERENCES

1. Mohs FE. Chemosurgery: A microscopically controlled method of cancer excision. Arch Dermatol. 1941;42:279-95.
2. Tromovich TA, Stegman SJ. Microscopically controlled excision of skin tumors: Chemosurgery (Mohs). Fresh tissue technique. Arch Dermatol. 1974;110:231-2.
3. Ad Hoc Task Force: Connolly SM, Baker DR, et al. AAD/ACMS/ ASDSA/ASMS 2012 appropriate use criteria for Mohs micrographic surgery: A report of the American Academy of Dermatology, American College of Mohs Surgery, American Society for Dermatologic Surgery Association, and the American Society for Mohs Surgery. J Am Acad Dermatol. 2012;67:531-50.

4. Dinehart SM, Henry L. Dietary supplements: altered coagulation and effects on bruising. Dermatol Surg. 2005;31:819-26.

5. Wilson W, Taubert KA, Gewitz M, et al. Prevention of infective endocarditis: guidelines from the American Heart Association: a guideline from the American Heart Association Rheumatic Fever, Endocarditis, and Kawasaki Disease Committee, Council on Cardiovascular Disease in the Young, and the Council on Clinical Cardiology, Council on Cardiovascular Surgery and Anesthesia, and the Quality of Care and Outcomes Research Interdisciplinary Working Group. Circulation. 2007;116:1736-54.

6. Maragh SL, Otley CC, Roenigk RK, et al. Antibiotic prophylaxis in dermatologic surgery: updated guidelines. Dermatol Surg. 2005;31:83-93.

7. Wright TI, Baddour LM, Berbari EF, et al. Antibiotic prophylaxis in dermatologic surgery: Advisory statement. J Am Acad Dermatol. 2008;59(3):464-73.

8. Messingham MJ, Arpey CJ. Update on the use of antibiotics in cutaneous surgery. Dermatol Surg. 2005;31:1068-78.

9. Alam M, Lee A, Ibrahimi O, et al. A multistep approach to improving biopsy site identification in dermatology physician, staff, and patient roles based on a Delphi Consensus. JAMA Derm. 2014;150(5):550-8.

10. Butler ST, Youker SR, Mandrell J, et al. The importance of reviewing pathology specimens before Mohs surgery. Dermatol Surg. 2009;35(3):407-12.

11. Weber PJ, Moody BR, Dryden RM, et al. Mohs surgery and processing: novel optimizations and enhancements. Dermatol Surg. 2000;26(10):909-14.

12. Lee KC, Higgins HW II, Dufresne RG Jr. Tumor recurrence after Mohs micrographic surgery. J Am Acad Dermatol. 2014;70:385-6.

13. Zabielinski M, Leithauser L, Godsey T, et al. Laboratory errors leading to non-melanoma skin cancer recurrence following Mohs micrographic surgery. Dermatol Surg. 2015;41:913-6.

14. Campbell T, Armstrong AW, Schupp CW, et al. Surgeon error and slide quality during Mohs micrographic surgery: is there a relationship with tumor recurrence? J Am Acad Dermatol. 2013;69:105-11.

15. Ridha H, Garioch JJ, Tan EK, et al. Intraoperative use of Mohs surgery for the resection of major cutaneous head and neck cancer under general anesthetic: initial experiences, efficiency and outcomes. J Plast Reconstr Aesthet Surg. 2015;68(12):1706-12.

16. Sines DT, Polomsky M, Dutton JJ. Predicting the surgical margin of resection in periocular cutaneous neoplasms and the significance of reconstruction following mohs micrographic surgery. Opthal Plastic Reconstr Surg. 2016; 32(4):284-91.

17. Sniezek PJ, Prodland DG, Zitelli JA. A randomized controlled trial comparing acetaminophen, acetaminophen and ibuprofen, and acetaminophen and codeine for postoperative pain relief after Mohs surgery and cutaneous reconstruction. Dermatol Surg. 2011;37(7):1007-13.

18. Rowe DE, Carroll RJ, Day CL. Long-term recurrence rates in previously untreated (primary) basal cell carcinoma: implications for patient follow-up. J Dermatol Surg Oncol. 1989;15:315-28.

19. Rowe DE, Carroll RJ, Day CL. Mohs surgery is the treatment of choice for recurrent (previously treated) basal cell carcinoma. J Dermatol Surg Oncol. 1989;15:424-31.

20. Rowe DE, Carroll RJ, Day CL Jr. Prognostic factors for local recurrence, metastasis, and survival rates in squamous cell carcinoma of the skin, ear, and lip. Implications for treatment modality selection. J Am Acad Dermatol. 1992;26(6):976-90.

21. Fleischer AB Jr, Feldman SR, Barlow JO, et al. The specialty of the treating physician affects the likelihood of tumor-free resection margins for basal cell carcinoma: results from a multi-institutional retrospective study. J Am Acad Dermatol. 2001;44(2):224-30.

22. Delaney A, Shimizu I, Goldberg LH, et al. Life expectancy after Mohs micrographic surgery in patients aged 90 years and older. J Am Acad Dermatol. 2013;68:296-300.

23. Paradela S, Pita-Fernández S, Peña C, et al. Complications of ambulatory major dermatological surgery in patinets older than 85 years. J Eur Acad Dermatol Venereol. 2010;24(10):1207-13.

24. Cook J, Zitelli JA. Mohs micrographic surgery: a cost analysis. J Am Acad Dermatol. 1998;39:698-703.

25. Kauvar AN, Arpey CJ, Hruza G, et al. Consensus for Nonmelanoma Skin Cancer Treatment. Part II: Squamous Cell Carcinoma, Including a Cost Analysis of Treatment Methods. Dermatol Surg. 2015;41(11):1214-40.

26. Kauvar AN, Cronin T Jr, Roenigk R, et al. Consensus for Nonmelanoma Skin Cancer Treatment: Basal Cell Carcinoma, Including a Cost Analysis of Treatment Methods. Dermatol Surg. 2015;41(5):550-71.

27. Bialy TL, Whalen J, Veledar E, et al. MMS vs traditional surgical excision: A cost comparison analysis. Arch Dermatol. 2004;140(6):736-42.

28. Essers BA, Dirksen CD, Nieman FH, et al. Cost-effectiveness of Mohs Micrographic Surgery vs. Surgical excision for basal cell carcinoma of the face. Arch Dermatol. 2006;142(2):187-94.

29. Tierney EP, Hanke CW. Cost effectiveness of Mohs micrographic surgery: review of the literature. J Drugs Dermatol. 2009;8:914-22.

30. Lee DA, Ratner D. Economic impact of preoperative curettage before MMS for basal cell carcinoma. Dermatol Surg. 2006;32(7):916-22.

31. Butler DF, Parekh PK, Lenis A. Imiquimod 5% cream as adjunctive therapy for primary, solitary, nodular nasal basal cell carcinomas before MMS: A randomized, double blind, vehicle-controlled study. Dermatol Surg. 2009;35(1):24-9.

32. Cook JL, Perone JB. A prospective evaluation of the incidence of complications associated with Mohs micrographic surgery. Arch Dermatol. 2003;139:143-52.

33. Lewis KG, Dufresne RG Jr. A meta-analysis of complications attributed to anticoagulation among patients following cutaneous surgery. Dermatol Surg. 2008;34:160-4.

34. West SW, Otley CG, Nguyen TH, et al. Cutaneous surgeons cannot predict blood-thinner status by intraoperative visual inspection. Plast Reconstr Surg. 2002;110:98-103.

35. Cook-Norris RH, Michaels JD, Weaver AL, et al. Complications of cutaneous surgery in patients taking clopidogrel-containing anticoagulation. J Am Acad Dermatol. 2011;65:584-91.

36. Bordeux JS, Martires KJ, Goldberg D, et al. Prospective evaluation of dermatologic surgery complications including patients on multiple antiplatelet and anticoagulant medications. J Am Acad Dermatol. 2011;65:576-83.

37. Syed S, Adams BB, Liao W, et al. A prospective assessment of bleeding and international normalized ratio in warfarin-anticoagulated patients having cutaneous surgery. J Am Acad Dermatol. 2004;51:955-7.

38. Chang TW, Arpey CJ, Baum CL et al. Complications with new oral anticoagulants dabigatran and rivaroxaban in cutaneous surgery. Dermatol Surg. 2015;41(7):784-93.

39. Kovich O, Otley CC. Thrombotic complications related to discontinuation of warfarin and aspirin therapy preoperatively for cutaneous operation. J Am Acad Dermatol. 2003;48:233-7.

40. Whitaker DC, Grande DJ, Johnson SS. Wound infection rate in dermatologic surgery. J Dermatol Surg. 1988;14:525-8.

41. Rogues AM, Lasheras A, Amici JM, et al. Infection control practices and infectious complications in dermatologic surgery. J Hosp Infect. 2007; 65(3):258-63.

42. Heal CF, Buettner PG, Drobetz H. Risk factors for surgical site infection after dermatologic surgery. Int J Dermatol. 2012;51(7):796-803.

43. Widmer AF, Rotter M, Voss A, et al. Surgical hand preparation: state-of-the-art. J Hosp Infect. 2010;74(2):112-22.

44. Ang GC, Roenigk RK, Otley CC, et al. More than two decades of treating atypical fibroxanthoma at Mayo Clinic: what have we learned from 91 patients? Dermatol Surg. 2009;35:765-72.

45. Snow SN, Gordon EM, Larson PO, et al. Dermatofibrosarcoma protuberans: a report on 29 patients treated with Mohs micrographic surgery with long-term follow-up and review of the literature. Cancer. 2004;101:28-38.

46. O'Connor WJ, Lim KK, Zalla MG, et al. Comparison of Mohs micrographic surgery and wide excision for extramammary Paget's disease. Dermatol Surg. 2003;29:723-7.

47. Boyer JD, Zitelli JA, Brodland DG, et al. Local control of primary Merkel cell carcinoma: review of 45 cases treated with Mohs micrographic surgery with and without adjuvant radiation. Dermatol Surg. 2002;47:885-92.

48. Chiller K, Passaro D, Scheuller M, et al. Microcystic adnexal carcinoma: 48 cases, their treatment and their outcome. Arch Dermatol. 2000;136:1355-9.

49. Spencer JM, Nossa R, Tse DT, et al. Sebaceous carcinoma of the eyelid treated with Mohs micrographic surgery. J Am Acad Dermatol. 2001; 44:1004-9.

50. Bene NI, Healy C, Coldiron BM. Mohs micrographic surgery is accurate 95.1% of the time for melanoma in situ: a prospective study of 167 cases. Dermatol Surg. 2008;34:660-4.

CHAPTER 11

Elliptical Excision

Derek Hsu, Lara E Rosenbaum, Ashish C Bhatia

HISTORY

Dermatologic surgery has had a long history and was even performed in ancient civilizations, such as Babylon and Greece.[1] Indeed, physicians from these civilizations performed a wide range of dermatologic procedures from excisions to cautery. Celsus, a Roman philosopher and author of *De Re Medicina* in the early first century, wrote that skin cancer could be treated in multiple ways, including "caustic medicaments, some the cautery, some excision with a scalpel."[2] Although it is difficult to verify that physicians in these times were actually excising carcinomas, their descriptions of these lesions as "nonhealing ulcers" and other various keywords likely represented basal or squamous cell carcinomas. It is fascinating that even in the earliest parts of recorded human history skin excisions were being performed.

More recently, the invention of anesthesia has also undoubtedly facilitated the process of elliptical excisions. One of the first uses of local anesthesia was cocaine administered to the eye in 1884, although physicians and patients alike soon discovered that the other effects of the cocaine made it a less than optimal choice for an anesthetic.[3] Soon other local anesthetics were developed, such as tropocaine and benzocaine, which provided a safer yet effective way to perform surgery. Techniques in dermatologic surgery have clearly progressed since the ancient eras, but the principles remain the same: excise the lesion completely while minimizing scarring.

DESCRIPTION OF PROCEDURE

Objective

The objective of the elliptical excision is to remove a skin lesion while providing optimal cosmetic results. The elliptical excision is among the most critical and fundamental components of cutaneous surgery, as knowledge of this procedure sets the foundation for other more advanced procedures. Skin specimens that are removed can either be malignant or benign. The elliptical excision can also serve to biopsy lesions while providing sufficient tissue for histopathologic evaluation.

Preoperative Evaluation

Before proceeding with the actual design and excision, it is crucial to perform a thorough history and physical examination, with emphasis on medications or conditions that may increase risk of infection or bleeding. The clinician must be aware of the type of lesion being removed, as this will affect the margins (Table 1). If the lesion is a melanoma, squamous cell carcinoma or other cancer at risk for metastasis, care should be taken to evaluate the draining lymph node beds during the physical examination. In general, discontinuation of prescription medications, including anticoagulants or antithrombotics, is not recommended prior to an elliptical excision.[4,5]

> Discontinuation of anticoagulants or antithrombotics before the elliptical excision is not recommended.[4,5]

Table 1: Commonly excised skin lesions and typical margins.

Basal cell carcinoma	3–5 mm
Squamous cell carcinoma	3–5 mm
Melanoma	5–20 mm (margin based on Breslow depth)
Dysplastic nevus (severe)	5 mm
Dysplastic nevus (mild, moderate)	2–3 mm
Benign lesion (e.g. cyst, lipoma, etc.)	0–1 mm

Design

The design of the ellipse is critical for the success of the procedure and can be performed in a few simple steps. There are three steps to the drawing. The first outlines the lesion to be removed, the next outlines the margin of additional tissue you want to excise, and the last is the ellipse itself (Fig. 1). The direction of the long axis of the ellipse should be parallel to that of the maximal skin tension lines (MSTL) (Figs. 2A and B). A strong light and magnification may be utilized to enhance the precision of skin markings. Establishing a routine, such as drawing a dotted line around the periphery of the lesion and a continuous line at the margin and ellipse, has been demonstrated to reduce the rate of incomplete excision of lesions.[6]

Take your fingers and pinch around the lesion in different directions. The orientation of the long axis of the ellipse will be along the lines of greatest laxity. This will help produce the most cosmetically appropriate scar. Wrinkling will be maximal with pinching in the direction of the short axis.

Since the MSTL folds as a result of contraction of the muscles underlying them, one can have the patient attempt to move the underlying muscles (flexing, frowning) to help assess the direction of the lines. In areas of high skin tension such as the forearm or back—the long axis of the ellipse may be oriented along the axis of greatest tension. One can have patients flex the muscles underneath

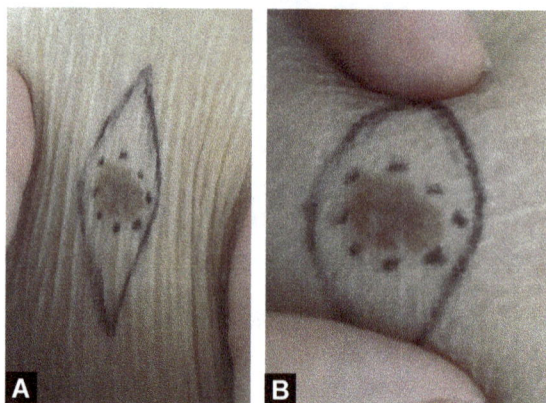

Figs. 2A and B: Pinching the skin can help determine the appropriate orientation of the skin ellipse. Wrinkling will be maximal with pinching in the direction of the short axis and this will help produce the most cosmetically appropriate scar. (A) Pinching in short axis. (B) Pinching in the long axis.

(assume maximal tension) when determining the orientation in these locations.

> Marking the lesion under strong light and magnification will provide more meticulous markings.

> Establishing a routine, such as drawing a dotted line around the periphery of the lesion and a continuous line at the margin and ellipse, has been demonstrated to reduce the rate of incomplete excision of lesions.[6]

The most common design of the ellipse is a 3:1 long axis to short axis ratio. The reason it is called a "fusiform" ellipse rather than just an ellipse is because it is not actually ovaloid in nature. Thus, there is generally an apical angle of 30° between the lines that makeup the fusiform ellipse.

Excision

The ideal choice of local anesthesia is 1% lidocaine with epinephrine extending about 1.5 cm beyond the planned incision site. The epinephrine will increase the anesthesia's duration of action as well as lessen bleeding. Dosing should not exceed 7 mg/kg. Patients should be in a comfortable position during the procedure but at the same time care must be taken to minimize tension at the incision site. Before the incision, the site should be thoroughly cleaned with an antiseptic, such as povidone iodine.

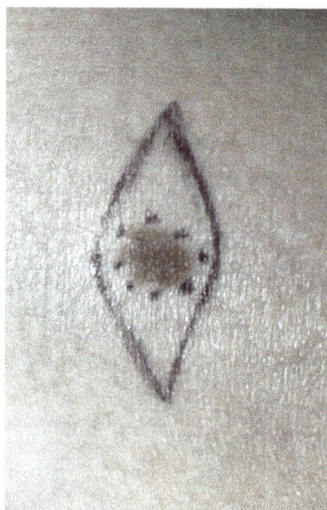

Fig. 1: Establish a routine and mark both the clinical lesion and the margin/ellipse prior to anesthetizing the skin.

Inject the anesthesia after the incision lines are drawn, as the vasoconstrictive effects of epinephrine can make it difficult to visualize the edges of the lesion.

Three-point counter tension can help facilitate a smooth initial incision.

Inject the anesthesia after the incision lines are drawn, as the vasoconstrictive effects of epinephrine can make it difficult to visualize the edges of the lesion. Additionally, the volume of anesthetic can also cause distortion of the tissue and make it impossible to appreciate the MSTL's. Three-point counter tension can help facilitate a smooth initial incision. The initial incision should extend through the dermis and be approximately perpendicular to the skin surface. Cross-hatching at the apices should be avoided. Cross-hatching is when the incision extends beyond the apices of the ellipse, and thus care should be taken to meet at the apex without going further. Precision of the apical portion of the incision can be made easier by initially penetrating the skin at a 90° angle, then pivoting the scalpel's cutting edge to a 45° angle while performing the remainder of the incision until the end where the incision can be done with the scalpel edge back at a 90° angle (Fig. 3). Depth depends on the excision location, although in most cases the upper adipose layer is the intended depth. Attempt to aim for uniform thickness during the excision process.

Undermining, the process of cutting the fibers that connect the skin to the subcutaneous tissue and fascia underneath, should typically be performed. Undermining facilitates wound edge approximation, and alleviates wound edge tension upon suturing. It also facilitates wound edge eversion and may improve cosmetic outcome. However, it is sometimes avoided in patients on anticoagulants due to increased dead space and thus increased risk of developing a hematoma. The amount of tissue to be undermined is up to the clinician's judgment but should be based on the ability to perform proper wound closure and eversion without compromising the healing process. It is imperative to undermine around the whole defect, including the apices. To determine whether undermining will be effective, one can slightly tug the wound edges toward each other. If the underlying fibers restrict mobility, undermining will likely help.[8] Undermining should be carried out using blunt-tipped scissors to avoid damage to surrounding tissue.[7] Care must be taken not to crush wound edges, if using forceps to hold the edges while undermining. Crushing the tissue can ultimately negatively affect the cosmetic outcome.

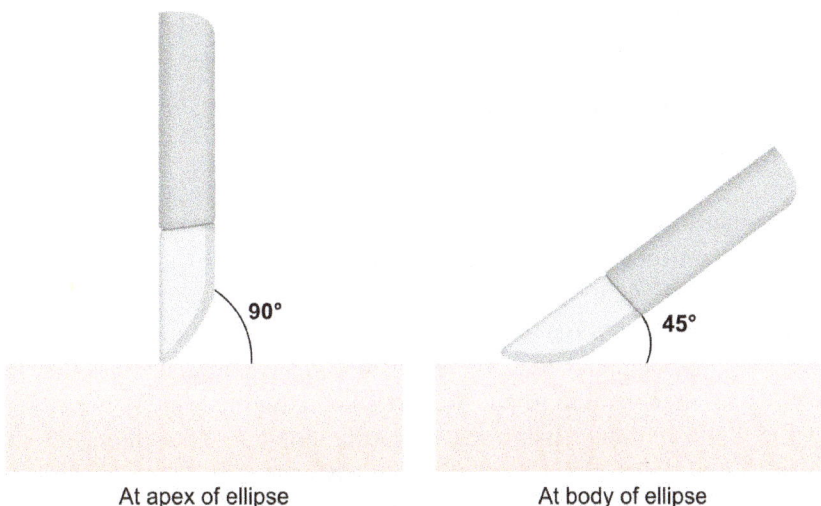

At apex of ellipse 90°

At body of ellipse 45°

Fig. 3: Precision of the apical portion of the incision can be made easier by initially penetrating the skin at a 90° angle, then pivoting the scalpel's cutting edge to a 45° angle while performing the remainder of the incision.

To determine whether undermining will be effective, one can slightly tug the wound edges toward each other. If the underlying fibers restrict mobility, undermining will likely help.[8]

Hemostasis should be performed next. Look for actively bleeding vessels after excision and undermining. Hemostasis can be performed with electrodessication, electrocoagulation, or even clamping and ligation of larger vessels. If this is not performed with precision, healthy tissue may be damaged unnecessarily. On the other hand, if hemostasis is performed inadequately, then there can be outward hemorrhage or a hematoma may form postoperatively.

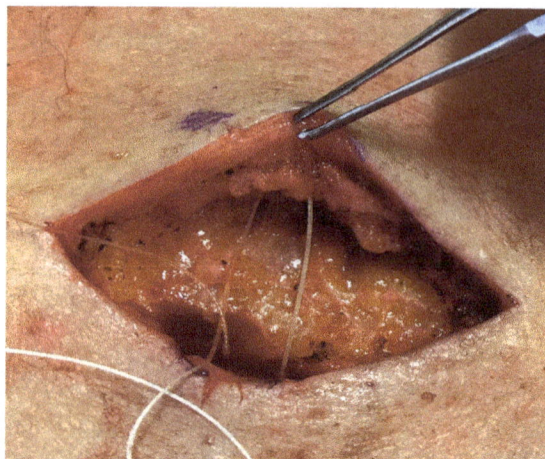

Fig. 4: The setback suture utilizes the undermined surface of the subcutaneous tissue to approximate the tissue and lessen wound edge tension. One study showed better cosmetic outcomes and wound eversion with this suture.

Wound Closure

The closure of the excision is of critical importance insofar that the skills of the surgeon will affect the healing and the ultimate cosmetic outcome. When performed correctly, closure should form a smooth line without deformity. In many cases, two layers of sutures will be placed—a subcutaneous layer approximating the subcutaneous tissue and dermis as well as a superficial layer to ensure the epidermis is even and closely approximated and to further assist with eversion. The most common sutures utilized to approximate the dermis and subcutaneous tissue includes polyglactin-910 (Vicryl) or poliglecapone-25 (Monocryl). A recent prospective study evaluated 140 patients after use of either of those sutures at 1-week and 3-month intervals on a visual analog scale and observed that poliglecaprone-25 had significantly less extruded sutures than polyglactin-910.[9] However, the overall cosmetic appearance of the scars was similar.

The issue of whether to evert the skin during closure has been a recent topic of controversy. Classically, eversion was thought to offset the scar's natural depression due to contractile forces during healing. A 2015 randomized trial which employed a split-scar intervention—half the wound being everted and the other half undergoing planar repair—was evaluated at 3-month and 6-month follow-up with the Patient Observer Self-Assessment Scale (POSA). There were no significant differences between everted and planar repair in terms of cosmetic appearance.[10]

Another point to consider during the repair is the actual suture technique. The current gold standard is the buried vertical mattress suture (BVMS) although recently another technique known as the set-back suture has also come into favor. The set-back suture utilizes the undermined surface of the subcutaneous tissue to approximate the tissue and lessen wound edge tension (Fig. 4). The set-back technique leads to increased eversion as well. A 2015 prospective study of 46 patients who had undergone elliptical excisions was randomized to either the BVMS or set back suture and evaluated at 3 months with the POSA.[11] The set-back suture provided statistically significant better cosmetic outcomes and wound eversion.

Postoperatively, cleaning the surgical site should be performed to remove any residual tissue, antiseptic or blood. Dressings typically consist of some form of ointment and a pressure dressing, which is composed of gauze and an absorbent cushion. This dressing can be removed 24–48 hours later. After removal of the dressing, the site is often cleansed daily. General restrictions include avoiding strenuous physical activity as well as submerging the wound in any water (including baths, pools, lakes, and oceans). Removal of the sutures should take place after proper epithelization of the wound. On the face, this is typically around 7 days, and on the extremities and trunk this is typically between 10 days and 14 days.[7]

COMPARISON TO VARIOUS PROCEDURES

Mohs micrographic surgery (MMS) is a more specialized surgical technique typically utilized for removing locally invasive, aggressive or recurrent skin malignancies. One of the primary differences between a standard elliptical excision and MMS is that the histological evaluation of an elliptical excision only evaluates a small portion of the margin in comparison to the much more thorough evaluation of margins after MMS. Additionally, the margins taken in MMS are much narrower than with excisions, allowing sparing of as much normal tissue as possible. As such, MMS is more often used for locally aggressive skin cancers, and lesions in higher risk locations with a paucity of extra skin. High risk locations include embryonic fusion planes, such as the temple, nose, nasolabial fold, periorbital area, and preauricular and postauricular skin.[12] Mohs is the preferred choice in cases where clinicopathologic management of the cancer is needed, if more precise margins are needed, and if maximal preservation of normal tissue is of critical importance. Standard elliptical excisions are significantly less labor-intensive and less costly than MMS because performing MMS requires a dermatologic surgeon with a certified laboratory, a histotechnician, and knowledgeable ancillary staff. MMS also takes significantly longer in terms of time in the office, so it may not be ideal for a patient that is not able to tolerate that. For more information on MMS please see Chapter 10.

The choice of shave or punch biopsy versus excision is something that should be kept in mind. If a lesion needs to be removed completely—whether for diagnostic or therapeutic purposes—an excision should be performed. Excisions should also be performed; if a punch or shave biopsy cannot adequately sample a lesion. Another advantage of an excisional biopsy is that it provides more tissue for histopathologic examination or other testing.

Another alternative to excision for certain skin lesions is electrodessication and curettage. As a treatment modality, electrodessication and curettage is usually reserved for small, less aggressive skin cancers as well as various benign lesions. Disadvantages of electrodessication and curettage include scarring and potential interactions with pacemakers. Advantages of an excision include the ability to evaluate the pathology as well as the margins for clearance, achieving a higher cure rate and less chance of recurrence for the skin cancer.

COMPLICATIONS

Complications after an elliptical excision can include infection, hematoma, and dehiscence. Hematomas usually occur due to inadequate hemostasis and will typically present within 24–72 hours. Swelling of the wound site with erythema and tenderness point toward a hematoma. To confirm the presence of a hematoma, one can visually inspect for a hematoma by removing the sutures. Aspiration for blood is another option, though it may be difficult, if the pool of blood has congealed. To surgically explore and evacuate a hematoma, lidocaine without epinephrine may be used. If one visualizes active bleeding after evacuation of the hematoma, hemostasis is the next step. Antibiotics can be considered to prevent infection. Complete reclosure is often delayed to allow for further drainage.

Infections after excisions are rare, occurring around just in 1% of cases. They usually develop 3–5 days after the excision has taken place. The patient and caretaker should be educated about the signs and symptoms of infection, such as erythema, pain, and warmth. Signs of overt infection may be present, such as pus, which can be expressed; if one applies pressure with the fingers around the wound. Bacterial cultures should be obtained in this scenario. Antibiotics should be prescribed in a presumed infection, which can be changed once sensitivities are available from the bacterial culture. The most common microorganism causing infection after excision is *Staphylococcus aureus*, and thus empiric treatment with dicloxacillin or cephalexin is often advisable.

If dehiscence of a closed excision occurs, the first step is to evaluate whether infection

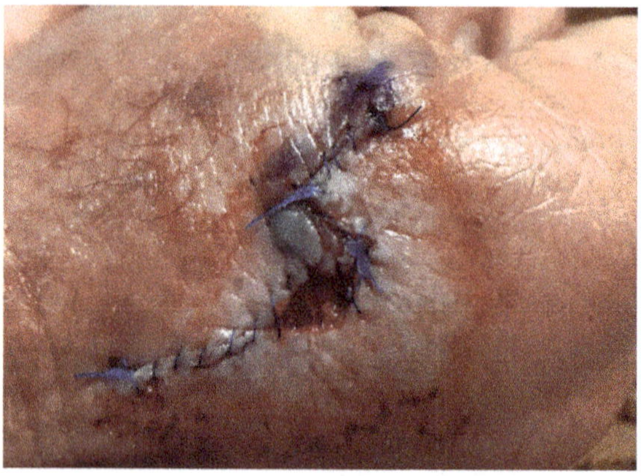

Fig. 5: Wound dehiscence is a possible complication and the wound should be evaluated for infection or hematoma. Typically a dehisced wound is allowed to heal by second intention.

or hematoma may have contributed (Fig. 5). Patients should also be asked about any physical activity or manipulation that may have contributed to the dehiscence. Typically, a dehisced wound is not closed. Rather, the underlying cause is treated and the wound is often allowed to heal by secondary intention. In this scenario, the cosmetic outcome may be less than optimal. Wound edge necrosis is another rare complication of excisions with closures. It most often occurs in the setting of vascular compromise due to significant wound edge tension during closure. Opening and debriding the wound edge, and then letting it heal by secondary intention are the next steps.

REFERENCES

1. Coleman WP, Hanke CW, Orentreich N, et al. A history of dermatologic surgery in the United States. Dermatol Surg. 2000;26(1):5-11.

2. Crouch HE. History of basal cell carcinoma and its treatment. J R Soc Med. 1983;76(4):302-6.

3. Ruetsch YA, Boni T, Borgeat A. From cocaine to ropivacaine: the history of local anesthetic drugs. Curr Top Med Chem. 2001;1(3):175-82.

4. Wright TI, Baddour LM, Berbari EF, et al. Antibiotic prophylaxis in dermatologic surgery: advisory statement 2008. J Am Acad Dermatol. 2008; 59(3):464-73.

5. Callahan S, Goldsberry A, Kim G, et al. The management of antithrombotic medication in skin surgery. Dermatol Surg. 2012;38(9):1417-26.

6. Hussain W, Mortimer NJ, Salmon PJ. Optimizing technique in elliptical excisional surgery: some pearls for practice. Br J Dermatol. 2009;161(3): 697-8.

7. Leshin B. Proper planning and execution of surgical excisions. In: Wheeland RG (Ed). Cutaneous Surgery. Philadelphia: WB Saunders Company; 1994. pp. 171-7.

8. Miller CJ, Antunes MB, Sobanko JF. Surgical technique for optimal outcomes: Part I. Cutting tissue: Incising, excising, and undermining. J Am Acad Dermatol. 2015;72(3):377-87.

9. Regan T, Lawrence N. Comparison of poliglecaprone-25 and polyglactin-910 in cutaneous surgery. Dermatol Surg. 2013;39(9):1340-4.

10. Kappel S, Kleinerman R, King TH, et al. Does wound eversion improve cosmetic outcome? Results of a randomized, split-scar, comparative trial. J Am Acad Dermatol. 2015;72(4):668-73.

11. Wang AS, Kleinerman R, Armstrong AW, et al. Set-back versus buried vertical mattress suturing: results of a randomized blinded trial. J Am Acad Dermatol. 2015;72(4):674-80.

12. Dim-Jamora KC, Perone JB. Management of cutaneous tumors with Mohs micrographic surgery. Semin Plast Surg. 2008;22(4):247-56.

CHAPTER 12

Nail Procedures: Tips and Tricks

Ashley Nault, Sreya Talasila, Shuai "Steve" Xu, Simon Yoo, Aleksandar L Krunic

INTRODUCTION

This chapter focuses on specific tips and tricks related to nail procedures. First, it is necessary to discuss the proper tools and anesthesia techniques that maximize the potential for successful outcomes. Then, a general overview of specific procedures is presented highlighting the tips and tricks. These techniques allow the operator to efficiently and effectively perform nail surgery with reproducible results. A discussion of nail procedure danger zones is presented in an effort to prevent serious sequelae that can result from nail procedures. Finally, approaches to postoperative wound care are essential to minimize pain and promote healing.

HISTORY OF NAIL PROCEDURES

Nail procedures have a long history dating back to the ancient Egyptians, ancient Babylonians, and Ming dynasty of China where nails were colored and trimmed for cosmetic effect. Descriptions of nail surgery for medical conditions have begun to appear in the literature over the past 70 years with two publications in 1946 ballooning to 23 in 2014. Many providers perform nail procedures including podiatrists, hand surgeons, and dermatologists.

INSTRUMENTATION: TOOLS OF THE TRADE

Dental syringe with a 30-gauge needle: A "30-gauge ¼" needle is utilized for injecting anesthesia to minimize the pain associated with larger needles. The dental syringe is recommended because it produces the higher pressure required when injecting into the highly resistant dermal tissue of the digit.

> Try using a 3 mL Luer-Lock syringe, if you are working on smaller fingernails and toenails. The smaller profile can make it easier to use than the dental syringe.

Sterile surgical glove used as a tourniquet: A sterile glove with the respective fingertip removed can be placed on the patient. The remaining part of the glove on the respective digit is rolled down to the base of the digit, which creates a tourniquet. This "glove technique" also creates a clean field surrounding the nail.

> The "glove technique" creates a tourniquet while creating a clean field around the operative site.

Nail plate elevator: This tool is used to release the nail plate. A freer septum elevator is most commonly used for complete nail plate avulsion whereas a smaller 2–3 mm curved or flat nail plate elevator works effectively for partial avulsions.

Mosquito hemostat (blunt end): After the nail plate has been dissected from the nail bed, the hemostat positioned so that the grooved surface is under the nail plate. The hemostat is clamped down and traction is used to free the nail plate from any adhesions at the matrix.

Double-action nail nippers: Useful for cutting through thick nail plates.

Nail splitter: This tool is used in partial longitudinal nail avulsions. The flat lower blade slides along the nail bed while the upper blade cuts through the nail plate.

Single- and double-pronged skin hooks: Skin hooks are used to retract the proximal nail fold in order to visualize the nail matrix.

Surgical blade: Used for shave biopsies of the nail bed or nail matrix and for resection of periungual nail tissue. The 15-blade is the most commonly utilized.

Nail spatula: The nail plate elevator comes in one size; however, nail spatulas can vary from 4.5 inches to 7 inches in length. The width can also vary from 3 mm to 5 mm. The nail spatula can also be flexible or rigid. The variation in size can make the nail spatula useful for avulsion of smaller nail plates on the 5th digit or 5th toe. Both the nail spatula and the nail plate elevator can be used for nail plate avulsions.

ANESTHESIA TECHNIQUES

Choosing a Local Anesthetic

The author's preferred anesthetic is 1% ropivacaine. This has a rapid onset (3–15 minutes) and a long duration (up to 8–12 hours). The long duration is helpful for postoperative pain control and for nail procedures that are expected to last longer than 1.5 hours. One should be aware, however, that long-acting anesthesia can mask symptoms of acute postoperative complications. Ropivacaine also has inherent vasoconstrictive properties, which may improve hemostasis and duration of anesthetic. Lidocaine 1–2%, is readily available in most offices, and is also an option. It offers faster onset (1–3 minutes) but with a shorter duration (1–2 hours). This varies between suppliers and geographic location, but typically ropivacaine is more expensive than lidocaine.

Alternative local anesthetics include:
- Mepivacaine 1%: Fairly rapid onset (2–5 minutes), shorter duration (1–2 hours)
- Bupivacaine 0.25%: Intermediate onset (5–10 minutes), longer duration (4–8 hours).

> Ropivacaine is good option for anesthesia. It is more potent, but also more expensive.

Digital Nerve Block for Nail Procedures

For nail procedures, the author's digital anesthesia technique of choice is the digital nerve block. Alternatives include a distal wing block, transthecal nerve block, or distal digital infiltration.

Advantages

The advantages of digital nerve block include:
- The digital nerve block is useful for all types of nail surgery as it provides anesthesia to the entire digit.
- The anesthetic does not interfere with the nail anatomy or affect the surgical approach.
- Anesthesia is usually more prolonged with the added benefit of postoperative pain control.
- The technique can be used when there is infected tissue in the surgical region, such as in paronychia, as the needle punctures are made in the proximal digit.
- The block can also be supplemented with addition of local anesthetic directly in the surgical area.

> **Expert Tip**
> We recommend waiting for 15–30 minutes after the block before performing nail procedures. Schedule another patient at this time to avoid feeling rushed.

Disadvantages

The disadvantages of digital nerve block include:
- A digital nerve block requires a waiting period up to 15–20 minutes for the block to completely anesthetize the surgical area. Alternatively, a distal infiltrative wing block provides nearly immediate anesthesia.
- The block requires two needle punctures as compared to one puncture for the transthecal or subcutaneous nerve block.
- There is potential for incomplete anesthesia, which may require additional infiltrative anesthesia.

> **Expert Tip**
> The transthecal block can injure metacarpal bones, and is generally not necessary for nail surgical procedures.

Caution

When performing digital blocks, special attention special attention should be paid to:

- Use the smallest amount of anesthetic to avoid compression on nearby nerves and vasculature. Higher concentrations of anesthetic can decrease the total volume of anesthetic necessary to achieve a nerve block.
- Avoid injecting directly into the nerve. Disproportionate pain or paresthesias may alert you that your needle is inserted in or pressing on the nerve.
- Limit prolonged use of the tourniquet. It should be removed after 20–30 minutes.

Is epinephrine safe in a digital nerve block?
Epinephrine causes local, transient vasoconstriction, which can reduce bleeding and increase the duration of anesthetic. There is no evidence of harm caused by the use of epinephrine in digital nerve blocks. It is prudent to avoid the use of epinephrine in patients at increased risk for digital ischemia, such as patients with peripheral vascular disease, thromboangiitis obliterans, Raynaud's phenomenon, or vasospastic disease. Of note, epinephrine has not been shown to lengthen the duration of action for either ropivacaine or bupivacaine.

Proper Injection Technique for Digital Nerve Blocks

The volar and dorsal digital nerves run in parallel along each side of the digit and terminate just beyond the distal interphalangeal (DIP) joint where they branch to supply the nail and surrounding tissue. With the palmar (plantar) surface of the hand (foot) facing downward, slowly insert a 27–30-gauge needle perpendicularly into the web space at the metacarpophalangeal (metatarsophalangeal) joint. Slowly inject the anesthetic into the subcutaneous tissue, forming a small wheal. Then, slowly advance the needle toward the palmar (plantar) direction while injecting anesthetic. Finally, massage the anesthetic down to the level of the digital nerves.

Expert Tip
We prefer the lateral approach or the superior approach. The inferior approach increases the risk of damage to the digital tendons.

This technique, as compared to advancing the needle to bone and then withdrawing, avoids potentially coming into contact with the nerve or any nearby vasculature. Withdraw the needle and repeat on the other side of the digit. Wait at least 10–15 minutes after the final injection and then test for anesthesia. If there are areas of sensation present, additional waiting time or local infiltrative anesthesia may be required. Of note, it is important to inject slowly to reduce the amount of pain experienced by the patient during this part of the procedure.

COMMON NAIL PROCEDURES

Nail Avulsion

Nail avulsion is the most common nail procedure. This entails freeing all or part of the nail plate from its surrounding structures and then detaching it from the nail bed. The procedure can be performed using either a distal or proximal approach. Nail avulsion can be diagnostic and/or therapeutic as it allows for visualization, sampling, and manipulation of the underlying nail bed and matrix. The procedure is most frequently indicated for ingrown nails (onychocryptosis), chronic onychomycosis, and periungual warts.

The need for a total versus a partial nail avulsion depends on the nail condition. For nail matrix or nail bed biopsies, only a partial avulsion may be necessary. Similarly, onychocryptosis requires only a partial nail avulsion. Total nail dystrophies will typically require a total nail avulsion. If clinically appropriate, partial nail avulsion is favored over complete avulsion, as it avoids unnecessary trauma to surrounding tissue and results in fewer postoperative complications (Figs. 1A and B).

Proximal Nail Avulsion

The proximal approach is preferred when the distal nail is dystrophic and fibrotic, firmly attached to hyponychium/nail bed, or there is difficulty in separating the nail plate from the nail bed. This

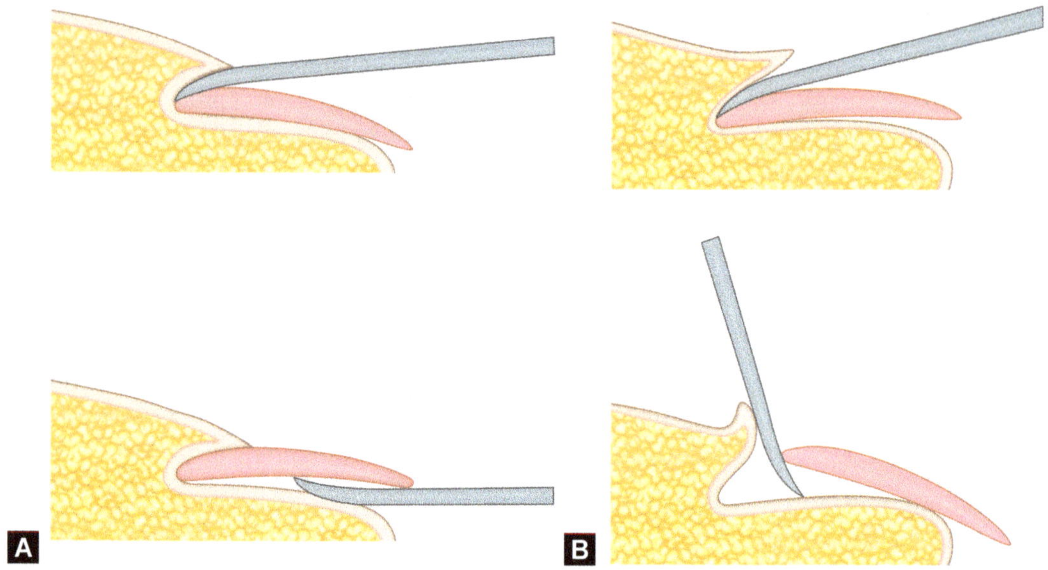

Figs. 1A and B: Illustration of both the distal (A) and proximal (B) nail avulsion techniques.

commonly is the case in onychogryphosis, distal subungual onychomycosis, or pachyonychia congenita.

- Prior to the procedure, ensure adequate anesthesia is achieved using a digital nerve block
- Gently slide the nail elevator under the proximal nail fold
- Leaving the tip of the nail elevator inserted under the proximal nail fold, rotate the nail elevator 180° and insert under the proximal edge of the nail plate, with the concave surface facing upwards
- With the tip of the nail elevator now pointing distally, push distally in back-and-forth motions to free the nail plate from the matrix and nail bed
- Repeat the procedure along the width of the nail root
- Continue to progress distally until the hyponychium or, in a partial nail avulsion, the selected stopping point is reached
- For a partial avulsion, nail splitters are used to cut the desired part to be removed
- Using a hemostat, grasp as much as the nail plate as possible and lift up to release the nail plate from the nail bed.

Tip 3.2: Distal Nail Avulsion

Distal nail avulsion is the classic technique for nail avulsion. In most cases, it is performed unless

the distal edge is unmovable from the underlying hyponychium.

- After adequate anesthesia is achieved via a digital nerve block, insert the nail elevator under the distal-free edge of the nail plate and separate it from the underlying hyponychium
- Slide the elevator facing downward with its concave side proximally with a back-and-forth motion and continue this motion along the entire width of the nail plate to release the entirety of the nail
- There will be a decreased amount of resistance upon reaching the matrix.
- Perform several longitudinal sweeps with the nail elevator to completely free the nail plate from the underlying nail bed.
- To release the nail plate from the proximal nail fold, gently slide the nail elevator under the proximal nail fold to free the eponychium from the nail plate.
- Using a hemostat or platypus nail forceps, grasp the nail plate and pull in an upward motion to avulse the nail (Fig. 2).

Chemical Nail Avulsion

Chemical nail avulsion with urea paste is a non-surgical alternative for nail debridement and avulsion in the treatment various nail diseases. It is indicated for symptomatic nail dystrophy in

Fig. 2: In this image, the surgeon is removing the nail plate after a partial nail avulsion.

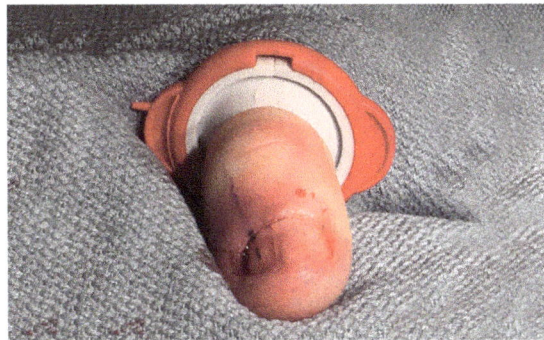

Fig. 3: Partial nail avulsion is used to reveal a melanocytic lesion in the proximal nail matrix.

patients with diabetic neuropathy, peripheral vascular disease, or patients with immunosuppression. Chemical nail avulsion can provide similar pain relief as surgical avulsion without the need for local anesthesia and with less risk of infection, hemorrhage, and intraoperative pain. The urea softens the nail plate as well as dissolves the adhesive bond between the nail bed and nail plate. This method requires compliance from the patient, as the area needs to remain occluded and dry for 1 week. The most common adverse effect is irritation of the surrounding tissue.

- Place adhesive tape on the surrounding soft tissues to avoid irritation. We frequently use Blenderm™.
- Generously apply urea paste to the nail plate. The adhesive felt (i.e. moleskin) or waterproof stretchable tape (e.g. Blenderm™) can be used to create a barrier and confine the paste to the treated area.
- The nail should then be occluded and kept dry for 1 week.
- After 1 week, a blunt dissection of the dystrophic nail is performed with a nail elevator and nail snippers.

Nail Matrix Biopsy

After successful nail avulsion, often the clinical indication is to conduct a biopsy of an underlying tumor or melanocytic lesion. A nail matrix biopsy involves retraction of the proximal nail fold for visualization followed by shave or punch biopsy of the underlying diseased matrix (Fig. 3).

The most important indication for a nail matrix biopsy is unexplained longitudinal melanonychia,

which raises the clinical suspicion for malignancy. Other indications include tumors of the nail matrix and nail abnormalities involving the length of the nail. The latter is often secondary to inflammatory processes such as psoriasis or lichen planus. Because the proximal matrix supplies a majority of the nail plate, including the dorsal surface of the nail plate, biopsies from the proximal matrix are more likely to result in permanent nail dystrophy. This should be taken into consideration and discussed with the patient prior to starting the procedure.

> The most important indication for a nail matrix biopsy is unexplained longitudinal melanonychia to rule out melanoma.

To start, incisions are made on both sides of the eponychium (periungual skin) at the intersection of the proximal and lateral nail folds. The proximal nail fold is then retracted with a skin hook to expose the entire matrix. Upon completion of the nail matrix biopsy, retract the proximal nail fold, which can be pulled back, and the incisions sutured with simple 5-0 nylon interrupted sutures. This chapter includes a video demonstrating the nail matrix biopsy procedure (📹 1).

There are various options for biopsy technique and the decision to perform one is commonly based on the size and clinical suspicion of malignancy of the lesion. For longitudinal melanonychia or other lesions, where the width of the pigmented band or lesion in other cases, is 3 mm or less, a 3 mm diameter punch biopsy is recommended. The punch should go through the matrix

Fig. 4: The surgeon is using a 15-blade to biopsy the melanocytic lesion.

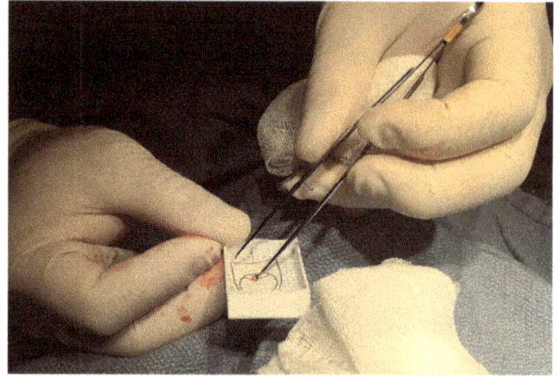

Fig. 5: The lesion is oriented correctly to ensure adequate tissue processing and histopathological analysis.

down to the level of bone. Using fine-tipped scissors carefully cut the base of the biopsy specimen. This should be adjacent to the periosteum. Do not use forceps for this step as this can easily crush the delicate matrix. Usually, it is not necessary to close the defect created by the biopsy; it will heal by secondary intention.

A shave biopsy of the nail matrix can also be performed and typically heals with minimal scarring or nail dystrophy. This technique is most commonly used to sample benign-appearing, wide bands of longitudinal pigmentation. Using a 15-blade, an incision is made surrounding the lesion with a 1–2 mm margin. Then, a shave biopsy of the entire lesion is performed with the scalpel blade parallel to the tissue surface (Fig. 4).

> A shave biopsy of the nail matrix typically heals with minimal scarring or nail dystrophy.

To decrease the likelihood of postoperative nail abnormalities, the resulting specimen should be approximately 1 mm or less in thickness.

After the biopsy specimen is removed, we recommend correctly orienting the biopsy sample for further histopathological processing. The specimen should be placed on a piece of paper or cardboard to keep from curling, inserted in a cassette and placed in a container of formalin (Fig. 5).

Other variations of nail matrix biopsies include transverse elliptical excisions for lesions greater than 3 mm involving the distal matrix or lateral longitudinal biopsies for wide pigmented bands located on the lateral edge of the matrix.

If a partial avulsion was performed, the elevated nail plate should be returned to its original position and sutured to the lateral nail fold using a horizontal mattress stitch.

The proximal nail fold is then returned to its position overlying the nail matrix and proximal nail plate. At each incision of the proximal nail fold, the tissue should be sutured with 6-0 absorbable sutures.

Nail Matricectomy

Ingrown or dystrophic nails are a common problem frequently presenting to dermatologists. A nail matricectomy is a technique used to destroy the area of the nail matrix where the abnormal nail is growing from. The entire nail matrix can also be destroyed in this manner as well, if clinically indicated. There are three main methods to destroy the nail matrix. The first involves the use of phenol, an aromatic organic compound. The second method involves the use of cryotherapy with liquid nitrogen. The third method is surgical removal (e.g. Vandenbos procedure). After a digital block as described above, the toe is cleansed. We typically recommend the use of a constriction band distal to the nail. The risk of tissue necrosis is low given the relative speed of the procedure.

Exposing the Nail Matrix

Exposing the nail matrix for the purposes of matrixectomy can be accomplished in a similar manner to a proximal nail avulsion, which is detailed above. Once the nail matrix is exposed, we prefer the use of either phenol or liquid nitrogen. Although it is possible to remove the nail matrix surgically, we recommend the use of chemical or cryotherapy as these methods achieve the intended outcome with a smaller wound.

Chemical Matricectomy

Once the nail matrix is exposed, we use a cotton-tipped applicator soaked in phenol. We typically recommend using at least three cotton-tipped applicators applied evenly and completely in the matrix in order to prevent the risk of spicules.

Cryotherapy Matricectomy

An alternative to phenol is a cryotherapy matricectomy. In this instance, we recommend 15–20 second applications of liquid nitrogen with at least three freeze-thaw cycles.

Electrosurgery Matricectomy

Another alternative is to use electrocautery to destroy the nail matrix. We typically recommend starting at low power (setting of 10–12 W) and increasing as needed. If a patient has a pacemaker or implantable cardiac defibrillator, bipolar leads should be used.

Digital Myxoid Cyst Treatment

Digital myxoid cysts are benign, dome-shaped, translucent or skin-colored nodules located on the dorsal aspect of the digit between the DIP joint and the proximal nail fold. Rarely, they may also arise under the nail matrix or on more proximal joints. They predominate on the middle and index fingers of the dominant hand. Only 5–10% of digital myxoid cysts appear on the toes. Digital myxoid cysts most commonly occur between the ages of 40 years and 70 years old and are twice as frequent in females than males. Digital myxoid cysts are in fact pseudocysts as they do not have a true epithelial lining. Nail dystrophy is the most common complication, and occurs in 24% of patients with digital myxoid cysts. Dystrophy can often precede the gross detection of the pseudocyst for months. A longitudinal nail plate depression is the most common finding as a result of the pressure from pseudocyst on the nail matrix.

Digital myxoid cysts can also cause pain, tenderness, decreased range of motion of the joint, and recurrent discharge of its fluid contents.

Although controversial, it is hypothesized that digital myxoid cysts evolve from one of two different mechanisms. The first theory describes a superficial type, which is due to metaplasia of dermal fibroblasts resulting in excess production of hyaluronic acid. A second theory suggests a ganglion or deep type of digital myxoid cyst. This type is associated with osteoarthritis of the DIP joint and Heberden's nodes. The hyaluronic acid within the pseudocyst originates from the degenerative joint and connects via a pedicle to the pseudocyst. The pedicle can be visualized via intra-articular injection of methylene blue; this is often used during surgical resection. Although there are several treatment options ranging from conservative measures to surgical excision, the recurrence rate can often be high (>10%) depending on the treatment modality used.

Cryotherapy for Digital Mucous Cysts

- First, drain the digital myxoid cyst using a 21- or 25-gauge needle to puncture the cyst and express its contents.
- Then spray the cyst with liquid nitrogen in a freeze-thaw cycle with 15–30 seconds of freezing and 60–90 seconds of thawing.
- There should be at least a 2 mm margin of treated skin around the cyst to ensure the cyst base and pedicle are treated to prevent further fluid movement from the joint.

Sclerotherapy for Digital Mucous Cysts

Sclerotherapy damages the endothelial lining and occludes the blood vessels supplying the digital myxoid cyst. A variety of sclerosing agents are available including chemical agents (iodine, alcohol), osmotic agents (salicylates, hypertonic saline), or detergents (sodium tetradecyl sulfate, polidocanol, diatrizoate sodium):

- Drain the cyst as described earlier
- Using a 25- to 29-gauge needle, inject the sclerosing agent into the cyst until there is complete whitening of the cyst, indicating sufficient filling

- Immediately apply a compression dressing on the lesion and leave in place for 24 hours
- Additional injections may be required for complete treatment.

Nail Clippings

Nail clippings can be of useful diagnostic yield. Most commonly, nail clippings are used for the histopathological assessment of onychomycosis with the periodic acid-Schiff (PAS)-diastase stain. In some cases, confirmation of onychomycosis by PAS stain occurs when previous fungal cultures and potassium hydroxide (KOH) were negative. However, nail clippings can provide useful information beyond onychomycosis. For inflammatory conditions, nail clippings may help in diagnosis of psoriasis or lichen planus. Nail clippings may help differentiate subungual hemorrhage versus melanin. Finally, nail clippings can be useful for nail matrix tumors, such as an onychomatricoma.

- For thick, hard nails consider double-action nail nippers
- Always wear a protective eye shield and mask
- We recommend placing the patient's hand or foot on a large, preferably solid-colored (blue) fabric. This provides a useful background for the clipped nail.
- When clipping the nail, use your other hand to cover the digit with gauze to prevent losing the clipped nail.
- Ensure you have a sufficiently large clipping to ensure accurate histopathological analysis. We recommend a nail clipping of 5 mm in length and at least 2 mm in width (preferably 4 mm).

> Nail clippings may help differentiate subungual hemorrhage versus melanin.

ANATOMICAL DANGER ZONES

Vasculature

Although the lateral digital arteries and nerves and flexor and extensor tendons are potentially at risk from surgical procedures, most dermatologic surgeons limit their activity to the nail unit and thus should be able to avoid harm to these structures.

The blood supply to the nail unit primarily comes from the lateral digital arteries that send branches to the dorsal aspect of the distal phalanx. The arteries anastomose and form arcades with the respective contralateral artery and send parallel longitudinal branches in the connective tissue of the nail bed and matrix. Thus, severing an artery on one side results in compensation by the contralateral side. Venous drainage parallels arterial drainage. Large collecting veins lie in the lateral nail folds on either side of the nail plate and form an arch in the proximal nail fold.

> Limiting surgery to the nail unit minimizes the potential for harm to vascular structures.

Innervation

The fingers and toes have paired sensory dorsal and volar digital nerves; the dorsal nerves reach the distal phalanx of only the 1st and 5th digits. The palmar and plantar nerves lie to the side of the flexor tendon and the volar artery. The three branches that innervate the distal phalanx divide just distal to the DIP. Innervation follows the arterial supply. A branch of the digital dorsal nerve courses over the DIP joint; it then trifurcates, supplying branches to the nail unit, the tip, and the pulp.

Tendons

Extensor and flexor tendons extend across the DIP to the distal phalanx. The extensor tendon attaches proximal to the matrix.

> **Expert Tip**
> The extensor tendons insertions project approximately 6–12 mm proximally from the cuticle. The section above this line should be avoided, due to the risk of severing the tendon and hyperflexion of the DIP joint leading to mallet finger.

WOUND CARE

A bulky dressing should be used for at least 48 hours, which limits and also absorbs any excessive bleeding, and provides protection against trauma. Avoid dressings that are too tight. The associated limb should be elevated for 48 hours.

We suggest Xeroform dressing as a balled-up pressure dressing directly on the surgical site, followed by multiple 2 × 2 gauzes folded in half and wrapped over the nail unit transversely and longitudinally. These can be secured with silk tape (circumferential taping should be avoided as this can inadvertently function as a tourniquet).

The original dressing can be removed after 48 hours, after which the patient can change the dressing, cleanse the wound, and apply a padded dressing.

AVOIDING COMPLICATIONS

Nail Dystrophy

The most important complication of nail surgery is permanent nail dystrophy, the expectation of which should be discussed with the patient preoperatively. This may be in the form of split nails, nail plate thinning, grooving, distortion, and distal or proximal pterygium. When performing a matrix embolization, the lateral matrix horn should be removed to prevent a nail spicule.

Bleeding

Bleeding is common after removal of the tourniquet. Holding pressure is usually sufficient to staunch moderate blood flow. If an artery can be seen after releasing the tourniquet, it may be ligated using 5-0 absorbable suture material. For limited bleeding, application of cotton-tipped applicator dipped in 35% aluminum chloride is sufficient. For moderate bleeding, calcium alginate or oxidized cellulose dressings will suffice. For severe postoperative bleeding, a 0.5 cc injection of anesthetic as a wing block is suggested as a chemical tourniquet until the hemorrhage ceases.

Pain

Individual pain thresholds are variable. The digits have one of the high densities of free C-fiber nerve endings, which relay pain stimuli to the central nervous system. Vagal reactions from pain are avoided by advising the patient eat 2 hours prior to surgery. Preoperative sedation can be helpful to reduce operative pain and anxiety. Prior to surgery, a 30-gauge needle should be used along with slow infusion of anesthesia. Ropivacaine or bupivacaine are recommended for their long-term analgesia, even postoperatively. If the patient is in pain during surgery, it is due to insufficient administration of anesthesia. Postoperatively, an appropriate dressing is necessary to avoid injury. The patient should be recommended to elevate the extremity to reduce both edema and pain. For toenail surgery, the foot should be elevated to 30° and the patient should be recumbent for 48 hours. Analgesics are usually necessary for optimal pain control.

Infection

The potential for nfection can be minimized by adhering to strict antisepsis guidelines. However, the subungual space cannot be completely sterilized and antibiotic prophylaxis should be considered, if it is appropriate. The phalanx lies directly below the nail unit with little interspersed dermis—and no subcutaneous tissue. Pain after 24–48 hours may be indicative of infection. The dressing should be removed, and the digit inspected; if redness and edema are present, the overlying stitches should be removed. Postoperative infection can be complicated by felon, compartmental cellulitis, lymphangitis, osteomyelitis, DIP joint pyarthrosis, and terminal osteitis. Risk factors include diabetes mellitus, peripheral arterial impairment, and immunosuppression. The patient should be recommended to wash the digit twice daily with antiseptic soap prior to the surgery. If infection occurs, sample the pus, and administer antibiotics that are effective against *Staphylococcus* and adapt according to the culture sensitivities.

> **Expert Tip**
> Nail surgeries are at high risk of infection, particularly toenails. We typically recommend 1-week duration of antibiotic prophylaxis for all toenail surgeries as well as digital myxoid cyst procedures.

Tissue Necrosis

Necrosis is an unpredictable complication. It can occur if the sutures are placed too tightly or not removed in time. It can occur when flaps are used for closure. It may also be a result of poor peripheral circulation due to prolonged ischemia after injection of epinephrine. Again, epinephrine may need to be avoided in patients with peripheral vascular disease, diabetes mellitus, or connective tissue disease. Patients should be encouraged to discontinue smoking, as this can be detrimental to healing after nail surgery. Avoid infiltration of excessive volume during anesthetic administration; only the minimum amount necessary should be used. If necrosis occurs, a hand surgeon should be consulted for debridement. Systemic antibiotics should be initiated to avoid potential infection, and peripheral vasodilators such as calcium channel blockers and blood thinners such as aspirin should be considered to increase blood flow.

Joint Stiffness

Stiffening of the DIP joint is common. This may be due to prolonged splinting. Patients tend to hold the operated finger stiffly and in an extended position. Patients should be informed to keep the affected finger in physiologic flexion.

Other Complications

Reflex sympathetic dystrophy (RSD) is rare, but has been reported after various surgical procedures. It occurs more commonly in the upper extremities, and is more commonly in women and those above the age of 50 years. Pain after 10 days may indicate RSD and may require treatment to prevent it from becoming a chronic issue. Referral to a specialized pain clinic should be sought.

VIDEO LEGEND 📹

Video 1: Lateral incisions and exposure of the nail matrix.

FURTHER READING

1. Abimelec P. Tips and tricks in nail surgery. Semin Cutan Med Surg. 2009;28(1):55-60.
2. Fleckman P, Allan C. Surgical anatomy of the nail unit. Dermatol Surg. 2001;27(3):257-60.
3. Haneke E. Nail surgery. Clin Dermatol. 2013;31 (5):516-25.
4. Jellinek NJ, Vélez NF. Nail surgery: best way to obtain effective anesthesia. Dermatol Clin. 2015; 33(2):265-71.
5. Keramidas EG, Rodopoulou SG. Ropivacaine versus lidocaine in digital nerve blocks: a prospective study. Plast Reconstr Surg. 2007;119(7):2148-52.
6. Krunic AL, Wang LC, Soltani K, et al. Digital anesthesia with epinephrine: an old myth revisited. J Amer Acad Derm. 2004;51(5):755-9.
7. Richert B, Dahdah M. Complications of nail surgery. In: Nouri K (Ed). Complications in Dermatological Surgery. Philadelphia, PA, USA: Elsevier Health Sciences; 2008. pp. 137-58.
8. Robinson JK, Haneke CW, Siegel D, et al. Surgery of the Skin: Procedural Dermatology, 3rd edition. Philadelphia, PA, USA: Elsevier; 2015. pp. 755-80.
9. Vandenbos KQ, Bowers WP. Ingrown toenail: a result of weight bearing on soft tissue. US Armed Forces Med J. 1959;10(10):1168-73.

CHAPTER 13

Flaps and Grafts

Michael W Pelster, Ashish C Bhatia

HISTORY

The history of cutaneous surgery began over 4,000 years ago. Dated to 2100 BC, the Edwin Smith Papyrus first discussed the reconstruction of traumatic wounds in ancient Egypt.[1] The first reference to cutaneous flaps is thought to date to c. 700

> Edwin Smith Papyrus first discussed the reconstruction of traumatic wounds in ancient Egypt in 2100 BC.

BC in ancient India by the surgeon Sushruta, who described a variety of local flaps, primarily for nasal reconstruction. In the 1st and 2nd centuries AD in ancient Rome, Celsus and Galen separately described the use of advancement and island pedicle flaps in the reconstruction of facial defects.[2] In 16th century Italy, surgeons further advanced the use of local and pedicle flap reconstructions on the head and neck. In the early 18th century, European surgeons, borrowing from the techniques of Indian practitioners, first described the use of interpolated forehead flaps for the correction of large defects of the nasal tip and ala,[2,3] the foundation of the modern-day paramedian forehead flap. Modern use of flaps and grafts dates to World War I. Large numbers of injured soldiers necessitated advancements in facial reconstruction.

Advanced cutaneous surgery was handled primarily by general surgeons, plastic surgeons, and otolaryngologists for many centuries.[2] However, dermatologists assumed greater responsibility for cutaneous tumor extirpation and the immediate reconstruction of the oncologic deficit using flaps and grafts after the invention of the Mohs technique by Frederic Mohs in the 1930s and the subsequent introduction of the fresh tissue technique

in 1958. Accordingly, over the last 50 years, dermatologic surgeons have been at the forefront of innovation in facial reconstruction given the high volume of skin cancers and resultant oncologic cutaneous defects in technically challenging anatomic sites, such as the nose, ear, and periorificial skin.

DESCRIPTION OF PROCEDURES

Many schemas have been utilized to conceptualize flap design, which focus on location, eponym, designations, and blood supply (axial pattern relying on a named artery versus random pattern flap).[2] However, the most useful classification system is based on the primary motion of the flap: advancement, rotation, transposition, and interpolation. Hereafter, we will discuss a few general principles of flap design followed

> The most useful classification system is based on the primary motion of the flap: advancement, rotation, transposition, and interpolation.

by several illustrative examples of common flaps organized by primary flap motion.

Several important principles must be followed to ensure optimal flap and graft execution. First, effective preoperative patient counseling and informed consent are critically important. The surgeon must ascertain each patient's preference with respect to cosmesis, wound care, and the time commitment and expense required for follow-up visits and revision procedures. For example, some patients who value convenience over cosmesis may prefer an immediate full-thickness skin graft (FTSG) on the nose when a bilobed flap or other more complicated closure might produce a better aesthetic outcome. Secondly, high-quality preoperative and postoperative photographs from several angles are critical for interval reassessment at follow-up visits. These photographs also document any preexisting facial asymmetry or other unique patient characteristics. Review of these images can enhance patient satisfaction since some individuals take notice of longstanding minor imperfections only after their attention is directed to their face following tumor removal and repair.

Another general principle of flap design requires the preoperative localization of tissue reservoirs. Although not an inviolable rule, laxity most often occurs laterally for defects on the medial face and inferiorly for defects on the lateral face. Therefore, when designing a flap, the

> Laxity most often occurs laterally for defects on the medial face and inferiorly for defects on the lateral face.

cutaneous surgeon's first instinct should be to look in these locations to isolate the area(s) of greatest tissue laxity.

Determining the proper depth for undermining prior to flap elevation is absolutely vital to maximize the potential for flap survival and produce optimal surgical outcomes. This appropriate depth of this plane varies depending upon the anatomic site and is impacted by the clinical

> The plane of flap elevation and undermining is absolutely vital to ensure flap survival and optimal surgical outcomes.

scenario. Briefly, undermining in areas other than the head and neck region should ideally take place in the deep subcutaneous fat. On the scalp, the subgaleal plane is preferred, while on the nose, undermining should take place immediately above the perichondrium. Elsewhere on the face, undermining ideally takes place in the superficial

> On the scalp, subgaleal plane undermining is preferred, while on the nose, it should take place immediately above the perichondrium. Elsewhere on the face, undermine at the level of superficial subcutaneous fat.

subcutaneous fat to avoid damage to neurovascular structures; however, in areas of hair-bearing skin (e.g. the eyebrows), it is preferred to undermine in the deeper subcutaneous fat to avoid trauma to the hair bulbs that can produce alopecia. Furthermore, delicate tissue handling is very important. Toothed forceps are less traumatic than flat-edged forceps and skin hooks even less so, leading many dermatologic surgeons to use hooks for hemostasis, flap elevation, and at times even for dermal suturing. This will minimize any subtle tissue trauma that may adversely affect scar outcome.[4] Similarly, precision of flap design is critical. Especially for more complicated transposition flaps, the angle of takeoff and sizing of the primary (and sometimes secondary) lobes are crucial to avoid complications, such as pincushioning and flap necrosis.

Finally, patient factors play a crucial role. Patients undergoing Mohs micrographic surgery and subsequent flap and graft repair are very frequently on one or more anticoagulant or antiplatelet agents. Currently, the generally accepted principle is to maintain patients on any medically indicated anticoagulation, as it is felt that any increased operative risk related to poor hemostasis is far outweighed by the increased risk of myocardial infarction or stroke conferred by stopping these medications.[5,6] That being said, failures of hemostasis contribute to a large number of graft failures,[7] therefore, meticulous intraoperative hemostasis is absolutely critical.

> Meticulous intraoperative hemostasis is absolutely critical to prevent graft failure.

Additionally, smokers have known worse outcomes after flap and graft repair,[8,9] so it is critical to provide counseling regarding smoking cessation and appropriate informed consent, so that patients are aware of their personal responsibility to prevent poor outcomes. Finally, postoperative wound care should utilize plain petroleum jelly only, as it has been demonstrated to have equal infection rates when compared with topical antimicrobials while decreasing the risk of contact dermatitis.[10]

The first type of primary flap motion is advancement. Many textbooks begin their discussion with a consideration of classic unilateral and bilateral rectangular advancement flaps. These repairs, however, are used quite infrequently in cutaneous surgery. This chapter will focus on the more-commonly used A to L and A to T advancement flaps. This nomenclature is derived from the shape of the defect and ultimate lines of closure.

> "A to L" and "A to T" are the most commonly utilized advancement flaps.

For example, an A to L flap consists of a circular defect combined with a standing cone (the A), which is repaired with an advancement flap that will ultimately consist of connecting perpendicular lines (the L). The inferior forehead immediately superior to the eyebrow is a common location for the utilization of these A-L or A-T advancement flaps. To execute this flap, a standing cone is excised superiorly to the defect as if the wound were to be closed in a vertically-oriented linear fashion perpendicular to the superior margin of the brow. Subsequently, incisions are made laterally (A to L) or laterally and medially (A to T) along the brow at the level of the base of the wound. The flap and surrounding skin are then elevated and undermined in the appropriate plane, taking care to minimize damage to neurovascular structures and to undermine deep to the hair bulbs of the eyebrow to diminish the risk of alopecia. Sometimes, dog-ears need to be excised to eliminate tissue redundancy along the horizontal arm(s); however, most often this redundancy can be "sewn out" with meticulous suturing technique utilizing the rule of halves (Figs. 1A to D).[11]

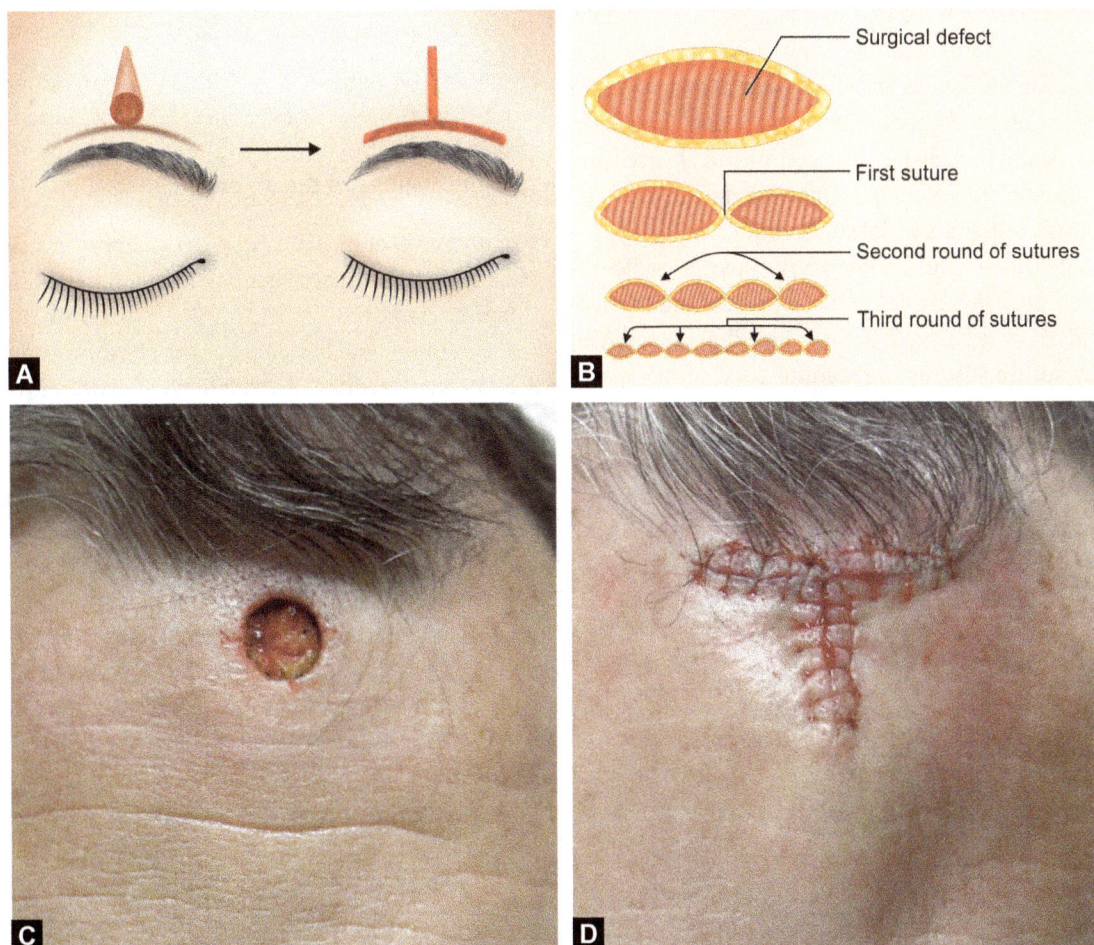

Figs. 1A to D: (A) Diagram of an A to T flap above the eyebrow; (B) Visual representation of sewing out tissue redundancy utilizing the "rule of halves"; (C and D) Before and after photographs of surgical defect closed using A to T advancement flap.

These same principles can be applied to defects in other locations near free margins, most notably in wounds of the lateral upper cutaneous lip just superior to the vermilion border.

A commonly-utilized and versatile variant of the standard advancement flap is the island pedicle flap (also known as the V-Y advancement flap).[12,13] The distinctive feature of the island pedicle flap is that its vascular supply is derived from a deep subcutaneous and/or muscular pedicle rather than through lateral dermal connections to the adjacent dermis and subcutis as in the vast majority of surgical flaps. A healed island pedicle

> The distinctive feature of the island pedicle flap is that its vascular supply is derived from a deep subcutaneous and/or muscular pedicle.

flap is easily identified by its unique scar shape, which has been likened to a kite (Figs. 2A and B). Two commonly used locations for island pedicle flaps are for defects within the lateral eyebrow and the superior cutaneous lip near the nasolabial fold.[2] The island pedicle flap is accomplished by incising a triangle of tissue adjacent to the defect. The surrounding tissue is widely undermined in the appropriate plane, and the deep tether of the pedicle is freed only slightly at the distal apex of the triangle and in some cases, at the leading edge as well. The key suture secures the leading edge of the island to the distal edge of the wound, and the result-

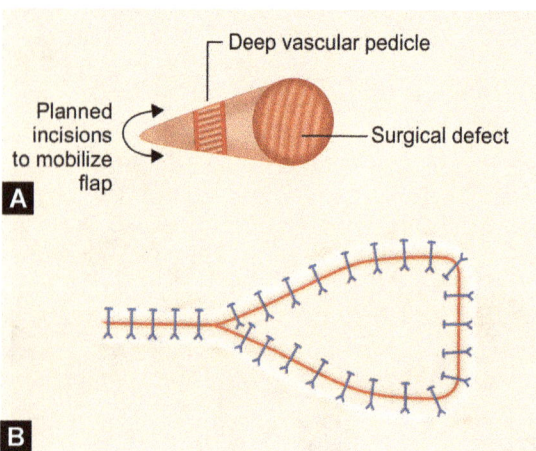

Figs. 2A and B: (A) Diagram of incision plan for an island pedicle flap; (B) Kite-shaped sutured lines of executed island pedicle flap.

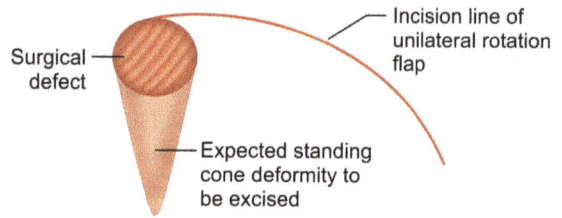

Fig. 3: Diagram for planning a unilateral rotation flap.

ant defect at the original site of the island's apex is closed linearly (hence, the kite-shaped pattern).

The second type of primary flap motion is rotation. Rotation flaps share many of the same design concepts as advancement flaps. The executed incision, however, takes a curvilinear form rather than the straight lines employed in advancement flaps (Fig. 3). Because of this, the tension of wound closure is directed away from the original defect. Additionally, a curvilinear incision/flap recapitulates facial rhytides or cosmetic

> Rotation flaps have a curvilinear form rather than the straight lines employed in advancement flaps. This directs the tension of wound closure away from the original defect.

subunits and/or displaces dog-ears to more favorable anatomic locations, leading to better cosmesis. Rotation flaps are most commonly used on the scalp, temple, medial cheek, and chin, but have also been described in a variety of more novel scenarios.[14] Larger defects or those in areas of particularly tight skin often require bilateral rotation flaps (the so-called O-Z flap). The O to Z flap requires the incision of two opposing rotational arcs with take-off points on opposite sides of the circular defect, after which each flap is raised and rotated in to each cover half of the defect (Figs. 4A and B). Two commonly utilized location-specific eponymous rotation flaps are also worthy of mention: the Rieger dorsal nasal rotation flap[15] (Figs. 5A and B) for large distal nasal defects and the Mustarde rotation flap for large defects on the superomedial cheek and/or lower eyelid (Figs. 6A and B).[16]

The third type of primary flap motion is transposition. Transposition flaps are unique in two primary ways. First, they move ("transpose") skin crossing over intervening normal skin into the defect. Additionally, transposition flaps place

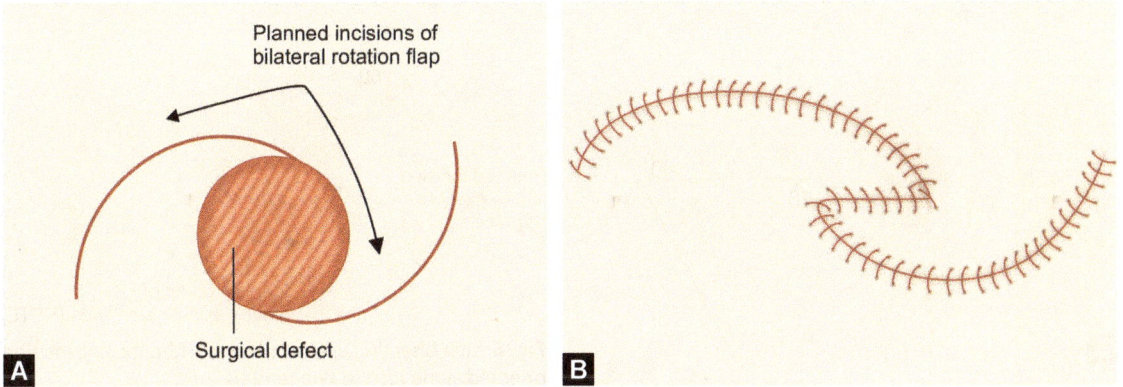

Figs. 4A and B: (A) Diagram of surgical defect and plan for bilateral rotation flap; (B) O to Z shape of sutured lines of executed bilateral rotation flap.

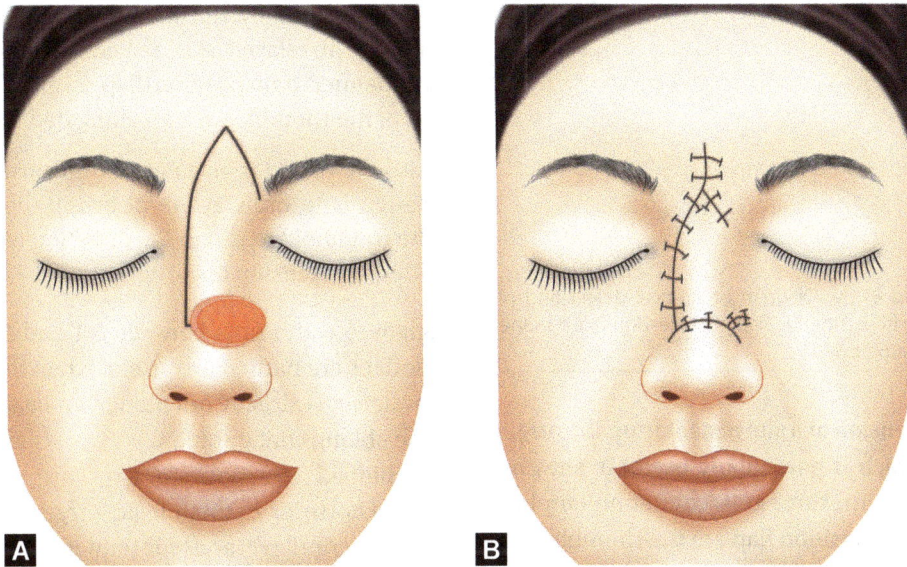

Figs. 5A and B: (A) Diagram of surgical defect and plan for dorsal nasal rotation flap (Rieger flap) with backcut; (B) Sutured lines of executed dorsal nasal rotation flap.

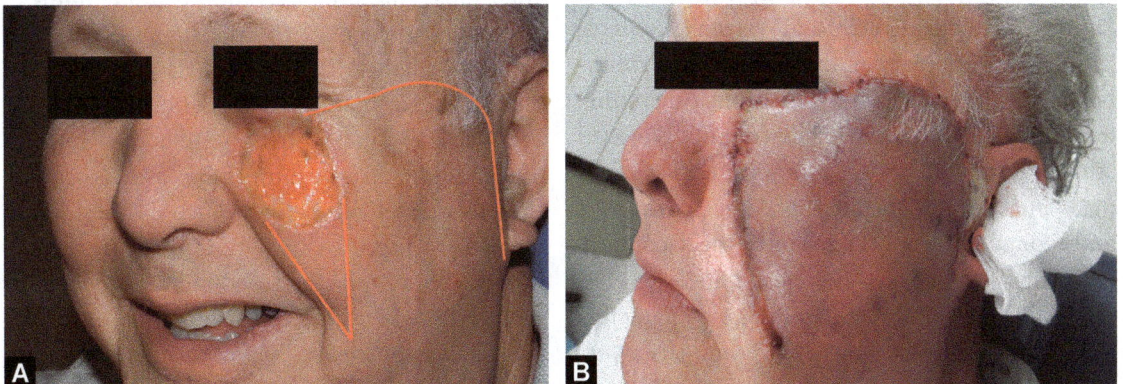

Figs. 6A and B: (A) Large medial cheek defect with planned incisions for Mustarde flap superimposed; (B) Mustarde flap sutured into place.
Source: Ian Maher

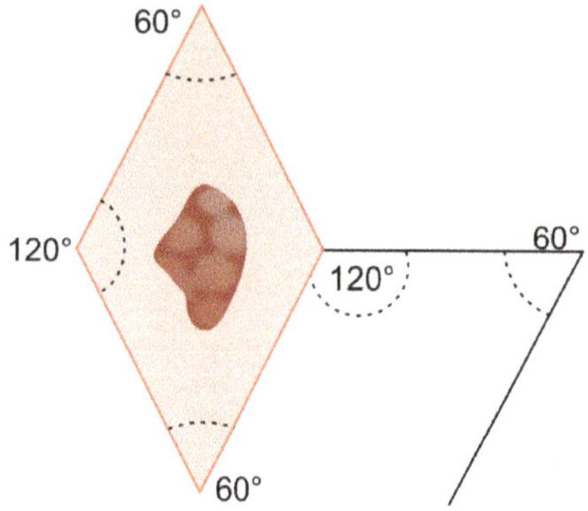

Figs. 7A and B: (A): Diagram of surgical defect and plan for closure with a rhombic flap; (B) Question mark shape of executed rhombic flap.

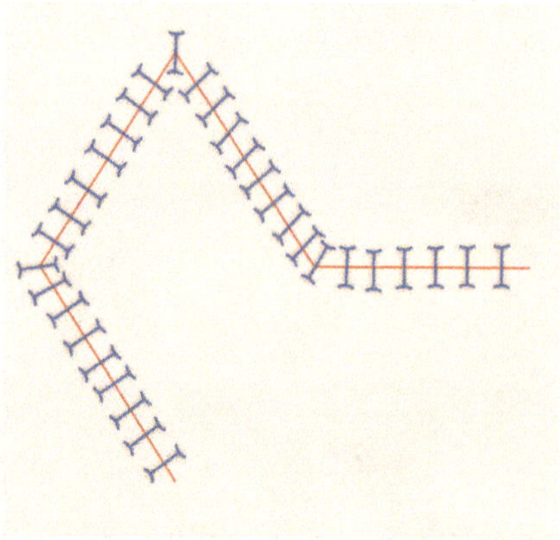

Fig. 8: Line bisecting apex of planned rhombic flap incision oriented along resting skin tension lines.

transposition flap design; one particularly useful pearl is that a line bisecting the apex of the rhombic should ideally run in the same direction as rhytides or relaxed skin tension lines (Fig. 8).[23] The banner transposition flap is merely a variant of the rhombic with an elongated lobe with a

> A useful pearl for visualizing transposition flap design is to draw a line bisecting the apex of the rhomboid to run in the direction of the rhytides/skin tension lines.

length to width ratio between 3:1 and 5:1.[24] Banner flaps are particularly useful when the cutaneous defect is already oriented in an oval or otherwise oblong configuration.

Bilobed transposition flaps are considered a workhorse of dermatologic surgery. The original description[25] and subsequent Zitelli modification[26] are considered classic texts of flap design (Figs. 9A and B). Bilobed flaps consist of two adjacent and connected transposition flaps. Their most common utilization is in medium- to large-sized defects of the distal nose, although use of the bilobed flap has been described in sites on the cheek, hand, and posterior ear as well.[2] Trilobed flaps, conceptually similar designs with the addition of one more lobe, are also occasionally utilized on the very distal nose for larger defects or when the skin is particularly inelastic.[27] Of note, both Z-plasties (used most frequently for scar revision) and interpolation flaps (e.g. paramedian forehead flap, melolabial interpolation flap, Abbe flap) are also variants of transposition flaps, but a detailed discussion of their mechanics is outside of the scope of this chapter.

maximal tension at a site distant from the original wound, which is particularly useful in sites near free margins. The three most commonly employed types of transposition flap are the rhombic transposition flap, the bilobed transposition flap, and the banner transposition flap.

Rhombic flaps vary in design and have several eponymous geometric variants, including the Limberg,[17] Dufourmentel,[18] and Webster.[19] Regardless of the particular variant, creation of a rhombic flap requires two angled incisions originating from the defect. This flap is subsequently elevated and undermined in the appropriate plane and then "pushed" into the original defect, covering it and redirecting wound tension to the secondary (or tertiary) defect, which is closed linearly (Figs. 7A and B). The rhombic flap leaves a characteristic "question-mark" scar. The rhombic is a versatile closure that can be utilized in a variety of anatomic locations, mostly near free margins.[20-22] Novice surgeons often have difficulty visualizing

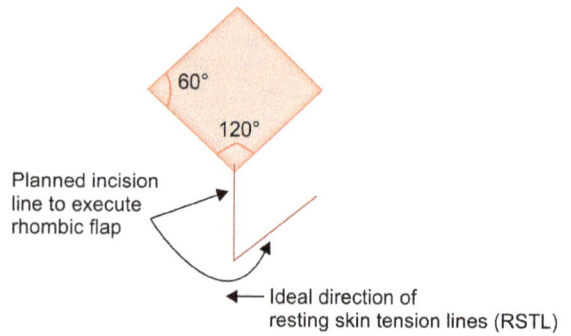

Figs. 9A and B: (A) Original bilobed flap; (B) Zitelli modification of bilobed flap.

Although generally not preferred when compared to linear closure and flaps, skin grafts are also an important component of the dermatologic surgeon's reconstructive repertoire. A FTSG consists of the epidermis plus the entire thickness of the dermis. It can be harvested from essentially any location, but a specific site is generally chosen to optimize tissue match with the recipient site and ideally, from an area where the

> Donor skin is harvested from sites to optimize tissue match ideally without creating cosmetic morbidity at this site.

donor site itself will not cause significant cosmetic morbidity. Common sites include the inner upper arm, the supraclavicular skin, the conchal bowl, the preauricular cheek, and the postauricular skin. To execute a FTSG, a template is first made using the size and shape of the wound to be repaired as a guide. This template is then utilized to draw out the planned area to be excised for the graft, with the area marked often being slightly oversized to account for graft contraction. The graft is then excised and subsequently "defatted" (i.e. all subcutaneous fat is removed) with scissors to ensure that it contains epidermis and dermis only. It is then sewn into the defect with epicuticular sutures and sometimes "basting" sutures to ensure good adherence to the graft bed. Depending on surgeon preference, a bolster may be sewn over the graft to further promote contact between the graft and wound base, although there are limited data supporting this practice.[28] Often a good pressure dressing can perform the role of the bolster. Critically, even if the graft appears necrotic or there is eschar formation in the postoperative period, it is important to avoid debridement, as a FTSG will provide a biologic dressing even if it does not fully take. Of note, a commonly used variant called a Burow's graft is merely a FTSG harvested from a standing cone adjacent to a given defect rather than from a separate donor site (Fig. 10).[29]

Two less commonly-used variants of skin grafts are split-thickness skin grafts (STSGs) and composite grafts. A STSG consists of epidermis and only the partial thickness of the der-

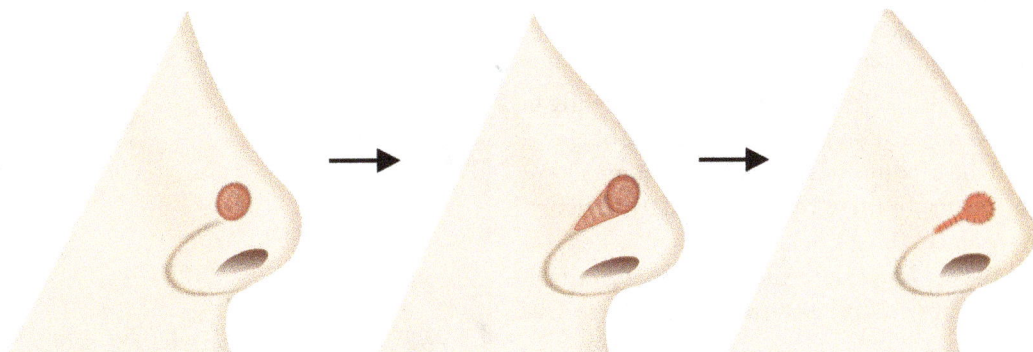

Fig. 10: Diagram of execution of a Burow's graft. Tissue from an adjacent Burow's triangle is used as a FTSG to close the defect.

mis. Because of lower metabolic requirements, STSGs can be used to cover a large surface area in which a FTSG would not viably function or there would not be enough donor tissue available without donor site morbidity. However, they are less commonly used due to inferior cosmesis at both sites and pain at the granulating donor site that may persist for a long time. Composite grafts are defined as a FTSG with one additional component

> Split-thickness skin grafts are less commonly used due to inferior cosmesis at both sites and pain at the donor site.

of the integument (most frequently cartilage but occasionally subcutaneous fat). Composite grafts are most often used for deep defects on the nose, especially in case where it is feared that alar rim collapse secondary to loss of cartilage might lead to functional morbidity.[30]

Benefits Compared to Alternative Approaches

Most surgical wounds are closed with an elliptical (or fusiform) excision, ellipse variants (e.g. crescent, S-plasty, M-plasty), or allowed to heal by secondary intention. Flaps and grafts, however, offer a variety of benefits compared to these methods, especially on the face, ears, scalp and digits.

First, flaps and grafts are often critical to prevent distortion of free margins. Repair of defects close to the eyelid, alar rim, columella, lips, and helices are at risk of distorting the free margin if tension vectors are directed perpendicularly to a free margin. For example, a defect just superior to the eyebrow cannot be closed linearly in a vertical fashion because the inferior standing cone would cross into the eyebrow and superior eyelid. Furthermore, this defect cannot be closed linearly in a horizontal fashion because of the risk of elevation of the eyebrow due to vertically oriented tension vectors. In these cases, a carefully designed advancement flap (A to L or A to T) provides sufficient laxity for closure without crossing critical structures or risking distortion of the brow (*see* Figs. 1A to D).

Additionally, flaps and grafts allow closure in sites where the inherent characteristics of the skin

prevent primary closure. Anatomic regions where there is little laxity include the scalp, the lower third of the nose, and much of the auricle, among other sites. Thus, on the scalp, when primary closure is, at times, impossible, large (often bilateral) rotation flaps (the so-called O to Z flap) (*see* Figs. 4A and B) or primary closure with a Burow's graft[29] [i.e. utilization of the excised standing cone(s) as a FTSG] enable patients to avoid the wound care inherent in second intention healing, another

> A full thickness skin graft allows patients to avoid the wound care inherent in second intention healing.

option on the scalp. On the inferior third of the nose, bilobed flaps (*see* Figs. 9A and B) or (in the case of larger defects) interpolation flaps such as the paramedian forehead flap and melolabial interpolation flap enable closure when sufficient laxity for primary closure is absent. Similarly, on the ear, full thickness skin grafts[31] (Figs. 11A and B) or (for specific defects) helical rim advancement flaps[32] enable closure in areas of very tight skin.

When faced with a deep defect which could allow for adjacent tissue distortion as the wound contracts through second intention healing, another option is partial granulation followed by a FTSG. This can allow the depth to fill sufficiently to place a FTSG without a depression in the repair site, and at the same time, provide an excellent bed of granulation tissue for good graft take. This method is often used in lieu of a bilobed flap on

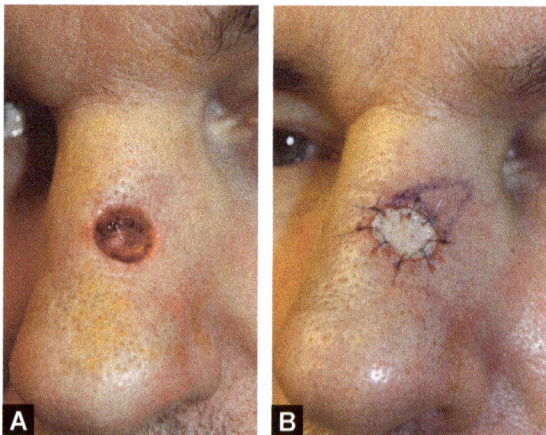

Figs. 11A and B: (A) Photograph of surgical defect on the nasal sidewall; (B) Repair with full-thickness skin graft.

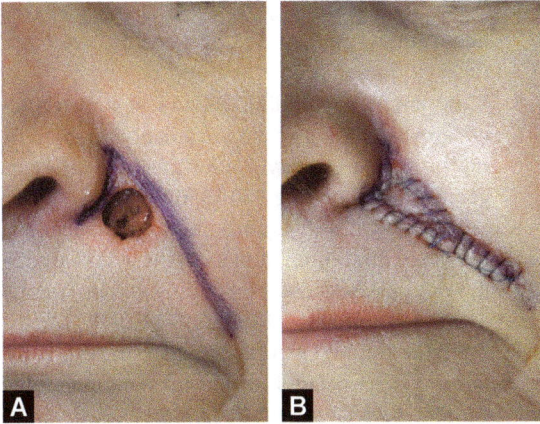

Figs. 12A and B: (A) Photograph of surgical defect of the upper cutaneous lip; (B) Sutured closure of executed island pedicle flap.

the lower one-third of the nose when a bilobed flap is not desired (e.g. actinic damage or scarring of flap donor site).

When compared to second intention healing, flaps and grafts can minimize wound care. With a flap or graft, daily application of Vaseline with or without an overlying bandage until suture removal is often sufficient, whereas granulating wounds can take weeks to months to heal. Especially for elderly patients or individuals who otherwise have difficulty performing their activities of daily living, appropriate care of a wound healing by second intention may be extremely difficult.

Flaps also sometimes allow the surgeon to hide scars in rhytides, resting skin tension lines, or along the boundaries of cosmetic subunits. Common examples illustrating this phenomenon include the use of the island pedicle flap on the superolateral cutaneous lip (Figs. 12A and B)[33] and the eponymous Mustarde rotation flap for large medial cheek defects (*see* Figs. 6A and B).[16]

RISKS AND LIMITATIONS

There are a number of risks and limitations to the use of flaps and grafts. Flaps carry an increased risk of necrosis compared to primary closure or second intention healing, especially, if inappropriately designed (i.e. flap length exceeding width by more than a ratio of 3–4:1) or when placed under undue tension. Similarly, the requisite wider area of undermining required for most flaps inc-

reases the risk of injury to nearby nerves or vessels as well as other complications, such as hematoma formation. In particular, for repairs on the head

> The requisite wider area of undermining required for most flaps increases the risk of injury to nearby nerves or vessels.

and neck commonly encountered after Mohs micrographic surgery, large flaps may place the relatively superficial temporal branch of the facial nerve, marginal mandibular nerve, and spinal accessory nerve at risk of temporary or permanent paresis. Another risk largely specific to flaps is the risk of pincushioning, also known as a trapdoor deformity.[34] Additionally, many interpolation flaps (e.g. paramedian forehead flap, melolabial interpolation interpolation flap, mastoid interpolation flap) require two or three stages, placing an additional burden on the patient, who has to come to the clinic multiple times for suture removal, takedown, and revision procedures. Finally,

> Interpolation flaps require two or three stages requiring multiple clinic visits.

in the case of repairs of defects created by skin cancers (especially those not cleared utilizing the Mohs technique, which offers the highest rates of tumor clearance in the vast majority of clinical settings), recurrence is often much harder to detect. In fact, recurrent tumor can track under a flap and become quite advanced prior to detection of

> Tumor recurrences following excisional surgery are more difficult to detect under a flap.

the recurrence. Along the same lines, if a defect is closed by a flap prior to definitive margin control and the tissue is found to have positive margins on frozen section pathology, it is often challenging to know exactly where to re-excise, and the patient often ultimately ends up with a less than optimal cosmetic outcome. Additionally, the incision lines required for some flaps can be quite long, and if poorly executed or designed, may be more esthetically conspicuous than a simpler side-to-side closure or FTSG. Finally, flaps require significantly increased operative time compared to a complex linear closure and certainly more so than allowing the wound to heal by second intention;

the cost to the healthcare system is also greater. Thus, it is important to restrict flap and graft closures to the clinical situations in which they are truly likely to deliver a superior functional and/or cosmetic outcome.

> Flaps and grafts are reserved for clinical situations where they are likely to deliver a superior functional and/or cosmetic outcome.

The utilization of grafts also comes with a number of risks and limitations. First, by their very definition, grafts do not carry their own blood supply and are thus at a relatively higher risk of ischemia and subsequent failure than most primary closures or local flaps. Furthermore, a graft introduces an additional wound and scar at the donor site. Grafts are also at relatively high risk of seroma or hematoma formation, if not sufficiently secured to the bed of the wound. Additionally, if inappropriately sized or placed in a suboptimal anatomic location, graft contracture can lead to ectropion, eclabion, alar distortion, or other cosmetically disfiguring distortions of free margins. Finally, there is a risk of inferior cosmesis for both FTSGs and especially for STSGs. Specifically, grafts tend to be hypopigmented relative to surrounding skin. While FTSGs can have excellent cosmesis, this requires donor tissue closely matched to the recipient site, which is not always possible; STSGs have known inferior cosmesis and are most often chosen for practical reasons in the setting of particularly large defects or a wound or patient unable to tolerate closure by another means.

REFERENCES

1. Zelac DE, Swanson N, Simpson M, et al. The history of dermatologic surgical reconstruction. Dermatol Surg. 2000;26:983-90.
2. Cook JL, Goldman GD, Holmes TE. Random pattern cutaneous flaps. In: Robinson JK, Hanke CM, Siegel DM (Eds). Surgery of the skin—procedural dermatology. London: Elsevier Saunders; 2015. pp. 252-85.
3. Carupe JC. Account of two successful operations for restoring a lost nose from the integument of the forehead. London: Longman; 1816. Plast Reconstr Surg (reprinted). 1966;37:167-83.
4. Boyer JD, Maino KL, Zitelli JA. Surgical Pearl: hemostasis assisted with two skin hooks. J Am Acad Dermatol. 2002;27:938-9.
5. Kirkorian AY, Moore BL, Siskind J, et al. Perioperative management of anticoagulant therapy during cutaneous surgery: 2005 survey of Mohs surgeons. Dermatol Surg. 2007;33:1189-97.
6. Kovich O, Otley CC. Thrombotic complications related to discontinuation of warfarin and aspirin therapy perioperatively for cutaneous operation. J Am Acad Dermatol. 2003;48:233-7.
7. Cook JL, Perone JB. A prospective study of complications associated with Mohs micrographic surgery. Arch Dermatol. 2003;139:143-52.
8. Rees TD, Liverett DM, Guy CL. The effect of cigarette smoking on skin-flap survival in the face lift patient. Plast Reconstruct Surg. 1984;73:911-15.
9. Goldminz D, Bennett RG. Cigarette smoking and flap and full-thickness graft necrosis. Arch Dermatol. 1991;127:1012-5.
10. Smack DP, Harrington AC, Dunn C, et al. Infection and allergy incidence in ambulatory surgery patients using white petrolatum vs. bacitracin ointment: a randomized controlled trial. JAMA. 1996;276:922-7.
11. Quatrano NA, Samie FH. Modification of Burow's advancement flap: avoiding the secondary triangle. JAMA Facial Plast Surg. 2014;16:364-6.
12. Tomich JM, Wentzell JM, Grande DJ. Subcutaneous island pedicle flaps. Arch Dermatol. 1987; 123:514-8.
13. Dzubow LM. Subcutaneous island pedicle flaps. J Dermatol Surg Oncol 1986;12:591-6.
14. Regula CG, Liu A, Lawrence N. Versatility of the O-Z flap in the reconstruction of facial defects. Dermatol Surg. 2016;42:109-14.
15. Rieger RA. A local flap for repair of the nasal tip. Plast Reconstr Surg. 1967;40:147-9.
16. Mustarde JC. Reconstruction of the eyelid. Minerva Chir. 1967;22:933-42 [in Italian].
17. Limberg AA. Design of local flaps. In: Gibson T (Ed). Modern trends in plastic surgery. London: Butterworth & Co.; 1966. pp. 38-61.
18. Dufourmentel C. Le fermeture des pertes de substance cutanee limitees: le lambeau de rotation en L pour losange' det "LLL". Ann Chirurgie Plast. 1962;7:61-6.
19. Webster RC, Davidson TM, Smith RC. The thirty degree transposition flap. Laryngoscope. 1978;88: 85-94.
20. Bullock JD, Flagg SV. Rhomboid flap in ophthalmic plastic surgery. Arch Ophthalmol. 1973;90:203-5.
21. Shotton FT. Optimal closure of medial canthal surgical defects with rhomboid flaps: "rules of

thumb" for flap and rhomboid defect orientation. Ophthalmolic Surg. 1983;14:46-52.

22. Gunter JP, Carder HM, Fee WE. Rhomboid flap. Arch Otolaryngol. 1977;103:206-11.

23. Borges AF. Choosing the correct Limberg flap. Plast Reconstr Surg. 1981;67:458-66.

24. Masson JK, Mendelson BC. The banner flap. Am J Surg. 1977;134:419-23.

25. Esser JS. Gestielte locale Nasenplastik mit zwei-plifgem Lappen, Deckung des sekundaren Defektes vom ersten Zipfel durch den zweiten. Dtsch Z Chir. 1918;143:385-90.

26. Zitelli JA. The bilobed flap for nasal reconstruction. Arch Dermatol. 1989;125:957-9.

27. Albertini JG. Trilobed flap reconstruction for distal nasal skin defects. Dermatol Surg. 2010;36:1726-35.

28. Langtry JA, Kirkham P, Martin IC, et al. Tie-over bolster dressings may not be necessary to secure small full thickness skin grafts. Dermatol Surg. 1998;24:1350-3.

29. Zitelli JA. Burow's grafts. J Am Acad Dermatol. 1987;17:271-9.

30. Gloster HM Jr, Brodland DG. The use of perichondrial cutaneous grafts to repair defects of the lower third of the nose. Br J Dermatol. 1997;136:43-6.

31. Trufant JW, Marzolf S, Leach BC, et al. The utility of full-thickness skin grafts (FTSGs) for auricular reconstruction. J Am Acad Dermatol. 2016;75:169-76.

32. Cavanaugh EB. Management of lesions of the helical rim using a chrondrocutaneous advancement flap. J Dermatol Surg Oncol. 1982;8:691-6.

33. Zitelli JA, Brodland DG. A regional approach to reconstruction of the upper lip. J Dermatol Surg Oncol. 1991;17:143-8.

34. Koranda FC, Webster RC. Trapdoor effect in nasolabial flaps. Causes and corrections. Arch Otolaryngol. 1985;111:421-4.

PART 4

Tips and Tricks: Cryosurgery and Cryotherapy

—*William Abramovits*

CHAPTER 14

Cryotherapy and Cryosurgery

William Abramovits, Hannah R Badon, Kimberly Dawn Vincent,
Hamad Patel, Stephen E Helms, Ronald Lubritz

> *"Let me introduce myself, I'm the cold hard truth"*
>
> —George Jones

INTRODUCTION

Cryosurgery describes treatments that utilize a low temperature gas, liquid, or solid to ablate tissue. The temperature of the tissue must be lowered to a critical level for a specific time to produce direct damage to its cells or to decrease blood flow to targeted lesions.

Many healthcare providers equate cryosurgery with cryotherapy.[1] Cryotherapy is to be used to describe procedures that lower the temperature of tissues without inducing a destructive response; examples would be the hypothermia used to treat patients during coma, the superficial desquamation of the epidermis for treating acne with "CO_2 slush," or the cooling of the skin to induce a mild anesthetic effect.[2]

Dermatologic cryosurgery comprises destructive procedures to destroy benign, premalignant, and malignant lesions.[1] Examples of benign lesions amenable to cryosurgery include skin tags, viral warts, seborrheic keratoses, benign lentigines, a variety of deep fungal and parasitic lesions, excessive adipose tissue, and keloids. Examples of premalignant lesions treated with cryosurgery include actinic keratosis, Bowenoid papulosis, leukoplakia, and actinic cheilitis. Cancerous lesions such as keratoacanthomas, squamous cell carcinomas, Bowen disease, basal cell carcinomas, lentigo maligna, melanoma, and even metastatic melanoma may also be amenable to cryosurgery under certain circumstances.[3] Over one hundred distinct dermatologic entities treatable with cryosurgery were listed in a recent, comprehensive textbook on dermatological cryosurgery and

> Cryotherapy affects tissues much less than cryosurgery and is used for superficial desquamation or a mild anesthetic effect.

cryotherapy.[4] Cryotherapy and cryosurgery are considered both a science and an art. A science because it is based on solid, physical fundamentals related to its cooling effects on different tissues measured through clinical, laboratory, and imaging methods, with careful statistical analysis. An art, because evidence-based medicine is not available to support every clinical situation where cryosurgery may be considered the "standard of care". Optimal practice requires knowledge, experience, and common sense.

Some physicians delegate cryosurgery to personnel without an in depth education of the physics behind cryosurgery or the clinical foundation of a dermatologist. This is possible because treatment with cryosurgery is fairly forgiving. If a lesion is undertreated there may be the option of retreating or treating it with an alternative modality. If a lesion is overtreated, healing mechanisms often repair the damage satisfactorily.

HISTORY OF CRYOSURGERY

Lowering temperatures for therapeutic purposes dates back to ancient Egypt and Greece where ice was purportedly used to relieve inflammation and pain. The first publication of the use of extreme cold to destroy skin tissue is credited to J Arnott in 1851. In the latter part of the 19th and the beginning of the 20th centuries, liquid air and carbon dioxide were part of the therapeutic armamentarium available to treat a variety of skin lesions from benign to malignant. Liquid nitrogen (LN) was introduced as the primary dermatologic cryogen in the middle and latter parts of the 20th century by HV Allington, IS Cooper, D Torre, S Zacarian, AA Gage, and GF Graham. Other distinguished contributors to the clinical and basic science knowledge base of cryosurgery include R Dawber, G Castro-Ron, E Kuflik, R Lubritz, JG Baust, JM Baust, GC Bischof, KR Diller, and MS Sabel.[4,5]

In the 21st century, advances in understanding cryotherapy and cryosurgery mechanisms, improvements in imaging methodology, and new forms of delivery equipment increased the effectiveness and safety of the technique.[6,7] In addition, cryotherapeutic procedures are being used in combination with other modalities. For instance, patients with multiple thin and thick actinic keratoses are often treated with a combination of cryosurgery and topical 5-fluorouracil for broader field effects.[8]

PRINCIPLES BEHIND CRYOSURGERY

There is a large body of fundamental knowledge critical to the proper use of cryosurgery. Each constituent of the skin is variably sensitive to cold; this is in contraposition to their similar sensitivity to heat, which destroys by terminal dehydration. Melanocytes are more sensitive to cold than epithelial cells, which in turn are more sensitive than connective and vascular tissues.[9,10] Viruses may actually be preserved at extremely low temperatures. Mechanisms by which low temperatures destroy cells and tissues include ice crystal formation in different types of tissue, the speed of freeze, osmolality changes, loss of electrolyte and pH balance, ischemic necrosis and immunity.

The capacity for different coolants or cryogens to lower temperatures varies significantly. Benign or very superficial lesions may be effectively treated with coolants that lower skin surface temperatures to –75° to –90°C (dimethyl ether and propane). A cryogen able to lower surface temperatures to –196°C (LN) is required for most malignant lesions.[4,11]

> Benign or very superficial lesions may be effectively treated with coolants only able to lower skin surface temperatures to –75° to–90°C while a cryogen able to lower surface temperatures to –196°C (liquid nitrogen) is required for malignant lesions.

Because speed of freeze and slowness of thaw are relevant to the destruction of all but the most superficial of lesions, LN is the cryogen selected by most dermatologists.

Current cryosurgery equipment utilizing LN can deliver temperatures below –50°C to a depth of 4–5 mm in an efficient and reproducible way (Figs. 1A to D). Less efficient cryogens, are available in canisters. There is little published data supporting the use of the latter and they are generally believed to be inadequate to destroy epithelial skin cancers and thicker lesions.[12,13] They are also much more expensive than LN when utilized in busy clinics that perform cryosurgery daily. We primarily mention these canisters because they may be successful for very thin seborrheic keratoses or warts and some are sold over-the-counter for home use.

Liquid nitrogen may be delivered using metallic or cotton tipped applicators dipped in the liquid, closed probes within which the gas circulates, or open probes that allow spray to be localized to the exact size of the opening at the skin surface. Spray is the most efficient way to deliver LN, but its spread may require precise localization with cones or chambers, particularly when working

> Spray is the most efficient way to deliver LN

around delicate structures such as the eyes. Closed probes occasionally may be a better choice in this latter circumstance (*see* later under *Equipment*).

Morbidity from extreme cold is characterized by erythema, edema, circumscribed necrosis and

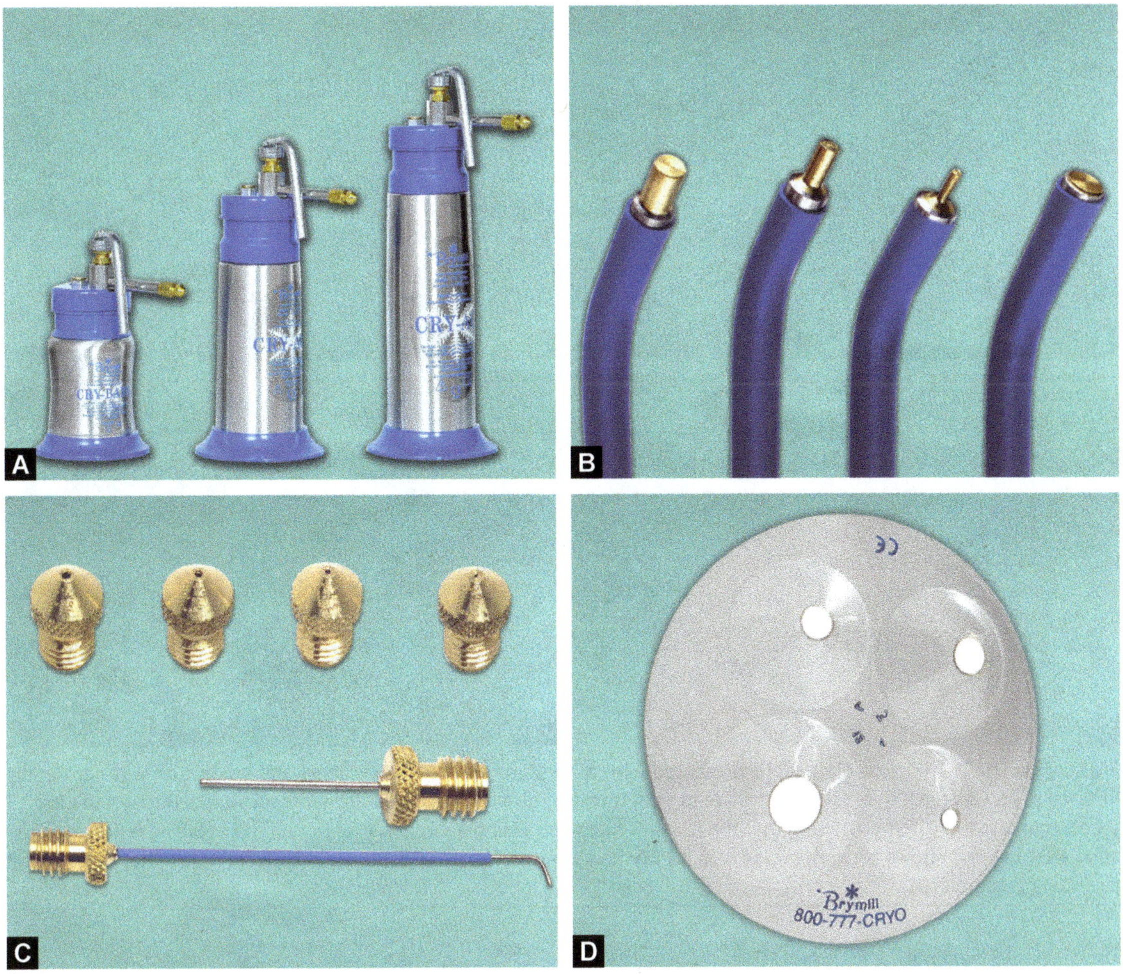

Figs. 1A to D: (A) Hand held cryosurgical instruments are available in various sizes. (B) Cryoprobes are available in a variety of sizes. These are utilized when the spray technique could affect surrounding structures, such as around the eyes. (C) Spray tips may deliver varying amounts of cryogen depending on the size of the orifice. (D) A plastic or rubber cone may also be used to contain spray to lesional skin while protecting normal surrounding skin and skin structures.

sloughing of devitalized cells. Relative stromal preservation provides a scaffold that permits fibroblasts to promote healing with reduced scarring. Bones and cartilage, even if devitalized, tend to resist sloughing. Vessels, in proportion to their size, may rewarm rapidly and survive. Nerves often tolerate cold and if damaged, can regenerate, provided the nerve sheath remains intact.[14]

For thick benign lesions, such as warts, hemangiomas, and seborrheic keratoses, LN can be sprayed in a manner that engulfs the entire lesion and creates a 2 mm halo. This treatment should produce a total freeze time of about 30 seconds. Recognizing that the type of equipment, diameter of the opening and the pressure on the trigger all contribute to the amount of LN delivered to the target. Thin lesions usually require lower spray times (Figs. 2A to D).[15]

> Freezing that produces a total thaw time of around 30 seconds should suffice for benign lesions.

A spray that produces a visible ice-ball extending 2–3 mm onto the perilesional skin and a total thaw time of 20–30 seconds should be adequate for premalignant thin lesions, such as actinic keratoses and some lentigines. However, for broader intraepidermal proliferations, two freeze thaw cycles may be necessary to ensure complete

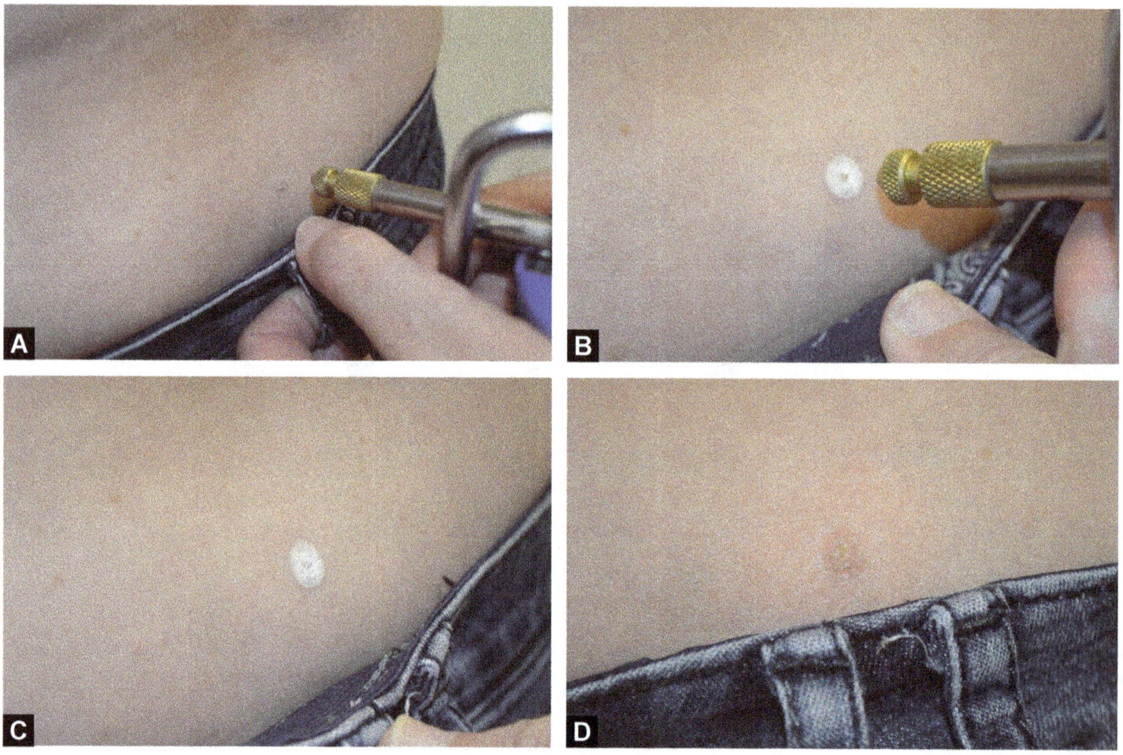

Figs. 2A to D: (A) A 45-year-old patient presented with a 7 × 7 mm brown, waxy, "stuck-on" lesion that was chronically irritated at his waistline. A decision was made to treat it cryosurgically. (B) Liquid nitrogen being applied to lesion after 15 seconds of cryospray demonstrating that the lesion is frozen including a 2 mm rim of normal skin. (C) The lesion immediately after freezing shows a persistent ice ball. (D) Erythematous, edematous papule is noted 5 minutes after cryosurgical treatment is completed.

destruction. Large lesions may be treated in sections, spraying segments of them at different sessions.[16]

> For premalignant thin lesions, a spray with a 2–3 mm margin and a total thaw time of 20–30 seconds is usually adequate.

For malignant lesions, such as basal and squamous cell carcinomas, at least two freeze thaw cycles (separated by 1 or 2 minutes after a complete thaw) resulting in a 4–5 mm halo that extends beyond the clinical margin and produces a thaw time of 60–90 seconds have been recommended. This will produce a sufficient depth of destruction and the eradication of over 95% of properly selected lesions (Figs. 3A to D). However, this clinical measurement will only be accurate provided the spray is kept centered in the lesion. This allows the ice ball to spread naturally outward until the lesion and surrounding halo are properly frozen. This is deemed appropriate because most epithelial cancer cells die at –30° to –50°C, most skin cancers do not extend more than 4 mm beyond the clinical margins, and most non-melanoma skin cancers do not invade to a depth of more than 3 mm below the skin surface.[17] When larger lesions are debulked by curettage, the tumor usually does not extend beyond 3 mm below the defect created.

> At least two freeze thaw cycles (separated by 1 or 2 minutes after a complete thaw) resulting in a 4–5 mm halo that extends beyond the clinical margin, and produces a total thaw time of 60–90 seconds should cure over 95% for malignant lesions

Cryosurgery may be monitored with thermocouples (needles with temperature sensing tips) carefully placed to detect low temperatures at the base of the lesion being treated. Thermocouple needles are placed at a 15–45° angle to a depth estimated to be 3 mm below the lesion. Experi-

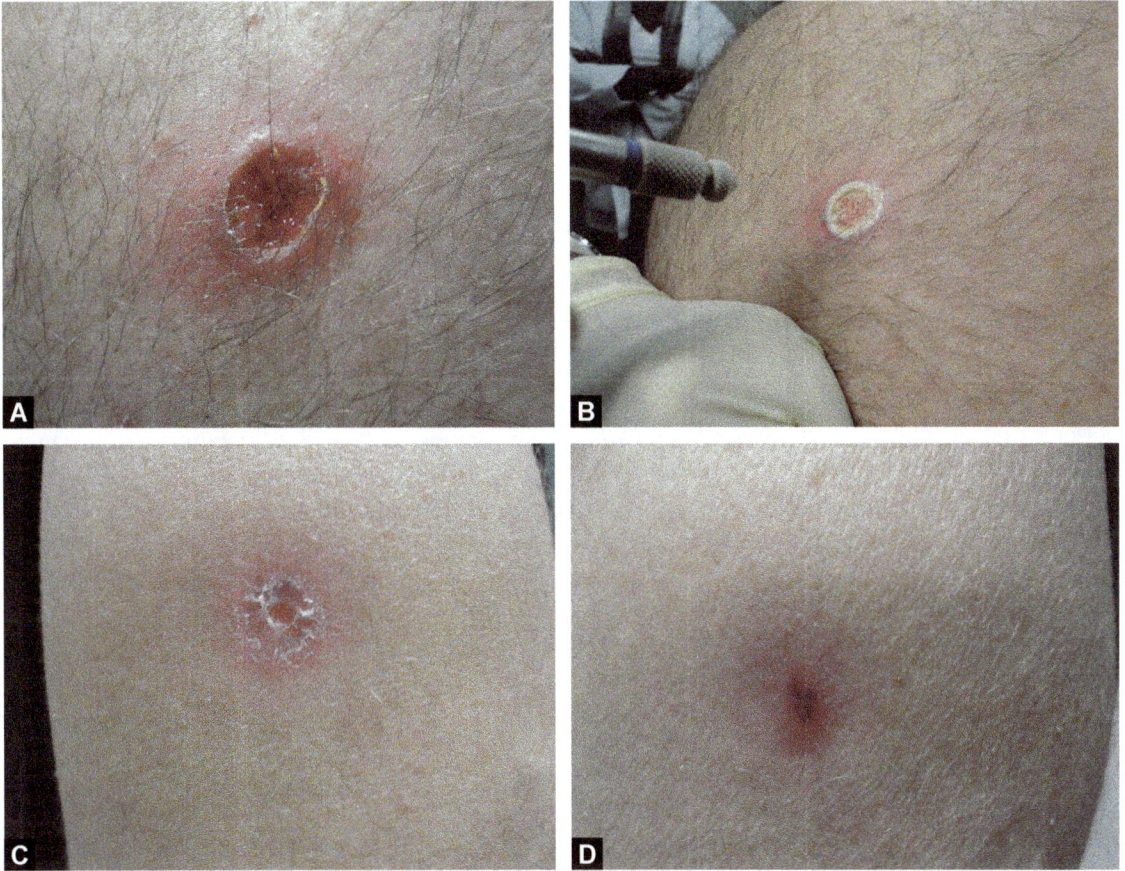

Figs. 3A to D: (A) Granulating base 2 weeks after a shave biopsy. Histopathology demonstrated squamous cell carcinoma extending to the deep margin. (B) Application of cryogen with spray technique showing a 1 mm margin. Spraying was then continued until a 5 mm margin was achieved. (C) Healing at site 1 month postcryosurgery. (D) Postinflammatory erythema 2 months after cryosurgical destruction.

mental and clinical data suggest that it is possible to accurately estimate the temperature at the base of a lesion without thermocouples. For every millimeter of halo on perilesional skin, the temperature is decreased by 10°C centripetally and beneath the lesion. Hence, a lesion frozen to a halo of 4–5 mm would have reached a temperature of approximately –40° to –50°C at the base and periphery.[18] In practice, experienced cryosurgeons monitor the halo visually and palpate the ice-ball formed around lesions being treated. The freeze time can then be extended, if it appears that the ice-ball has not reached an adequate depth.

CLINICAL DECISION-MAKING IN CRYOSURGERY

Cryosurgery results in high cure rates and excellent cosmetic results when competently performed.

Major components of the decision-making to choose cryosurgery or choose another modality relate to:
- Patient characteristics
- Lesion characteristics
- Location
- Size
- Operator experience
- Available alternative treatments

Components that may be less relevant, but are sometimes important, include:
- Cost of available treatment options
- Family and social issues
- Medical-legal risks
- Available facilities
- Available equipment

Regarding the Patient

The general health of the patient must be taken into account. An increase in complications due

Table 1: Conditions with intolerance to cold.

1. Cold urticaria, cold-agglutinin disease, cryoglobulinemia.
2. Autoimmunity: Systemic lupus erythematosus, scleroderma, Raynaud's syndrome or disease, rheumatoid arthritis, etc.
3. Lymphoproliferative disease: Some lymphomas, leukemias, Waldenström's macroglobulinemia, multiple myeloma, etc.

to cryosurgery may occur in conditions characterized by cold intolerance (Table 1).

Because spray gun units are portable, cryosurgery may be particularly useful to dermatologists making "house calls" and for patients in nursing homes, bedridden at home, or are otherwise unable to be transported to a dermatology office.

> Cryosurgery may be particularly useful for patients in nursing homes, bedridden at home, or otherwise unable to be transported to a dermatology office.

Cryosurgery is particularly useful in patients who are allergic to local anesthetics since most often no anesthesia is required. This approach is not possible with scalpel surgery or procedures that destroy tissue with heat, like electrodessication. In some cases, intradermal saline solution is injected under pressure beneath target lesions to decrease the pain of cryosurgery.

For large lesions, intradermal injection of anesthetic agents such as lidocaine may be required. In addition, topical anesthetic creams and ointments may reduce the pain of cryosurgery but generally do not provide the same degree of anesthesia as injectable agents.

Modern day pacemakers and cardiac defibrillators are better insulated than older ones. Still, when a clinical decision is made to avoid electrosurgery in patients with implantable devices, cryosurgery is often a useful alternative treatment option.

> Cryosurgery may be of choice over electrosurgery in patients with implantable devices

Dark-skinned individuals may experience hypopigmentation or depigmentation at the site of cryosurgery.[19] These changes can be short-lived or persistent. Similar changes may be seen on light-skinned patients treated within areas reddened or tanned by chronic actinic damage; it can be explained to them that the relative hypochromia is the result of a return to their background skin tone, usually matching that of the buttocks. Though much less common, hyperpigmentation occurs in some individuals.

Platelet function inhibitors and anticoagulants that prolong bleeding are not an absolute contraindication for cryosurgery though bruising may occur.[20] In non-melanoma skin cancer patients with normal immunity, higher rates of cure are reported than would be expected from destruction alone. While in severely immune-deficient patients, the cryosurgeon should warn the patient that recurrences may be more common than predicted. Such patients could be treated with more aggressive cryosurgery, combination therapies, or surgery with margin control.[21]

Regarding the Lesion

Knowledge of the anatomy and physiology of the skin on all the areas considered for cryosurgical treatment is of paramount importance.

Location

Lesions on the torso and extremities require no special considerations. In these areas, cryosurgery may be considered for even larger superficial malignancies greater than 2 cm in diameter. In the case of a large basal cell carcinoma, segmental treatments can be perfomed every few weeks; this reduces discomfort and makes care at home less difficult. Cryosurgery on the legs may require about three times longer to heal than those on the thighs and trunk.[22] Explaining this to patients will preempt concerns. Arguably, lesions in the nasolabial folds and periauricular locations may be particularly invasive. Referring these patients for Mohs micrographic surgery may be prudent.

Proximity to Organs and Structures

Lesions located in the periorbital region, even if malignant, may be effectively treated with cryo-

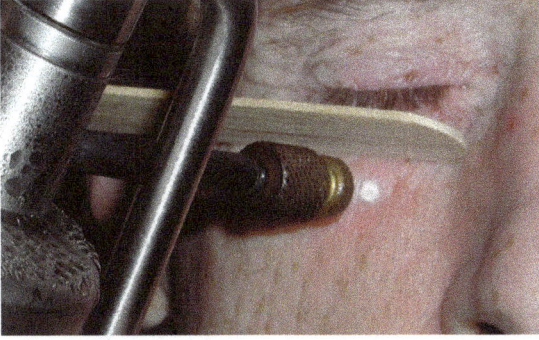

Fig. 4: Tongue blade is firmly pressed against the orbital rim to prevent the cryospray from damaging the eye.

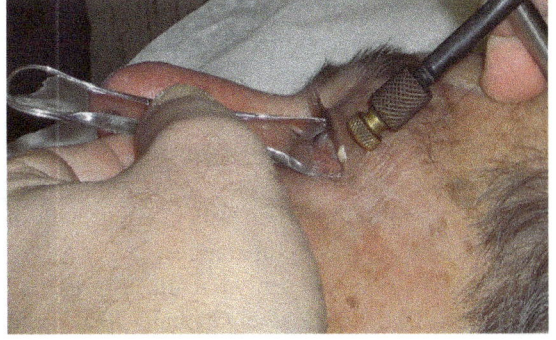

Fig. 5: Plastic Jaeger lid plate or other shield may be used underneath the eyelids to treat lesions on the thin skin of the eyelid.

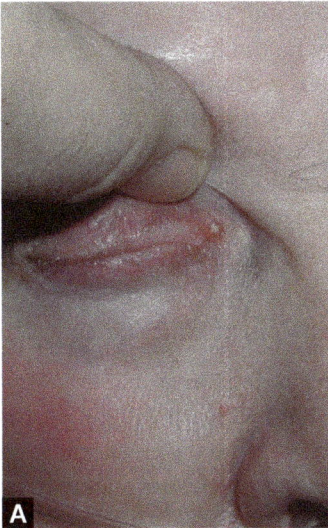

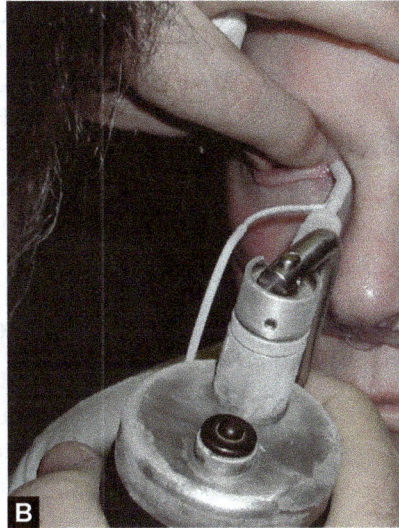

Figs. 6A and B: (A) A small keratinous cyst is present near the eyelid margin. (B) Application of liquid nitrogen utilizing a cryoprobe.

surgery. Protecting the eye is required. This can be accomplished with a tongue blade or plastic spoon (Fig. 4). When working on eyelids, plastic eye shields are preferred over metal ones since plastic conducts temperatures less efficiently.

> Lesions close to the eyes, even if malignant, may be effectively treated with cryosurgery by protecting the eye with a tongue blade or spoon.

A Jaeger plate may be placed underneath the upper or lower eyelid about 1 minute after 1–2 drops of an ophthalmic anesthetic is instilled onto the conjunctiva (Fig. 5). Using closed probes

avoids splatter and is another way to avoid complications from cryospray (Figs. 6A and B). After the probe freezes the skin, it may actually lift the skin away from the underlying structures. Cryosurgery of ear lesions can be accomplished safely and effectively. Even when the cartilage is damaged, it remains in place, serving as scaffold to support healing. In the authors' experience, the long-term results of ear cryosurgery surpass those of most wedge excisions.

> Cryosurgery of ear lesions can be effectively accomplished.

Pain may be intense in the early postoperative period, especially in areas, such as the ear. One must always be aware pain with cryosurgery may cause vasovagal reactions and the authors have noted this particularly when treating ears and fingers.

Periungual lesions, such as warts, may require repeated sessions a few weeks apart. Damage to the nail matrix can permanently affect growth of the nail plate in rare circumstances.

Aggressive cryosurgery of scalp lesions may cause localized hair loss but usually heal quite well.[23] Actinic keratoses usually respond and heal well. A recent article noted that precancerous lesions treated on the scalp have higher cure rates than facial lesions, speculating that this is because cryosurgeons tend to freeze more lightly on the face for fear of more noticeable scarring or pigmentary changes.[24]

Proximity to Vessels and Nerves

Smaller hemangiomas can usually be treated quite satisfactorily with cryosurgery. Intravascular thrombosis from extreme low temperatures causes endothelial damage, which explains the

> Hemangiomas can be nicely treated with cryosurgery.

surprisingly low incidence of bleeding following cryosurgery.[25] Compressing with a closed probe to exsanguinate vascular lesions increases the chance of success. Nearby midsize arteries, which rewarm quickly, may be spared. This explains delayed bleeding that rarely occurs postcryosurgery at shave biopsy sites.

In rare cases, cryosurgery has been reported to cause loss of part of a finger or toe. This may be due to overzealous freezing, particularly when individuals use cryochambers without proper experience. Similar concerns may apply to the penile shaft, however, the vascularity of the appendage may actually reduce such risks.[26,27]

It is possible to damage nerves with cryosurgery although this is usually transient. It may occur when treating large lesions at the base and side of a finger. Numbness may persist for months. Upper eyelid droop from deeply freezing around the temple and injuring the temporal and zygomatic branches of the facial nerve is extremely rare.[26,27]

Size

The American Academy of Dermatology (AAD) guidelines of Care for Cryosurgery, now decades old, suggests limiting the treatment of epithelial cancers of the skin to those less than 2 cm in diameter.[16] The theory behind this, resides in histologic evidence that these tumors are confined to within 4 mm beyond their clinical lateral margins and depth. However, competent cryosurgeons have successfully treated larger lesions for years.

Surrounding Tissues

It is possible to treat lesions in the midst of burn scars and irradiated skin. In fact, cryosurgery may be the best option when the mobility of the skin is too limited for a primary closure. Very thin skin, such as that of the scrotum, vagina, bald and actinically damaged scalp or face, and steroid atrophic skin on the extremities, may all be amenable to cryosurgery especially when compared to alternatives that take longer to heal.[26,27]

Lesion Characteristics

Thick lesions may require debulking by shave or curette before applying cryosurgery. Rarely electrodesiccation or chemical cauterization may be necessary to control superficial bleeding. Shaving

> Thick lesions may require leveling by shave or curettage.

and/or curetting malignant lesions to help the cryodestructive isotherms reach the desired depth and radial extent is commonly performed before the cryogen is applied.[28,29] Many malignant lesions are softer and more friable than the uninvolved surrounding skin. Thus, the tumor is easily debulked. Some lesions are firm, a property usually imparted by keratin, such is the case of squamous cell carcinomas. These lesions should be pared down or shaved off prior to cryosurgery. Other thick or firm lesions malignant or benign, may be treated with a technique referred to as intralesional cryosurgery in which a needle is passed through or below them and the freezing proceeds from the base of the lesion to the skin surface.[30]

Hard lesions should be pared or shaved off to the base to more effectively treat the base of the lesion.

The margins and depth of lesions are usually estimable visually and by palpation; their thickness resulting from the sum of what lies above and below the surrounding skin level. Ultrasound, confocal microscopy, and other imaging technologies may find practical use estimating lesion characteristics when they become price accessible.

Histology

Lesions where there is even a minimum of clinical suspicion for malignant potential should be biopsied prior to their destruction by heat or cold. Healthcare providers should be cautious when deciding proper treatment of basal cell carcinoma with morpheaform or desmoplastic features. The lateral margins and depth of these lesions may be difficult to estimate.

Lesions where there is even a minimum of clinical suspicion for malignant potential should be biopsied prior to their destruction by heat or cold.

Cellularity and immunohistochemistry may also be relevant tools in judging, if a lesion is likely to respond to cryosurgery.

The preferred type of biopsy to render underlying and surrounding tissues adequate for cryosurgery is the shave technique, particularly with the deep saucerization approach.

The preferred method of biopsy to render underlying and surrounding tissues adequate for cryosurgery is the shave or saucerization type.

Lesional architecture combined with clinical features permits an estimation of lesion volume, depth and width, and the type of invasive growth (pseudopods or semicircular). This also leaves a bed suitable for exploration and adaptation of tips that best meet the size and shape of lesional remnants.[26,27,31]

Biologic Aggressiveness

Many primary epithelial tumors are amenable to cryosurgery treatment. The cryosurgery guidelines of care list as relative contraindications unidentifiable margins and recurrences after excisions because scar tissue is less sensitive to cold than epithelial or melanocytic cells. Histologic aggressiveness, such as that of Merkel cell carcinomas and melanoma are best served by techniques utilizing real-time microscopically controlled margins and depth.[16]

Regarding the Physician

The ideal cryosurgeon has historically been the dermatologist because of their familiarity with the clinical behavior of lesions, differential diagnosis, awareness of cure rates and competence in all surgical (and medical) procedures of the skin and soft tissues. These procedures include electrodesiccation, laser or chemical surgery, superficial tangential or excisional surgery, and Mohs micrographic surgery. Chemotherapy agents and topical and systemic medications, such as hedgehog pathway inhibitors also play a role in the comprehensive care of patients. Dermatologists also have experience in the healing process and morbidity manifestations incumbent with each of these procedures as well as postoperative management. Finally, dermatologists are the experts in skin physiology, pathology, and the anatomy of its surrounding osseous, cartilaginous, vascular or neural tissues.

Regarding the Alternatives

Cryosurgeons have sometimes been accused of adhering to the dictum "to whoever only has a hammer, all problems look like nails". Recognizing that a wide range of lesions that can be treated effectively with cryosurgery, one should still keep in mind that in some instances, other options may be better, more efficient or effective. A discussion of risks, costs and benefits of available options allows patients help practitioners to choose the treatment that is best for them.

Table 2: Costs of equipping an office for cryosurgery treatment.

Cryosurgery equipment	Cost
1. Dewar	$800–$1,200
2. Cryosurgery gun	$1,200–$1,500
3. Assorted probes	$150
Total	$3,000*

*Monthly liquid nitrogen tank fill costs $75–100.

Regarding Cost and Economics

Cryosurgery is a very cost-effective procedure to perform. The investment in storage tanks (dewars—after James Dewar), delivery units, probes and ancillary equipment is rapidly recoverable (Table 2). LN is the only consumable requiring periodic replenishment, but it is readily available almost anywhere at a reasonable price. Large practices may afford the one-time investment in LN generators that consume only air and electricity.

One or many lesions can be rapidly treated in a single session thus making cryosurgery not only effective but also very efficient. This helps to minimize costs to the patient and/or insurance company. Support staff can readily be trained regarding cryosurgical instrumentation negating the need for specialized personnel.

Regarding Family and Social Issues

Besides being affordable, pre- and postoperative care is relatively straightforward and easily performed for the patients and caretakers. Most patients require no downtime from work or school, and only rarely does treatment interfere with social or family obligations.

Regarding Legal Risks

Just as with every procedure resulting morbidity or failure to cure, cryosurgery may invite litigious actions in societies like the United States. Though problems can arise from improper cryosurgical training, most relate to poor communication. It is important to set proper expectations before treatment is initiated. If issues like pain, swelling, blistering and sloughing are explained a priori,

> Most problems arise from improper cryosurgeon training, poor communication and inadequate setting of expectations.

patients usually do not overreact when they occur. The offer of free return visits for dressing changes as needed, or for the care of any perceived adverse event, usually avoids unnecessary calls from emergency facilities staffed with personnel unfamiliar with cryosurgical methods. This also may prevent improper prescription of antibiotics and needless psychological stress suffered by patients and relatives.

Regarding the Facilities

Cryosurgery is readily performed almost anywhere. Many dermatologists have a LN dispensing unit in every room or several spaces in key locations in their offices, filled at the beginning of the day and ready to use. Transporting LN in a dispensing unit to a nursing home, a prison, or the home of a bedridden patient is practical and safe as long as the unit is not dropped or tilted to where gas escapes the safety valve that seats on top of the lid.

Regarding the Equipment

Modern cryosurgery equipment can deliver sufficiently low temperatures in a predictable, consistent and reproducible manner. The ice balls they create reach adequate temperatures to destroy a range of benign and malignant lesions.

Liquid nitrogen may be stored in large capacity tanks called dewars, double-walled containers, with a vacuum or insulating material between walls.

> Modern cryosurgery equipment can deliver critically low temperatures in a predictable, consistent and reproducible manner.

Withdrawal devices may be adapted with a faucet to deliver LN out of the dewar into smaller thermos or other transporting equipment, such as metal vessels or even Styrofoam™ cups. Dewars may be kept capped and resting on a tilting base that facilitates pouring into dispensing equipment, if there is not a decanting device installed at the neck of the dewar.

Hand-held dispensing units are filled with LN to create enough pressure for the gas to flow out to the appropriate tips (*see* Figs. 1A to D). A trigger controls the release of the gas toward tips with an open pore to deliver a spray or a closed probe that cools as LN circulates through it and then exits via a relief hose.

If a closed probe is chosen, its tip should contact or be pressed onto the lesions to be frozen. The diameter of the lesion or its bed after debulking should match that of the probe tip for maximal control of freeze in depth and margins. Closed probe tips can be made to adhere to the base of the lesion which allows pulling lesional skin away from delicate underlying structures, such as vessels or nerves passing closely beneath the lesion. Probes are excellent for use around structures like the eyes where spray may accidentally damage the cornea, conjunctiva, or sclera.

If a spray tip is chosen, cones or chambers may be adapted to the diameter of the lesion to be treated. The spray method freezes more efficiently than all other modalities and is recommended for most lesions as the speed of freeze and consequent longer thaw time relates to destructive proficiency.[26,27] Caution must be used to avoid insufflation of the surrounding skin.

Cotton buds or metal tips dipped in vessels holding LN are less practical by virtue of lesser efficiency and carry the risk of contamination.

Units dispensing nitrous oxide, carbon dioxide and other refrigerants some of which are commercially available do not produce the temperature necessary for adequate destruction of all lesions. This is particularly important regarding the successful treatment of cancerous lesions.[12,13,23]

MANAGEMENT

Preoperative Care

Explanation of the procedure beforehand to patients and relatives should include the reasons for the choice of cryosurgery over its alternatives, the expectations of the cure rates, and the visible changes that will occur during the postoperative period. Standard antiseptic technique is

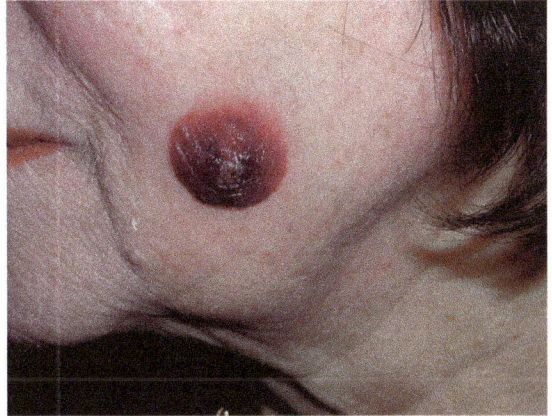

Fig. 7: A hemorrhagic bullae developed 3 days after cryosurgery.

adequate. Local anesthesia is preferable for deep or malignant lesions such as those requiring a double freeze-thaw cycle that penetrates deeply and widely enough for adequate destruction.

Postoperative Care

Postcryosurgery care is relatively simple. The fresh lesion induced by the freeze may be washed with gentle soaps or cleansers daily then covered with petrolatum or a hydroactive dressing and may or may not be bandaged. During the first few days edema, blistering and oozing is to be expected. As lesions begin to heal crusts may develop, petrolatum will soften them and aid in their gentle removal. Within 3–6, weeks, re-epithelialization should be complete and no further care required (Fig. 7).

Periodic evaluations are recommended to identify evidence of recurrence.

FAILURES

Failures with cryosurgery may be due to improper selection of patients or lesions, inexperience, improper training, or problems related to the equipment used. Access to back-up units is advisable.

> Failures with cryosurgery may be due to improper selection of patients or lesions, inexperience, improper training or equipment related problems.

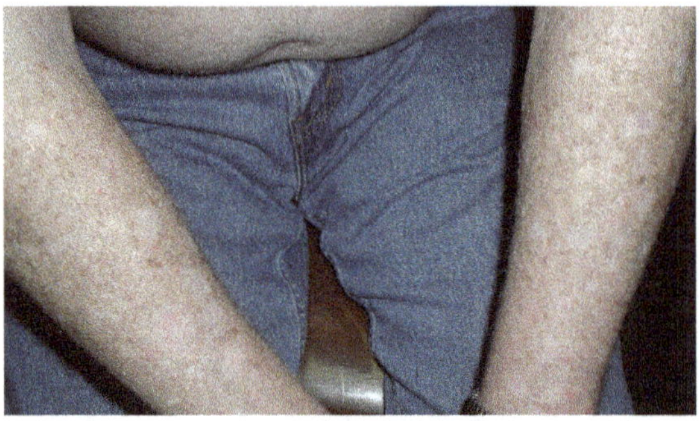

Fig. 8: Postinflammatory hypopigmentation remains 4 months after cryosurgery for actinic keratoses.

Complications of significance are rare. Acute pain and vasovagal reactions can occur. Delayed complications include blisters, sometimes hemorrhagic, bleeding, hypo- or hyperpigmentation, retraction, atrophy, hair loss, and scarring (Fig. 8). Most are easy to prevent and manage with proper education and training.

The balance of success (cure rates, expected improvement, etc.) over failure (relapse/recurrence, morbidity, mortality, costs, etc.) should always favor what is best for the particular lesion and what is most beneficial to the patient.

CONCLUSION

Cryosurgery in the right hands is a superb method to treat many well-selected skin lesions in well-selected patients. It has been an important part of the healthcare armamentarium for over a hundred years and has time and again demonstrated that "what is old can be new again".

FURTHER READING

1. Elton RF. Complications of cutaneous cryosurgery. J Am Acad Dermatol. 1983;8:513.
2. Gill W, Dacosta J, Fraser J. The control and predictability of a cryolesion. Cryobiology. 1970;6:347.
3. Kuflik EG, Gage AA, Lubritz RR, et al. History of dermatologic cryosurgery. Dermatol Surg. 2000; 26:715-9.
4. Lubritz RR, Torre D. Cutaneous cryosurgery for non-malignant and malignant lesions. In: Coleman WP, Colon GA, Davis RS (Eds). Outpatient Surgery of the Skin. New Hyde Park, New York: Medical Examination; 1983. pp. 188.
5. Torre D. Alternate cryogens for cryosurgery. J Dermatol Surg Oncol. 1975;1:56.

6. Torre D, Lubritz RR, and Kuflik E. Practical Cutaneous Cryosurgery. Norwalk: Appleton & Lange; 1988.
7. Zacarian SA. Cryosurgery for cancer of the skin. In: Zacarian SA (Ed). Cryosurgery for Skin Cancer and Cutaneous Disorders. St. Louis: C.V. Mosby; 1985. pp. 96.

REFERENCES

1. Themstrup L, Banzhaf C, Mogensen M, et al. Cryosurgery treatment of actinic keratoses monitored by optical coherence tomography: a pilot study. Dermatology. 2012;255(3):242-7.
2. Fox L, Csongradi C, Aucamp M, et al. Treatment modalities for acne. Molecules. 2016;21(8):1-5.
3. Peikert JM. Prospective trial of curettage and cryosurgery in the management of non-facial, superficial, and minimally invasive basal and squamous cell carcinoma. Int J Dermatol. 2011;50(9):1135-8.
4. Abramovits W, Graham GG, Har-Sai Y, et al. Dermatological Cryotherapy and Cryosurgery for Skin. London: Springer; 2016.
5. Cooper SM, Dawber RP. The history of cryosurgery. J Royal Soc Med. 2001;94(4):196-201.
6. Panagiotopoulos A, Chasapi V, Nikolaou V, et al. Assessment of cryotherapy for the treatment of verrucous epidermal naevi. Acta Dermato-Venereologica. 2008;89:292-4.
7. Raziee M, Balighi K, Shabanzadeh-Dehkordi H, et al. Efficacy and safety of cryotherapy vs. trichloroacetic acid in the treatment of solar lentigo. J Eur Acad Dermatol Venereol. 2008;22(3):316-9.
8. Dejaco D, Hauser U, Zelger B, et al. Actinic keratosis. Laryngorhinootologie. 2015;94(7):467-9.
9. Jakobiec FA, Iwamoto T. Cryotherapy for intraepithelial conjunctival melanocytic proliferations. Ultrastructural effects. Arch Opthamol. 1983;101 (6):904-12.
10. Gage AA, Meenaghan MA, Natiella JR, et al. Sensitivity of pigmented mucosa and skin to freezing injury. Cryobiology. 1979;16(4):347-61.
11. Abramovits W, Losorino M, Marais G, et al. Cutaneous cryosurgery. Dermatol Nurs. 2006;18(5): 456-9.
12. Nguyen NV, Burkhart CG. Cryosurgical treatment of warts: dimethyl ether and propane versus liquid nitrogen—case report and review of the literature. J Drugs Dermatol. 2011;10(10):1174-6.
13. Burkhart CG, Pchalek I, Alder M, et al. An in vitro study comparing temperatures of over-the-counter wart preparations with liquid nitrogen. J Am Acad Dermatol. 2007;57(6):1019-20.
14. El Ghalbzouri A, Hensbergen P, Gibbs S, et al. Fibroblasts facilitate re-epithelialization in wounded human skin equivalents. Lab Invest. 2004;84 (1):102-12.
15. Canadian Agency for Drugs and Technologies in Health. Cryotherapy systems for wart removal: a

review of clinical effectiveness, cost-effectiveness, and guidelines. Ottawa: Canadian Agency for Drugs and Technologies in Health; 2014.

16. Drake LA, Ceilley RI, Cornelison RL, et al. Guidelines of care for cryosurgery. J Am Acad Dermatol. 1994;31(4):648-53.

17. Lindgren G, Larko O. Cryosurgery of eyelid basal cell carcinomas including 781 cases treated over 30 years. Acta Opthalmologica. 2014;92(8):787-92.

18. Giuffrida TJ, Jiminez G, Nouri K. Histologic cure of basal cell carcinoma treated with cryosurgery. J Am Acad Dermatol. 2003;49(3):483-6.

19. Zimmerman EE, Crawford P. Cutaneous cryosurgery. Am Fam Physician. 2012;86(12):1118-24.

20. Elton RF. The appropriate use of liquid nitrogen. Primary Care. 1986;10(3):459-78.

21. Moutran R, Maatouk I, Stephan F, et al. Treatment of nodular basal cell carcinoma with cryotherapy and reduced protocol of imiquimod. Cutis. 2012;90(5):256-7.

22. Ranawaka RR, Weerakoon HS, Opathella N. Liquid nitrogen cryotherapy on Leishmania donovani cutaneous leishmaniasis. J Dermatol Treatment. 2011;22(4):241-5.

23. Ceilley RI, Del Rosso JQ. Current modalities and new advances in the treatment of basal cell carcinoma. Int J Dermatol. 2006;45(5):489-98.

24. Berman B, Qazi Shabbir A, MacNeil T, et al. Variables in cryosurgery technique associated with clearance of actinic keratosis. Dermatol Surg. 2017;43:424-30.

25. Chen WL, Zhang B, Li JS, et al. Liquid nitrogen cryotherapy of lip mucosa hemangiomas under inhalation general anesthesia with sevoflurane in early infancy. Ann Plast Surg. 2009;62(2):154-7.

26. Yaffe B, Shafir R, Tsur H, et al. Complications of liquid nitrogen cryosurgery for verrucae over bony prominences. Ann Plast Surg. 1986;16(2):146-9.

27. Goldberg LH, Landau JM, Moody MN, et al. Treatment of Bowen's disease on the penis with low concentration of a standard mixture of solasodine glycosides and liquid nitrogen. Dermatol Surg. 2011;37(6):858-61.

28. Spiller WF, Spiller RF. Treatment of basal-cell carcinomas by a combination of curettage and cryosurgery. J Dermatol Surg Oncol. 1977;3(4):443-7.

29. Abadir DM. Combined curettage and cryosurgery for treatment of epithelial cancers of the skin. J Dermatol Surg Oncol. 1980;6(8):633-5.

30. Har-Shai Y, Sommer A, Gil T, et al. Intralesional cryosurgery in the treatment of basal cell carcinoma of the lower extremities in elderly subjects. Int J Dermatol. 2016;55(3):342-50.

31. Andrews MD. Cryosurgery for common skin conditions. Am Fam Physician. 2004;15(10):2365-72.

PART 5

Tips and Tricks: Light-based Procedures

—*Robert T Brodell*

"Choose the biggest challenge you have and take action as focused and precise as a laser"
—James A Murphy, The Waves of Life Quotes and Daily Meditations

"I'm a big laser believer - I really think they are the wave of the future"
—Courteney Cox (2013)

CHAPTER 15

Vascular Lesion Lasers

Natalie Semchyshyn, Anastasia Kurta, Dee Anna Glaser

HISTORY

Laser surgery of vascular lesions has evolved over the years. The earliest studies of vascular laser treatment involved the argon laser, which improved the color of port-wine stain birthmarks (PWS), but resulted in unacceptable levels of scarring and dyspigmentation due to nonspecific heating of the superficial epidermis.[1]

The current era of laser treatment began in 1983 when Anderson and Parrish introduced the theory of selective photothermolysis and revolutionized the treatment of vascular lesions.[2] The flash lamp 585 nm pulsed dye laser (PDL) was developed to selectively treat the dermal vessels of PWS which can range from 10 μm to >100 μm in diameter, while sparing the epidermis from nonselective

> The flash lamp 585 nm pulsed dye laser (PDL) was developed to selectively treat the dermal vessels.

epidermal injury.[3] Subsequently, epidermal cooling devices were developed to protect the epidermis from overheating and allow the use of higher fluences to obtain greater treatment efficacy while decreasing the risk of pigmentary changes and scarring.[4] Cooling also makes the treatment more tolerable for patients. Various cooling devices are currently

> Cooling makes the treatment more tolerable for patients and decreases risk of adverse effects.

employed and include cryogen spray (dynamic cooling device), contact and forced-air cooling.

A wide variety of lesions including PWS, hemangiomas, cherry and spider angiomas, telangiectasia (including rosacea, poikiloderma of civatte),

striae, scars and postprocedural ecchymosis may all be successfully treated with lasers. Treatment for vascular lesions is usually pursued for a variety of reasons, including cosmesis, disfigurement, pain, and bleeding.

PROCEDURE

The main goal of utilizing lasers to treat vascular lesions is to induce vessel wall damage while minimizing injury to adjacent tissue. Carefully selecting the appropriate wavelength, pulse duration, and fluence-enables physicians to target the appropriate chromophore without damaging the surrounding structures, and as a result minimizing side effects such as dyspigmentation and scarring. The classic target chromophores for vascular lesions are oxyhemoglobin and deoxyhemoglobin (Fig. 1). The 585–600 nm PDL, long-pulsed 755 nm alexandrite and 1064 nm neodymium-doped yttrium aluminum garnet (Nd:YAG) and 532 nm potassium titanyl phosphate (KTP) lasers as well as intense pulsed light (IPL) devices have all been used to treat vascular lesions. Longer wavelengths penetrate more deeply. It is important to remember that melanin is a competing chromophore at shorter wavelengths and, if it absorbs the laser energy intended for hemoglobin, epidermal injury may occur, especially in darker skin types.

Selecting laser pulse width depends on the size of the target vessels; the larger the vessel, the longer the optimal pulse width. If the pulse width is too short, treatment will be ineffective; if it is too

> Selecting laser pulse width depends on the size of the target vessels.

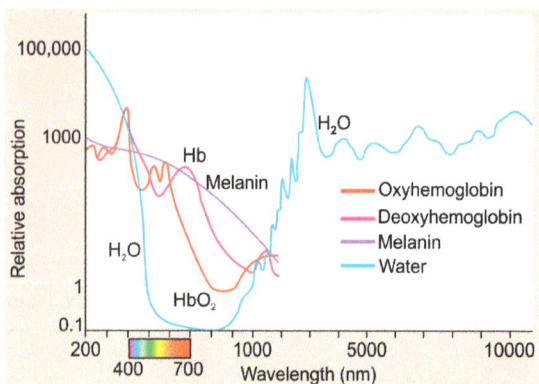

Fig. 1: Absorption spectrum of various chromophores.

long, bulk heating and unwanted tissue injury may occur. Choosing the right spot size is also important. Larger spot sizes have less scattering of the laser beam and deeper dermal penetration.

A good history and physical examination are essential and allow the physician to choose the appropriate laser treatment, and discuss patient expectations. It is important to ask about the use of medications that may increase risk of unwanted purpura, such as aspirin, nonsteroidal

> Always ask about the use of medications that may increase risk of unwanted purpura.

anti-inflammatory drugs (NSAIDs), vitamin E, *Ginkgo biloba*, and fish oil. If nonessential, these should be discontinued for 7–14 days prior to therapy. Discussing realistic expectations as well as expected side effects is crucial to patient satisfaction. The patient should understand, if multiple treatments and in certain cases, the utilization of more than one laser system may be needed to obtain optimum results. The patient should be informed, if there is a cost per treatment. Anticipatory guidance should be given in regard to expected appearance after treatment (purpuric vs nonpurpuric treatment) and care of the treated area. It is essential to discuss the use of sunscreen and avoiding sun exposure (no tan) to the area for at least one month before and after treatment to minimize adverse effects, such as epidermal injury and postinflammatory hyperpigmentation (PIH). PIH may occur with any laser treatment and the

> Avoid(ing) sun exposure (no tan) to the area for at least one month before and after treatment.

risk is increased in darker skin types. Laser treatment should be deferred, if a tan or PIH is present (Box 1).

PORT-WINE STAIN BIRTHMARKS

PWS lesions are vascular malformations that occur in 0.3–0.5% of newborns, equally prevalent in males and females. These lesions are composed of ectatic capillaries and postcapillary venules in the superficial vascular plexus. Associated syndromes may be present and are important to identify: Sturge-Weber in the facial V1 distribution and Klippel-Trénaunay when PWS occurs on an extremity. PWS are cosmetically disfiguring and may progress over time with soft tissue hypertrophy and development of vascular blebs which can cause bleeding and pain. When evaluating a patient with PWS, it is important to consider location and size of the lesion. For example, periorbital lesions, or those located on the forehead/temple, lateral aspect of the cheek, neck, and chin respond better than lesions in the centrofacial regions (medial aspect of the cheek, nose, and upper cutaneous lip).[5] An acquired PWS may respond more readily to treatment than one present since birth.

> An acquired PWS may respond more readily to treatment.

Infants may be safely treated and early treatment provides the best chance of improvement. Younger patients have thinner skin and less competing epidermal chromophore (from sun exposure), allowing for better penetration of the laser.

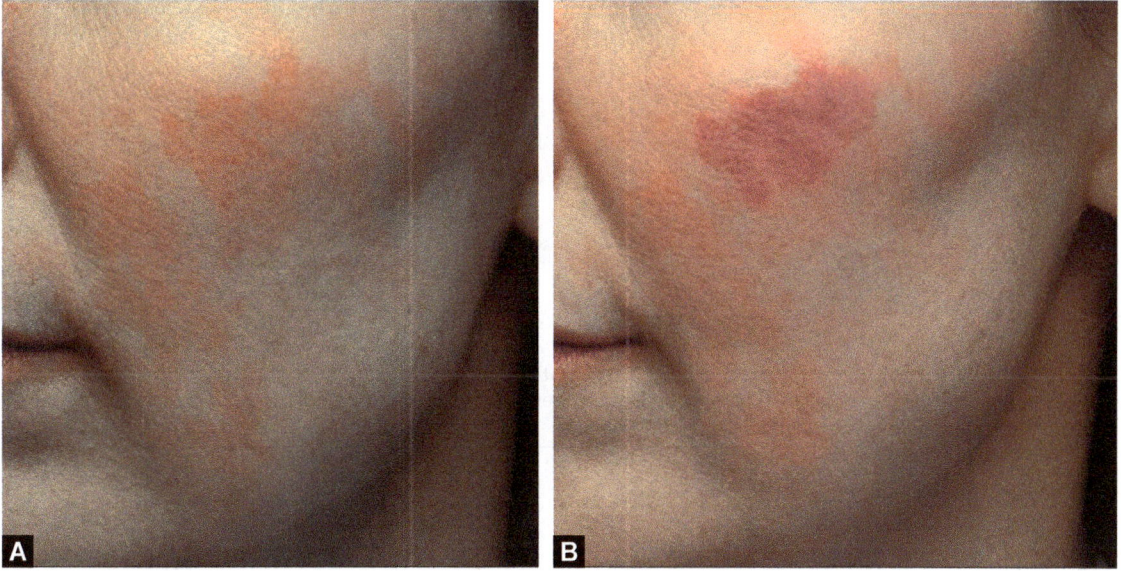

Figs. 2A and B: (A) Port-wine stain (PWS) prior to 595 nm pulsed dye laser (PDL) treatment; (B) Purpura is seen immediately after PDL treatment.

The PWS lesions are also thinner in the younger patient. Young infants may be safely treated in the office without general anesthesia. An assistant holds the swaddled infant firmly to prevent movement and holds eye protection in place while the treatment is performed. Excellent results were reported in a study by Geronemus et al. when treatment was initiated prior to 6 months of age with subsequent treatments at 3–4 weeks intervals.[6]

PDL is the laser of choice for PWS. Multiple treatments are necessary to see improvement, and patients should be prepared to have 10 or more treatments at monthly intervals. Patients

> Be prepared to have 10 or more treatments at monthly intervals.

should understand that the goal is improvement (not complete resolution) of the lesion and that the lesion will recur over time. Purpuric treatment is necessary and patients should be prepared. The immediate reddish-purple purpura will evolve to a dark eggplant color over the next 24 hours. Some patients may also experience significant edema in the treated area.

Pulsed dye laser with epidermal cooling is typically used with pulse durations from 0.45–6 milliseconds (ms) to induce purpura. It is important to determine the fluence threshold with a test

pulse on the darkest portion of the PWS before treating the entire malformation. Pulses should be

> Determine the fluence threshold with a test pulse on the darkest portion of the PWS before treating the entire malformation.

placed with approximately 10% overlap so that the purpuric spots are adjacent to (but not overlapping) each other. The fluence should be adjusted to achieve the desired end point, which is immediate purpura (wait 1-2 minutes to assess purpura) (Figs. 2A and B). If development of gray color is seen, the fluence is likely too high; scarring or blistering can occur. Clear aloe gel is applied over eyebrows or a (shaved) man's beard area to prevent singeing of the hairs. Although rare, allergic contact dermatitis may occur to aloe. Lower fluences are used for treatment on extremities and on darker skin types. Leg lesion treatment is challenging due to frequent occurrence of PIH.

Adverse effects are low with PDL, and consist of expected purpura that can persist for up to 14 days and PIH that can last several months. The risk of scarring is very low.

In our practice, we use a long-pulsed 595 nm PDL with cryogen dynamic cooling device (DCD) Vbeam Perfecta (Candela Corp, Wayland, MA). An appropriate starting setting for facial PWS

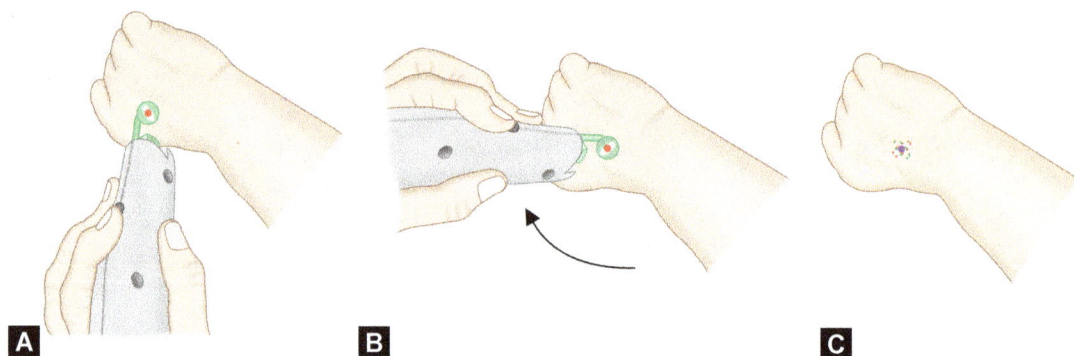

Figs. 3A to C: (A) The linear laser pulse is delivered once; (B) A 90 degree turn is made with the hand piece to deliver a second pulse overlying the first in a "criss-cross" pattern; (C) Dotted lines forming an "x" to demonstrate that the linear beams were delivered with a "criss-cross" technique.

treatment is to use a 10 mm spot at 7.5 J/cm² with a 1.5 ms pulse width, and 30/20 DCD.

> Typical starting settings for treatment of facial PWS are: 10 mm spot at 7.5 J/cm² with a 1.5 ms pulse width, and 30/20 DCD.

Alternatively, a 7 mm spot size may be used at 8–9 J/cm² and 0.45–1.5 ms pulse width. Cold aloe gel and cold packs are used immediately post-treatment for comfort. Aftercare consists of liberal use of sunscreen and sun avoidance. Patients are instructed to apply plain petroleum jelly to any area that blisters. They are given written instructions for aftercare and instructed to call, if extensive blistering, sores, or significant pain occurs.

If PIH occurs and retreatment is necessary, treatment should be deferred until the PIH resolves. The presence of PIH serves as a target for the laser and will result in decreased efficacy as well as epidermal injury that can lead to scarring.

> If PIH occurs, retreatment should be deferred until the PIH resolves because it can serve as a target for the laser.

Intense pulsed light devices have also been used to successfully treat PWS.[7] For PDL resistant PWS's or hypertrophic lesions in adults, the 755 nm alexandrite or the 1064 nm Nd:YAG lasers may be used to take advantage of the deeper penetration of these wavelengths. The use of these lasers carries an increased risk of bulk tissue heating with subsequent increase in risk of hypopigmentation and scarring, and should only be performed by experienced laser surgeons.[8,9]

Vascular blebs may occur within PWS and may be treated with PDL, long-pulsed alexandrite or Nd:YAG lasers. When treating with PDL, we have had good results using the "criss-cross" technique with the Vbeam Perfecta (Candela Corp, Wayland, MA) 595 nm laser: 3 × 10 mm spot at 17–18 J/cm² and 40 ms pulse width with 30/20 DCD; giving two pulses to form a "cross" ("x") with the lesion in the center (Figs. 3A to C and 🎥 1).

Topical rapamycin, an antiangiogenic agent, used adjunctively with PDL appears to be a promising method to improve treatment results; however, it remains investigational (Box 2).[10]

HEMANGIOMAS

Infantile hemangiomas (IH) are benign endothelial cell proliferations that express glucose transporter 1 (GLUT-1) and affect up to 10% of infants, predominantly females. These lesions typically present within the first month of life, proliferate for 6–8+ months, then, spontaneously involute over a period of several years. In critical anatomic sites, rapid proliferation can cause ocular complications including amblyopia, airway compromise, symptomatic hepatic involvement, or auditory canal obstruction. Perineal lesions may ulcerate and bleed.

Oral therapy with propranolol has become the treatment of choice for initial management of IH in critical anatomic sites.[11] The role of laser therapy in proliferative and involuting stages of IH remain controversial. PDL can be used to arrest the growth of IH. Due to the limited penetration of PDL, treatment is reserved for superficial hemangiomas and to treat residual telangiectasia. We treat superficial lesions to improve appearance, and lesions in the diaper area to improve/prevent ulceration and pain. Proliferating lesions are fragile and should be treated very carefully. Risks of treatment include ulceration, bleeding, scarring and hypopigmentation and parents should be advised of these risks. Treatment is performed every 2 weeks for lesions in the proliferative phase. Residual telangiectasia is treated with purpuric settings as we do for PWS. Loose, fibro-fatty tissue changes following hemangioma involution may be treated with fractional ablative or nonablative lasers.

Typical settings with the long-pulsed 595 nm PDL with DCD are 10 mm spot at 6–7.5 J/cm², and 1.5 ms pulse width with the goal of transient (purplish-blue color appears immediately after laser

> Typical settings with the long-pulsed 595 nm PDL with DCD are 10 mm spot at 6–7.5 J/cm², and 1.5 ms pulse width.

pulse, then fades) or "light" spotty purpura; a 10% overlap of pulses is performed. Treatment is gentler than for PWS to avoid ulceration. Aftercare consists of plain petroleum jelly and sun avoidance. An occlusive dressing may be used in the diaper area.

IPL devices and Nd:YAG lasers have also been used to treat infantile hemangiomas (Box 3).[12,13]

CHERRY ANGIOMAS AND SPIDER ANGIOMAS

Cherry angiomas are very common cosmetic concerns for both men and women. These benign,

nonblanchable red papules may appear anywhere on the body. Spider angiomas are most commonly seen on the face and consist of a central papular feeder vessel with radiating telangiectasia; these lesions blanch on diascopy. PDL is a good choice for treatment of these lesions. One to two treatments are usually needed.

In our office, we typically use the long-pulsed 595 nm PDL with DCD to induce a purpuric endpoint. Depending on the size of the lesion, 5–10 mm spot sizes may be used with 1.5 ms pulse width. For lesions 4 mm or larger, the 10 mm spot size is used to increase the depth of penetration.

> We typically use the long-pulsed 595 nm PDL with DCD to induce a purpuric endpoint; 5–10 mm spot sizes may be used with 1.5 ms pulse width, depending on the size of the lesion.

Alternatively, the previously-described "criss-cross" technique may be employed using the 3 × 10 mm spot, 17–18 J/cm², and 40 ms pulse width (*see* Figs. 3A to C). The endpoint is a darkening or graying of the lesion when cherry angioma is treated (Figs. 4A and B). The same technique may be used for spider angioma; in this case, the endpoint is reduction or clearance of the lesion (📹 1). If the spider angioma fails to respond to the "criss-cross" technique, standard purpuric settings may be employed. Post-treatment care includes sun protection/sun avoidance.

The 532 nm KTP laser is an excellent option for treating small lesions. Treatment is nonpuruic and typical settings with the 0.7 mm spot size are fluence of 14–19 J/cm², power of 3 watts, and frequency 3–6 Hz. The endpoint is a light graying of the lesions that will darken over the next day or

> KTP laser treatment is nonpurpuric and typical settings with the 0.7 mm spot size are fluence of 14–19 J/cm², power of 3 watts, and frequency 3–6 Hz.

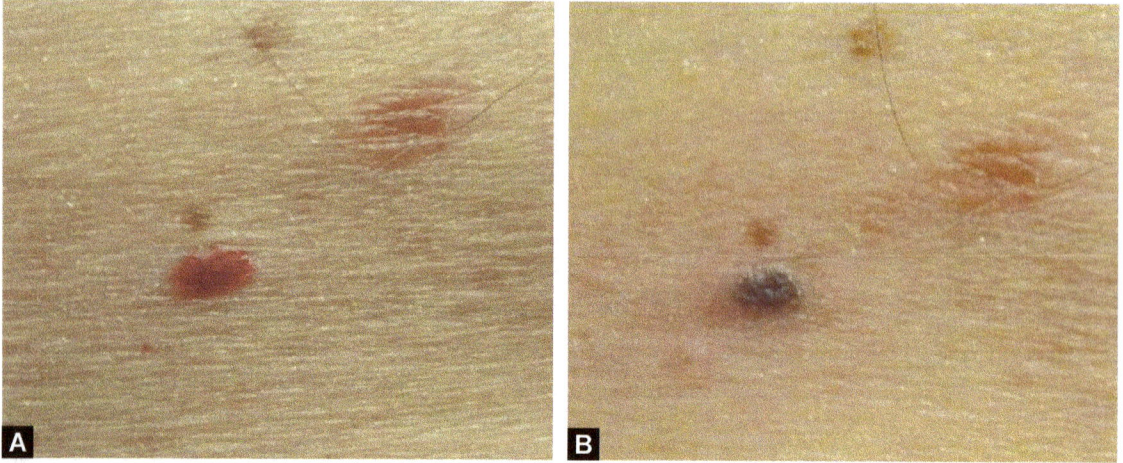

Figs. 4A and B: (A) Cherry angioma prior to 595 nm pulsed dye laser (PDL) treatment; (B) Darkening of lesion immediately post-PDL treatment.

two and flake off in 1–2 weeks for facial lesions, and 2–3 weeks for trunk/extremity lesions. Small lesions may resolve after one treatment; larger/ deeper lesions may require multiple treatments. Aftercare includes sunscreen/sun avoidance.

Long-pulsed Nd: YAG lasers, IPL devices and electrodessication may also be used to treat angiomas (Box 4).

TELANGIECTASIA: ROSACEA, POIKILODERMA OF CIVATTE, SUN DAMAGE

Telangiectasia are superficial vessels, approximately 0.1–1.0 mm in diameter and present either as a diffuse redness or as discrete red vessels. Telangiectasia are most often seen in the context of sun damage and rosacea, but they may also be associated with hormonal imbalances, connective tissue disease, genodermatoses, and hereditary hemorrhagic telangiectasia. In our experience, patients with such an underlying medical disorder tend to be less responsive to treatment and may not heal as well. Test spots with reevaluation after 1 month is prudent in patients with underlying medical conditions who may have numerous lesions.

Rosacea is clinically characterized by flushing, centrofacial erythema and telangiectasia; inflammatory lesions may also occur. PDL treatment can provide a good reduction in telangiectasia, background facial erythema, and decrease in

> **Box 4:** Clinical pearls for treatment of cherry and spider angiomas.
> - Pulsed dye laser (PDL) is a good treatment choice.
> - For lesions 4 mm or larger, use 10 mm spot size to increase depth of penetration.
> - Use the "criss-cross" technique with the 3 x 10 mm spot.
> - 532 nm KTP laser is a good choice for small lesions.

papules and pustules. Purpuric and nonpurpuric settings may be used. Approximately 3–4 monthly treatments are typically needed for significant improvement in redness (Figs. 5A and B).

> A purpuric treatment using 3 ms or 1.5 ms pulse width will give the patient more "bang for their buck",[14] if cost is a concern.

Patients are counseled that because the laser does not "cure" rosacea, the redness will likely recur in time, necessitating repeat treatment. If cost is a major concern and, if the patient is able to tolerate purpura, a purpuric treatment using 3 ms or 1.5 ms pulse width will give them a more "bang for their buck".[14]

In our practice, most patients are intolerant of purpura and are treated with nonpurpuric settings. Typical settings with the long-pulsed 595 nm PDL with DCD are 10 mm spot at 7.5 J/cm^2, and 6 ms pulse width. One pass is performed over the treatment area with a 30% overlap. If the patient is very red, they may experience

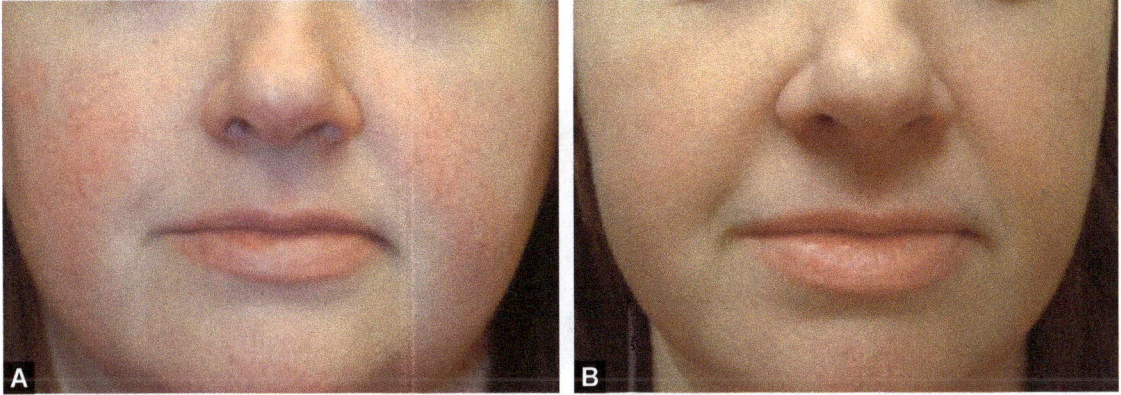

Figs. 5A and B: (A) Rosacea/telangiectasia prior to laser treatment; (B) Improvement in erythema and telangiectasia post 595 nm pulsed dye laser (PDL) treatment.

purpura even at these settings; a test spot in the reddest area will guide the treatment settings. Longer pulse width and lower fluences are used in darker skin types to reduce risk of adverse effects. Some patients experience significant periorbital edema that may last 3–5 days when the

> Longer pulse width and lower fluences are used in darker skin types.

full face/upper cheeks are treated. Many patients with rosacea have sensitive, reactive skin and some may develop a bumpy dermal edema which may manifest within minutes of treatment and evolve over 1–2 days to a general edema in the treated area (Fig. 6). This edema is temporary and will resolve. The treated areas appear redder immediately after treatment and this resolves over a few hours to 1–2 days. Ice packs may be used for posttreatment comfort. Sleeping in a more upright position (e.g. on 2–3 pillows or recliner) may help with posttreatment edema.

Individual telangiectases (e.g. perinasal) are often treated with a linear spot. Typical settings for perinasal telangiectasia with the long-pulsed 595 nm PDL with DCD are 3 mm × 10 mm spot at 17–18 J/cm² and 40 ms pulse width. The endpoint is a transient purpura of the vessel or disappearance of the vessel (Figs. 7A and B). Alternatively,

> Settings for treating perinasal telangiectasia with the long-pulsed 595 nm PDL with DCD are 3 mm × 10 mm spot at 17–18 J/cm² and 40 ms pulse width.

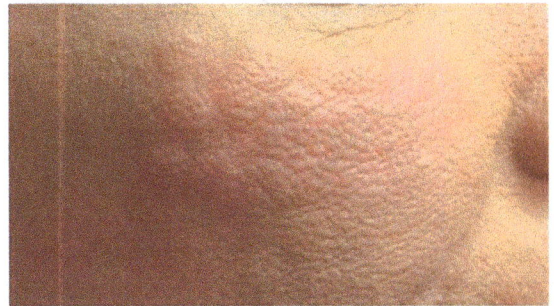

Fig. 6: Bumpy dermal edema development within minutes post-treatment with 595 nm pulsed dye laser (PDL).

individual vessels may be treated with a 10 mm spot at 7.5 J/cm² and 6 ms pulse width and double or triple pulse-stack achieving the same endpoints. Aftercare includes sunscreen/sun avoidance and patients are instructed to try to avoid activities that can cause facial flushing for at least 1 week (e.g. sauna, hot baths, intense exercise).

Poikiloderma of Civatte occurs on chronically sun-exposed skin, most commonly affecting the lateral neck, chest and lateral cheeks. Clinically, it presents as red-brown discoloration with associated telangiectasia. IPL can be used for treatment to target pigmentary and vascular components.[15] PDL can be implemented to treat the vascular component of poikiloderma of Civatte. To limit potential side effects, such as development of reticulated pattern and hypopigmentation, larger spot sizes and lower fluences are recommended. Patients should be counseled that multiple treatments are necessary and that they may initially

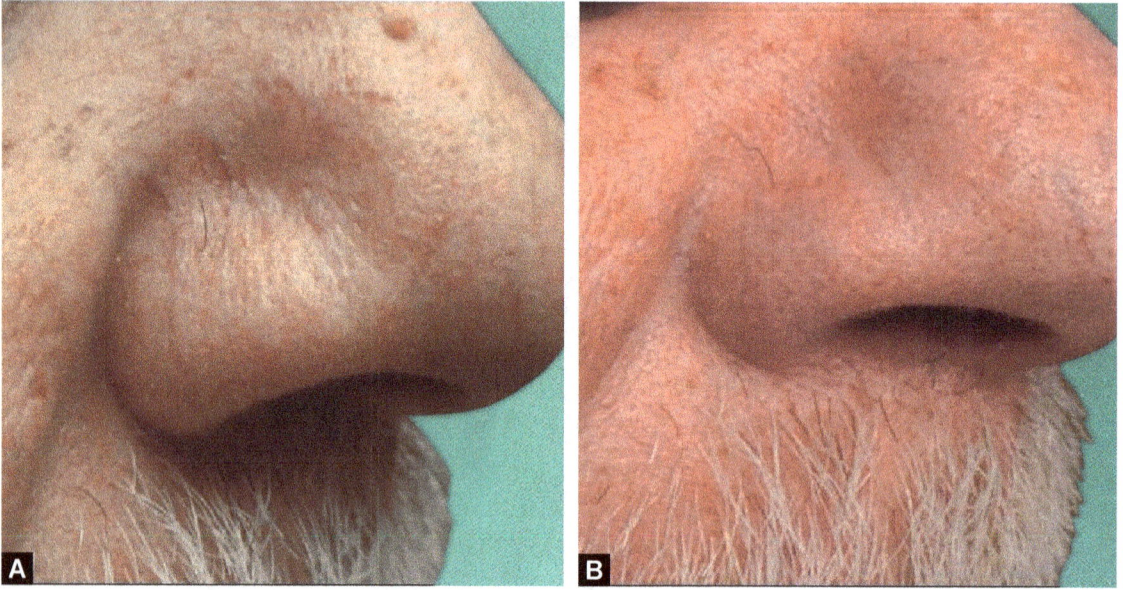

Figs. 7A and B: (A) Telangiectasia over right nasal ala; (B) Disappearance of telangiectasia post 595 nm pulsed dye laser (PDL) treatment using a linear spot.

To limit potential side effects, such as development of reticulated pattern and hypopigmentation [for the vascular component of poikiloderma of Civatte], larger spot sizes and lower fluences are recommended.

have a spotty or striped appearance, which will improve with subsequent treatments. We use the long-pulsed 595 nm PDL with DCD at settings of 5.5–7.5 J/cm^2, 6 ms pulse width with a 10 mm spot size to treat neck or chest areas. The desired endpoint is transient purpura. Even with this "nonpurpuric treatment", a few purpuric spots may occur in off-face areas and patients need to be counseled of this effect. A very low setting will avoid any purpura, but is not likely to be effective.

Several lasers and light sources can be used to treat telangiectasia, ranging from PDL, KTP, diode, Nd:YAG, and IPL (Box 5).[16]

Box 5: Clinical pearls for treating telangiectasia.

- Counsel patients that laser treatments will not "cure" rosacea.
- Warn patients of possible bumpy edema in treated area.
- Purpuric treatment may be more cost-effective.
- For poikiloderma of Civatte, start with low fluence on the reddest area to assess response.

STRIAE DISTENSAE

Striae distensae (rubra and alba) remain a treatment challenge. Both types may be treated with the PDL with modest results but short patient downtime. Treatment is more effective when performed on erythematous striae than on the hypopigmented type. Erythema and associated

Treatment with PDL is more effective when performed on erythematous striae.

telangiectasia improve due to selective photothermolysis. Skin texture improvement results from thermal injury to dermal vasculature initiating a cascade of events resulting in collagen remodeling.

Nonpurpuric settings are used and 3–6 treatments are performed at monthly intervals. The goal of treatment is improvement in erythema and skin texture, not resolution of the stretch marks. Typical settings with the long-pulsed 595 nm PDL with DCD include 10 mm spot at 6–7 J/cm^2 and 6 ms pulse width. Transient erythema resolves quickly and aftercare includes sun protection.

SCARS

The appearance of acne scars, surgical scars as well as traumatic scars has been improved with

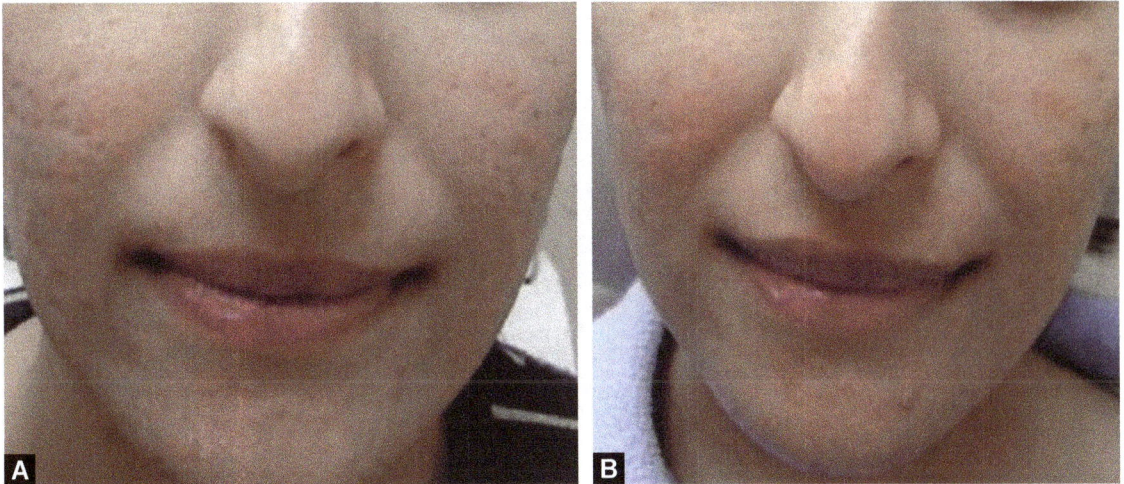

Figs. 8A and B: (A) Acne scarring prior to laser treatment; (B) Improvement in scars 1 month post 595 nm pulsed dye laser (PDL) treatment.

PDL (Figs. 8A and B). PDL is also effective in treating impending scars such as those that may be seen after ablative laser resurfacing or traumatic abrasion. In such cases, areas of persistent erythema and a subtle thickening may portend scar formation and are treated immediately. Three to six nonpurpuric treatments are performed on a monthly basis for scars.

As in the case of striae, the goals of treatment include improvement in erythema/telangiectasia as well as stimulation of collagen remodeling to normalize the scar appearance. Treatment is most effective if performed when erythema is still present. Typical settings in our office with the long-pulsed 595 nm PDL with DCD are 10 mm spot size at 7–7.5 J/cm^2 and 6 ms pulse width, using a 30% overlap. Laser treatment can be combined with intralesional triamcinolone injections to treat hypertrophic scars. In this case, the laser is

> To treat hypertrophic scars, laser treatment is combined with intralesional triamcinolone injections.

performed first as it induces some edema to soften the scar and allow for easier injection of the steroid. Laser treatment of keloids remains disappointing.

Ablative and nonablative fractional lasers are more effective in the treatment of striae and

> **Box 6:** Clinical pearl for treatment of scars.
> - Laser hypertrophic scars prior to performing intralesional steroid injection.
> - Resulting edema from the laser softens the scar and allows for easier injection of steroid.

established scars; however, cost and side effect profile are also increased (Box 6).

POSTPROCEDURAL ECCHYMOSIS

The PDL has been shown to decrease the time to resolution of postprocedural ecchymosis.[17] Cosmetic injectables, such as neurotoxins and soft tissue fillers are common and popular procedures. Post-treatment ecchymosis may occasionally occur, especially, if the patient is taking blood-thinning medications or supplements. While ecchymosis is temporary and self-resolving, it may cause undue distress in some patients. In these cases, we treat with the long-pulsed 595 nm PDL with DCD, 10 mm spot at 7 J/cm^2 and 6 ms pulse width. One pass is performed over the ecchymotic area with 30% overlap. Patients are informed that the laser will not immediately remove the bruise, but will typically cut the resolution time in half (Figs. 9A and B, Box 7).[18]

> Laser treatment will not immediately remove the bruise, but will typically cut the resolution time in half.

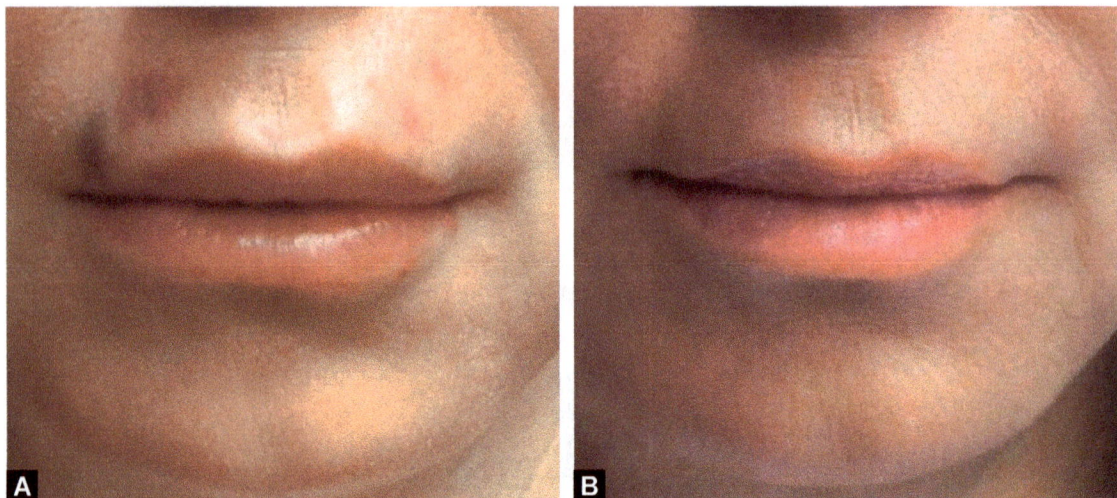

Figs. 9A and B: (A) Ecchymosis one day post lip augmentation with filler; (B) Ecchymosis resolution 72 hours post 595 nm pulsed dye laser (PDL) treatment.

Box 7: Clinical pearl for treating postprocedural ecchymosis.
- PDL treatment decreases ecchymosis duration by ~50%.
- Perform one pass with 30% overlap.

Conflict of Interest

Natalie Semchyshyn, Anastasia Kurta, and Dee Anna Glaser have no conflict of interest to disclose

VIDEO LEGEND

Video 1: "Criss-cross" technique using PDL for treatment of spider angioma; note the immediate clearance of the lesion at the end of the video.

REFERENCES

1. Dixon JA, Huether S, Rotering R. Hypertrophic scarring in argon laser treatment of port-wine stains. Plast Reconstr Surg. 1984;73(5):771-9.
2. Anderson PR, Parrish JA. Selective photothermolysis: precise microsurgery by selective absorption of pulsed radiation. Science. 1983;220:524-7.
3. Garden JM, Polla LL, Tan OT. The treatment of port-wine stains by the pulsed dye laser: analysis of pulse duration and long-term therapy. Arch Dermatol. 1988;124:889-96.
4. Chang CJ, Nelson JS. Cryogen spray cooling and higher fluence pulsed dye laser treatment improve port-wine stain clearance while minimizing epidermal damage. Dermatol Surg. 1999; 25(10):767-72.
5. Renfro L, Geronemus RG. Anatomical differences of port-wine stains in response to treatment with the pulsed dye laser. Arch Dermatol. 1993; 129(2):182-8.
6. Chapas AM, Eickhorst K, Geronemus RG. Efficacy of early treatment of facial port wine stains in newborns: a review of 49 cases. Lasers Surg Med. 2007;39(7):563-8.
7. Ho WS, Ying SY, Chan PC, et al. Treatment of port wine stains with intense pulsed light: a prospective study. Dermatol Surg. 2004;30(6):887-90.
8. Izikson L, Nelson JS, Anderson RR. Treatment of hypertrophic and resistant port wine stains with a 755 nm laser: a case series of 20 patients. Lasers Surg Med. 2009;41(6):427-32.
9. Yang MU, Yaroslavsky AN, Farinelli WA, et al. Long-pulsed neodymium: yttrium-aluminumgarnet laser treatment for port-wine stains. J Am Acad Dermatol. 2005;52(3 Pt 1):480-90.
10. Marqués L, Núñez-Córdoba JM, Aguado L, et al. Topical rapamycin combined with pulsed dye laser in the treatment of capillary vascular malformations in Sturge-Weber syndrome: phase II, randomized, double-blind, intraindividual placebo-controlled clinical trial. J Am Acad Dermatol. 2015;72(1):151-8.e1.
11. Drolet BA, Frommelt PC, Chamlin SL, et al. Initiation and use of propranolol for infantile hemangioma: report of a consensus conference. Pediatrics. 2013;131(1):128-40.
12. Li DN, Gold MH, Sun ZS, et al. Treatment of infantile hemangioma with optimal pulse technology. J Cosmet Laser Ther. 2010;12(3):145-50.

13. Vlachakis I, Gardikis S, Michailoudi E, et al. Treatment of hemangiomas in children using a Nd:YAG laser in conjunction with ice cooling of the epidermis: techniques and results. BMC Pediatr. 2003;3:2.

14. Alam M, Dover JS, Arndt KA. Treatment of facial telangiectasia with variable-pulse high fluence pulsed-dye laser: comparison of efficacy with fluences immediately above and below the purpura threshold. Dermatol Surg. 2003;29: 681-5.

15. Weiss RA, Goldman MP, Weiss MA. Treatment of poikiloderma of Civatte with an intense pulsed light source. Dermatol Surg. 2000;26(9): 823-8.

16. Bevin AA. Parlette EC, Domankevitz Y, et al. Variable-pulse Nd:YAG laser in the treatment of facial telangiectasias. Dermatol Surg. 2006;32(1):7-12.

17. Kassir R, Kolluru A, Kassir M. Intense pulsed light for the treatment of rosacea and telangiectasias. J Cosmet Laser Ther. 2011;13(5):216-22.

18. DeFatta RJ, Krishna S, Williams EF. Pulsed-dye laser for treating ecchymoses after facial cosmetic procedures. Arch Facial Plast Surg. 2009;11(2): 99-103.

CHAPTER 16

Fractionated CO_2 Laser

Ardalan Minokadeh, Elizabeth I McBurney

INTRODUCTION

Fractionated CO_2 laser (10,600 nm) is a surgical modality classically used for the management of photoaging, dyschromia, rhytides and scarring. In contrast to traditional scanned or pulsed CO_2 laser treatment that denudes 100% of the skin in a treated area, the fractionated laser induces microscopic columns of epidermal and dermal necrosis. Thus, a grid-like pattern of ablative columns on the skin is produced with residual viable tissue surrounding these focal areas of necrosis. The reservoir of undamaged skin enhances wound healing of the columns of necrotic skin and induces collagen formation, leading to rapid healing with a reduced potential for scarring when compared to the short-pulsed, high energy, rapidly scanned CO_2 laser.

The specific devices available for use vary in pattern of injury and the density of damaged skin (Figs. 1A and B). Energy density and the depth of injury can be adjusted. The primary tissue chromophore is water.

HISTORY

Patients are reluctant to undergo invasive laser treatments resulting in significant down time. The concept of focal microscopic treatment zones surrounded by islands of spared skin is the fundamental theme of fractional photothermolysis and is essential to the improved safety profile and shortened recovery time. This treatment was first used by Manstein et al. in 2004, as an alternative to the more established scanned or pulsed CO_2 and erbium-doped yttrium aluminum garnet (Er:YAG) lasers which ablate the entire skin

surface of a treated area.[1] There has been an explosion of information about the use of fractionated lasers. This has been summarized in numerous review articles.[2-5] There has been some thought that ablative fractional resurfacing may be superior to traditional CO_2 resurfacing devices for skin tightening, in that it is able to penetrate deeper into the dermis (>1500 μm).[2]

DESCRIPTION OF PROCEDURE

Consultation

It is critically important that physicians convey realistic expectations of the outcomes that are anticipated following fractionated CO_2 laser resurfacing. It is important to obtain verbal informed consent at the time of the original consultation, and written informed consent on the day of surgical procedure is also important for medical-legal reasons. This is best accomplished using photographs of representative patients who have undergone the procedure including preprocedure, immediate postprocedure, and 1 week postoperative follow-up (Figs. 2 to 4).

> Convey realistic expectations using preprocedure, immediate postprocedure, and 1 week postoperative follow-up.

The physician or staff should obtain frontal and oblique views using adequate lighting to highlight textural features of the face. Presenting a variety of cases including images of the best results, satisfactory results, and even rare patients with poor outcomes is a best practice.

It is important to discuss herpes virus prophylaxis on the initial visit since this should be started

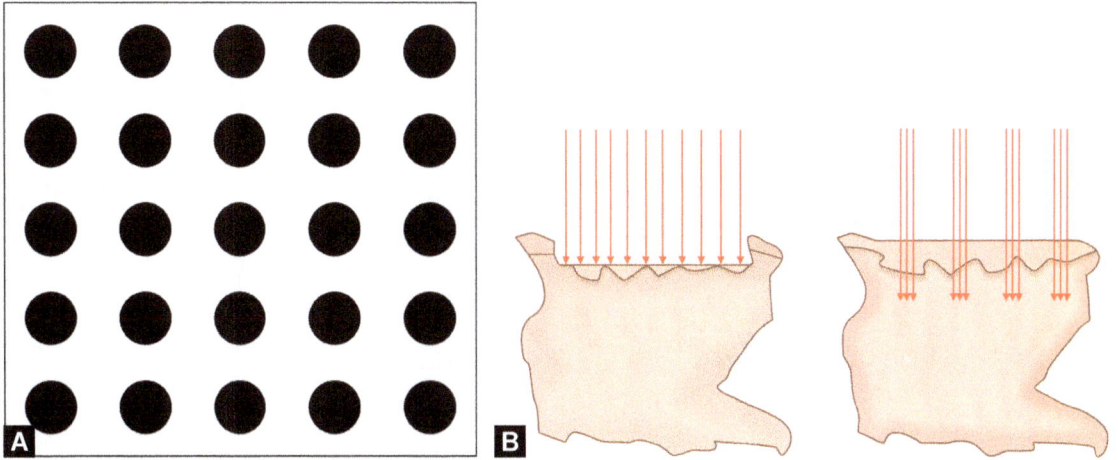

Figs. 1A and B: (A) Graphical representation of square-shaped laser beam profile. (B) Graphical representation of scanned or pulsed ablative and fractionated skin resurfacing.[1]

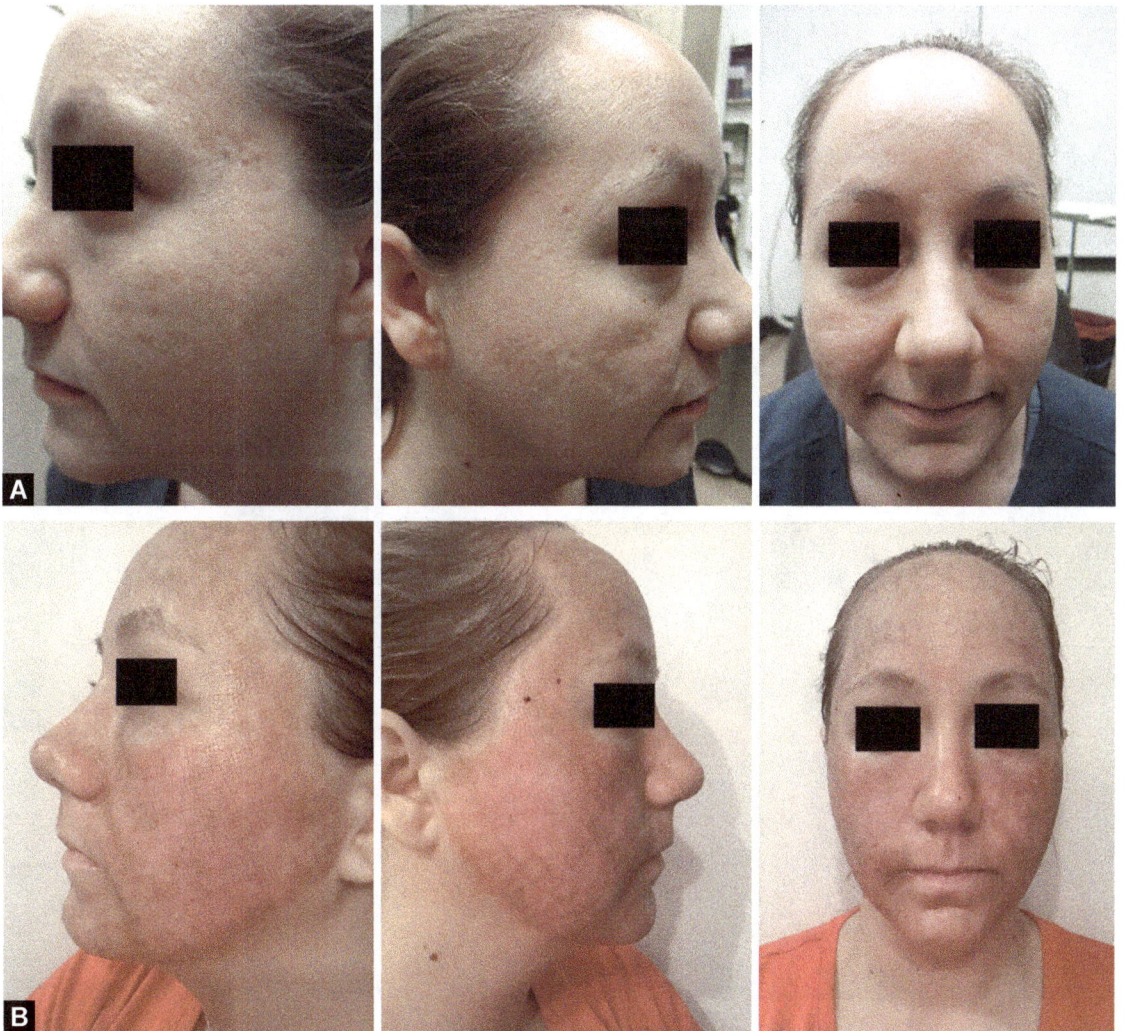

Figs. 2A and B

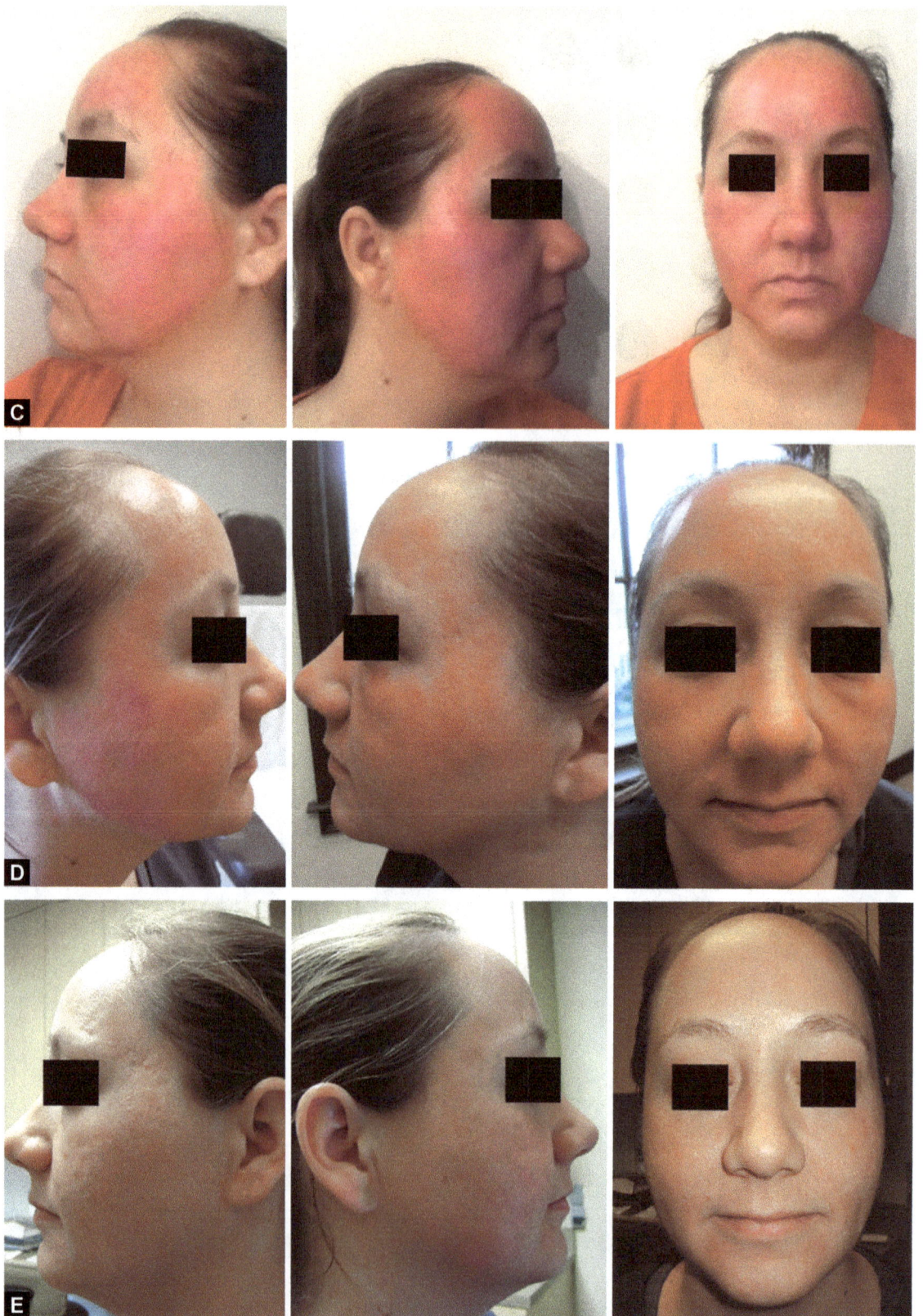

Figs. 2A to E: Treatment of acne scars in laser-naive patient with fractionated CO_2 laser. (A) Preprocedure, (B) after 24 hours, (C) 5 days, (D) 7 days and (E) 2 months photographs.

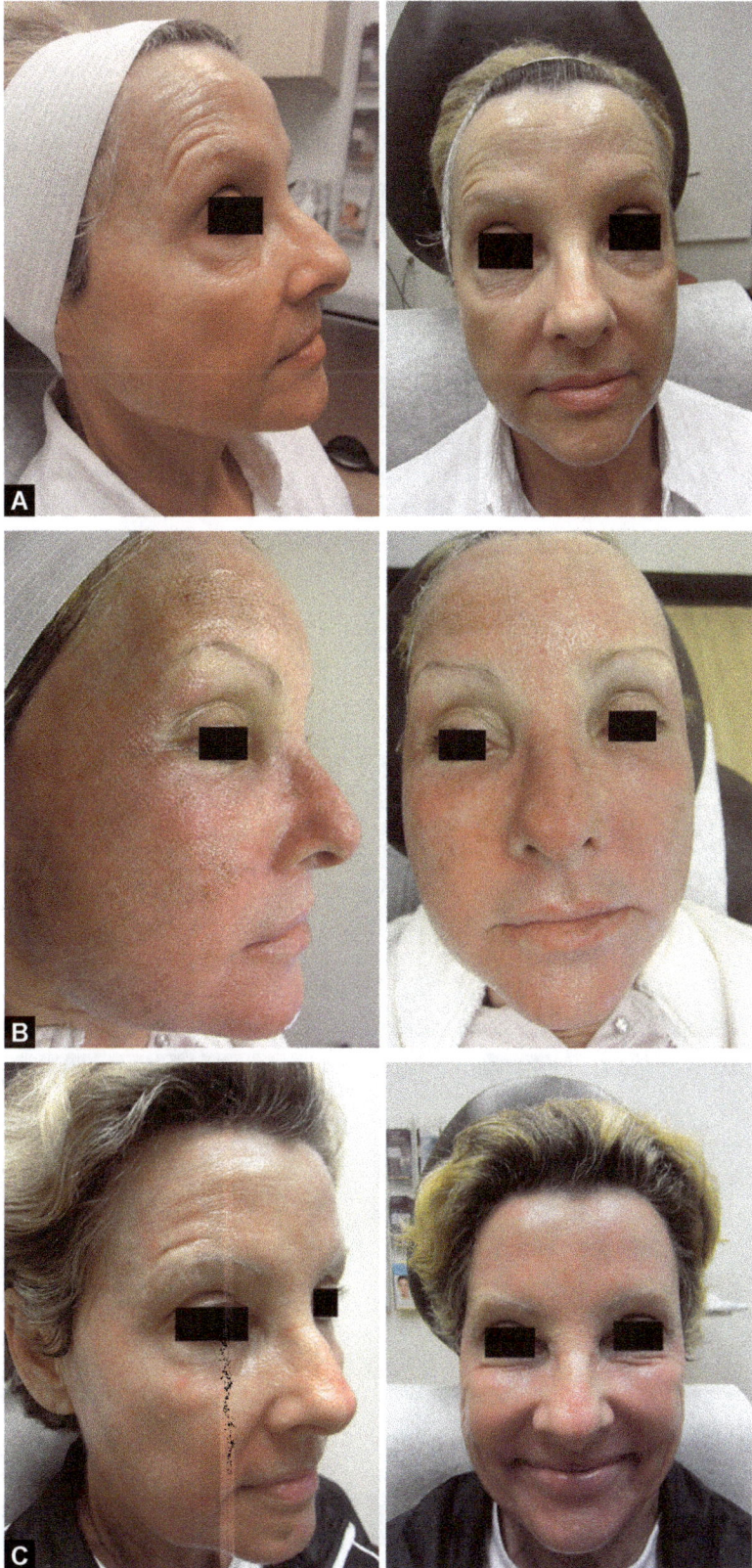

Figs. 3A to C: Treatment of rhytides and photodamaged skin with fractional CO_2 laser in a 62-year-old female. (A) Pretreatment (preoperative). (B) After 24 hours of treatment. (C) 6 days postoperative.

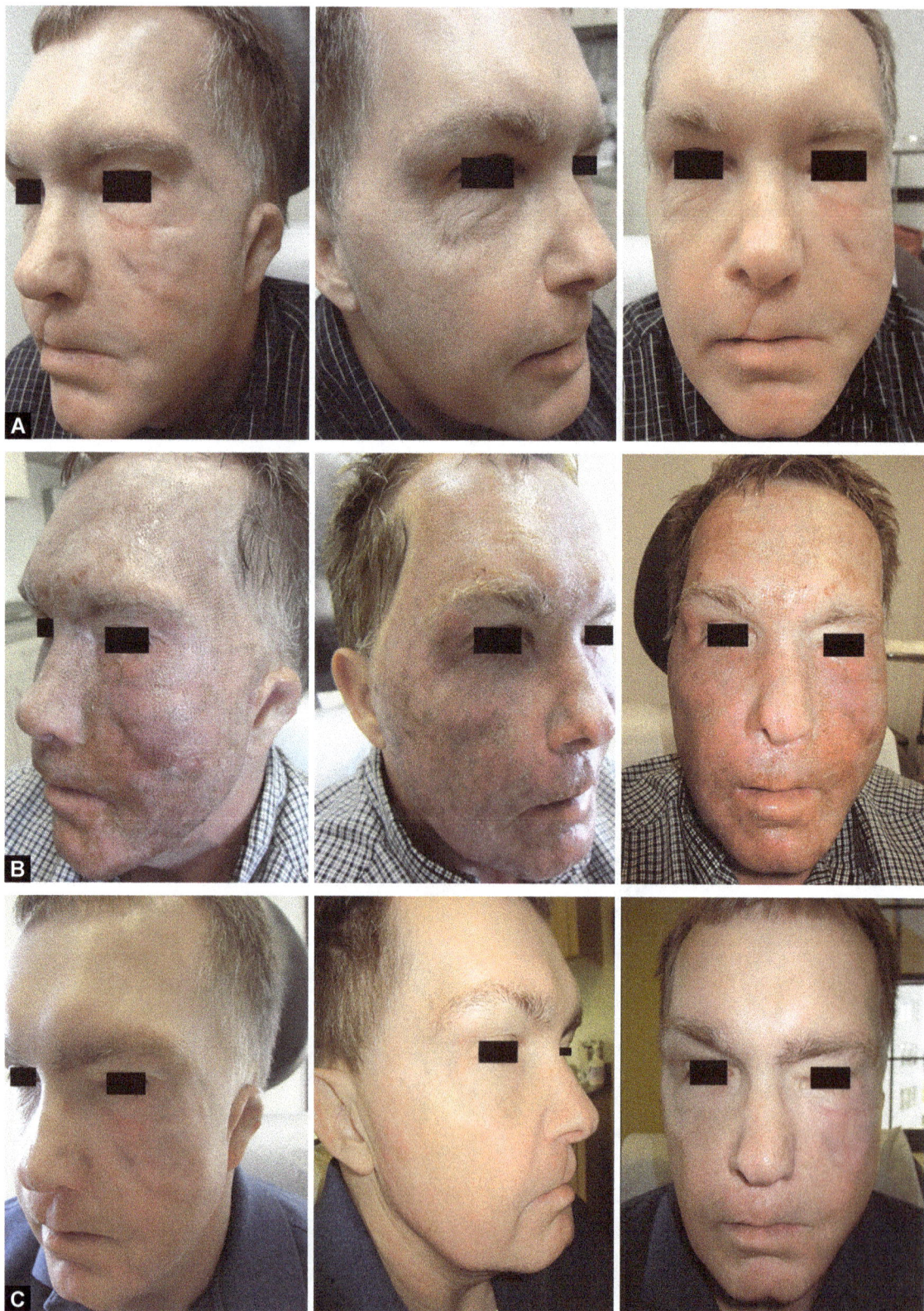

Figs. 4A to C: A 45-year-old male with congenital abnormalities of the left periocular area and also cleft palate. He had multiple facial implants with secondary infection in the implant and resulting scarring. (A) Pretreatment (preoperative). (B) After 24 hours of treatment. (C) 3 months postoperative.

the day before treatment is initiated in an effort to prevent eczema herpeticum induced by the trauma of this procedure. For patients with no history of cold sores, we use valacyclovir 1 g/day for 7 days. Patients with a history of herpes outbreaks are treated with a higher dose: 1 g three times daily.[6] Finally, patients should be told at the time of their initial visit to bring a driver on the day of the procedure.

Preprocedure

Review of written postoperative care instructions is an important exercise on the day of the procedure. Adherence to these instructions will improve outcomes and this serves as another opportunity for patient to understand risks and benefits of the procedure and ask any last minute questions (Fig. 5). Anxiolytics enhance the level of comfort and are accepted by the vast majority of our patients. We recommend diazepam 5 mg for full-sized adults, which is administered 1 hour prior to the start of the procedure. Hydrocodone/acetaminophen 5 mg/325 mg for pain control is also administered routinely to our patients 30 minutes prior to the procedure.

In-office Anesthesia

When patients arrive at the office 1 hour prior to the scheduled treatment, compounded topical lidocaine and prilocaine, equivalent to a 20% lidocaine preparation, is applied to the entire area to be treated. At the sites of planned intraoral

> 1 hour prior to the scheduled treatment topical lidocaine and prilocaine is applied to the entire area to be treated.

injections, a 1% xylocaine gel is utilized for topical anesthesia. Intraoral anesthesia for the medial upper cutaneous lip is achieved with two injection points immediately lateral to the superior labial frenulum. For full-face treatment, utilize infraorbital, mental, supratrochlear and supraorbital nerve blocks. Topical anesthesia is usually sufficient for the neck.

The areas of the lateral face are often inadequately anesthetized with the aforementioned nerve blocks. Anesthesia in these areas can be achieved using a *1-inch* 30-G needle inserting the needle in the pre-auricular space and using a fanning technique over the lateral cheek (*see online video*).

During Procedure

Eye protection is critically important prior to initiation of treatment with the fractionated CO₂ laser. Use moist eye pads for eye protection and use metal eye protection for treatment of the peri-

---

POSTOPERATIVE INSTRUCTIONS FOR CO₂ LASER TREATMENT

A full gauze dressing, in most cases, will be applied. You will return in 24 hours after the surgery to have this dressing change.

If you have no dressings applied, or after the dressings are completely removed:

- Soak the treated area for 15 minutes, 4 times a day using a solution of 1 tablespoon of white vinegar in 1 cup of cool water on a washcloth. Any scabs present should be gently soaked off, if possible. DO NOT PICK TO REMOVE DEAD SKIN OR SCABS.
- After soaking, pat the skin dry with a clean, soft towel and apply a layer of Veseline petroleum jelly over the entire area. Re-apply the ointment whenever the skin feels dry.
- Sleep on your back with your head elevated on a few pillows for the first 5–7 days.
- If the skin around the mouth is swollen or tight, drink from a straw.
- Avoid strenuous exercise for 2 weeks to prevent irritation of the skin.
- Do NOT expose the skin to the sun for 4 weeks. After complete healing of the skin, a sunscreen should be applied daily. Choose a sunscreen that has an SPF of 30 and is chemical free. Some suggestions are chemical-free sunscreen or physical blockers of titanium dioxide and zinc oxide.

Postoperative Expectations

- Mild-to-moderate redness is expected for 14–21 days after the procedure and will fade gradually over a 6–8-week period.
- Oozing of clear fluid from the surgical site may occur for 5–7 days.
- Mild-to-moderate swelling is normal and expected, and may last for 5–7 days.
- Do not apply make-up until skin is healed and there is no longer oozing of clear fluid from the surgical site.

Fig. 5: Post-treatment care instructions for fractionated CO₂-laser patients.

orbital region. Have the patient take out contacts before the eye shields are placed. Plastic shields are not appropriate in this setting as the heat from the laser can melt them. Everyone in the operating room should wear appropriate goggles. A smoke evacuator should be held within 2 cm of the

> Plastic eye shields are not appropriate.

laser beam throughout the procedure. Laser ultra-filtration masks are to be worn by all personnel. Forced cold air devices are used by some laser surgeons. The tip is held 2–3 inches above the skin surface during the procedure to diminish patient discomfort.[7]

The surgical site should be draped with moist towels. The thermal energy from the laser is a fire hazard. Have moist towels within reach. Prepare a basin filled with water and place towels in the basin to then place on the patient, if needed. Make sure that a fire extinguisher is available for use. Place a safety sign on the door of the treatment room warning of potential hazards with laser use (Fig. 6).

A moistened dental bolster is inserted underneath the upper lip in order to make the rhytides of the upper cutaneous lip accessible to the laser. Similarly, when treating the angles of the mouth, insert a wet tongue blade into the angles of the mouth to expose them to the treatment. Test the first pulse on a wet tongue depressor prior to applying pulses to the patient's skin to insure accuracy of the beam profile.

A video demonstrates the technique and the speed with which a fractionated CO_2 laser can be performed (📹 1).

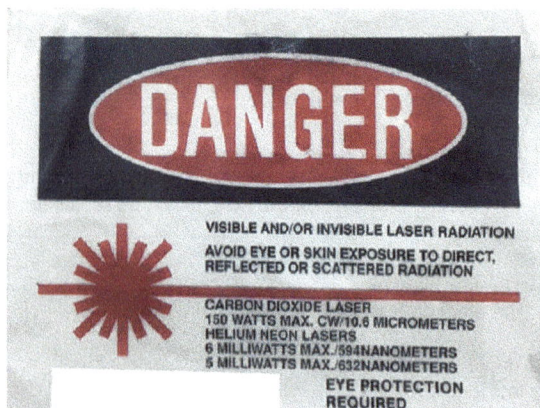

Fig. 6: Safety sign hanging on the door of the laser treatment room.

> A moistened dental bolster is inserted underneath the upper lip in order to make the rhytides of the upper cutaneous lip accessible to the laser.

The specific laser parameters of the procedure will vary based on the equipment. Four factors need to be considered:

1. *Density of the columns*: The density addresses how closely the columns of thermal injury are spaced.
2. *Fluence for depth of penetration*: The operator must be aware of the specific depth of penetration prior to use.
3. *Repetition rate*: Certain instruments require activation with a foot pedal and some have continuous regular firing rates.
4. *Number of passes*: Depending on the device used, either single or multiple passes may be needed.

When treating the neck in addition to the face, be sure to decrease the energy used relative to the settings for the face.

> When treating the neck, decrease the energy used relative to the settings for the face.

Postprocedure

Immediately, at the conclusion of the procedure, the person accompanying the patient is brought into the operating room and the written postoperative care instructions are reviewed. The preparation of ice packs is demonstrated. Prepare the packs by filling a regular balloon approximately three-fourths full with water. Add one tablespoon of regular alcohol (70% ethanol) is added to prevent solid freezing and this cold pack is placed in a freezer. The demonstration balloon can be taken home, placed in a plastic bag and then placed in the freezer multiple times for repeated use.

The patient and caregiver are also taught to prepare vinegar soaks [one tablespoon of 5% acetic acid (white vinegar) in one cup of water] to be used with gauze sponges. Apply the soaked sponges for 10 minutes, three or four times daily, and debride vigorously afterwards before liberally applying emollients such as Vaseline™, Aquaphor™ or Vaniply™ to the treated areas.

The patient and caregiver are also taught to recognize signs of infection including, expanding erythema, red streaks, fever, chills, and rigors. They should return to the office if any signs of infection appear, so that a culture can be performed immediately. Pending results, antistaphylococcal antibiotics should be started. If signs of infection persist despite antibiotic therapy, consider the possibility of candida and treat with a one-time oral dose of fluconazole 200 mg. We also encourage patients to send a digital photograph of the area for evaluation, via secure electronic means if they have any question about the appearance of the healing skin.

Patients should wear a full-face mask for 24 hours postprocedure and stay indoors for 5–7 days except for their office follow-up visits at 24 hr, 72 hr and 1 week. A wide-brimmed hat and a surgical mask over their lower face should be worn when traveling to the office for postoperative visits. Patients should be advised to adhere to strict sun protection efforts for 2 months following the laser treatment.

BENEFITS COMPARED TO ALTERNATIVE APPROACHES

The advantages of fractionated CO_2 relative to total ablative skin resurfacing include the significant decrease in social down time, risk of infection, pain, and a diminution of prolonged post-treatment erythema and hypopigmentation. There is little to no blood exposure during the fractionated laser procedure.

RISKS AND LIMITATIONS

Beware of this technique in patients with a history of acne since anecdotal cases of nodulocystic acne flares have been reported after fractionated laser treatment. The patient's acne should be well-controlled, with no regular flares of disease. Additionally, carefully consider treatment of patients with a history of recent use of isotretinoin. Some sources advocate avoiding laser procedures within the first year post-isotretinoin treatment, citing a concern for unusual scarring. More recent studies using modern instrumentation, however, demonstrate a lack of clinical and histopathologic evidence supporting post-treatment scarring in subjects previously treated with isotretinoin.[8,9]

Consider treatment of a test patch in patients with darker skin types, Fitzpatrick's skin type III-V, given the potential for pigmentary altera-

tion. Reassess the patient at a 4–6-week follow-up visit.

> Consider treatment of a test patch in patient with darker skin types.

A history of keloid scarring is an absolute contraindication for this procedure.

Given the use of the above mentioned medications, pregnancy is a contraindication for this procedure. Finally, always temper expectations. Use of the fractionated technique will not give the dramatic results seen with a single ablative carbon dioxide treatment. The patient may require two or three sessions.[5]

VIDEO LEGEND

Video 1: Demonstration of the fractionated CO_2 laser technique.

REFERENCES

1. Manstein D, Herron GS, Sink RK, et al. Fractional photothermolysis: a new concept for cutaneous remodeling using microscopic patterns of thermal injury. Lasers Surg Med. 2004;34:426-38.
2. Ortiz A, Goldman MP, Fitzpatrick RE. Ablative CO_2 lasers for skin tightening: Traditional versus fractional. Dermatol Surg. 2014;40:S147-51.
3. Aslam A, Alster T. Evolution of laser skin resurfacing: from scanning to fractional technology. Dermatol Surg. 2014;40(11):1163-72.
4. Peukert N, Bayer J, Becke D, et al. Fractional photothermolysis for the treatment of facial wrinkes: searching for optimal treatment parameters in a randomized study in the split-face design. JDDG. 2012;10:898-903.
5. Tierney E, Hanke W. Fractionated carbon dioxide laser treatment of photoaging: prospective study in 45 patients and review of the literature. Dermatol Surg. 2011;37(9):1279-90.
6. Gilbert S, McBurney E. Use of valacyclovir for HSV-1 prophylaxis after facial resurfacting: a randomized clinical trial of dosing regimens. Dermatol Surg. 2000;26(1):50-4.
7. Tierney E, Hanke CW. The effect of cold-air anesthesia during fractionated carbon-dioxide laser treatment: Prospective study and review of the literature. J Amer Acad Derm. 2012;67(3): 436-45.
8. Khatri KA, Iqbal N, Bhawan J. Laser skin resurfacing during isotretinoin therapy. Dermatol Surg. 2015;41(6):758-9.
9. Kim HW, Chang SE, Kim JE, et al. The safe delivery of fractional ablative carbon dioxide laser treatment for acne scars in Asian patients receiving oral isotretinoin. Dermatol Surg. 2014;40(12):1361-6.

CHAPTER 17

Pigmented Lesion Lasers

Evan Stiegel, Shilpi Khetarpal, Michelle B Tarbox, Jennifer Lucas

HISTORY

In 1960, an American engineer named Theodore Maiman developed the first working laser using a ruby crystal as its active medium.[1] Shortly after, Dr. Leon Goldman, who many refer to as the "Father of Laser Medicine", adapted the use of lasers to dermatology. During Goldman's early studies employing the ruby laser for ablation techniques, he observed that darker skin types absorbed more laser light than lighter skin types.[2] With this in mind, he hypothesized that melanin was a chromophore of the laser. Some years later, Goldman was among the first to investigate the use of a Q-switched ruby laser at a 50-microsecond pulse duration for treatment of pigmented lesions. Based on observations that destruction of pigmented lesions was independent of skin color, a more selective effect of the laser at the level of the melanosome was suggested. This new hypothesis was confirmed approximately twenty years later in several studies that revealed melanosome membrane disruption by electron microscopy in guinea pig skin irradiated with a Q-switched ruby laser.[3,4] Over subsequent years, the Q-switched ruby laser and many lasers with other wavelengths have demonstrated efficacy in targeting pigmented lesions of the skin, owing to the broad absorption spectrum of melanin. In the last two decades, investigators have primarily focused on studying Q-switched lasers for treatment of pigmented lesions due to their clear theoretical advantage over lasers with longer pulse durations in accordance with the theory of selective photothermolysis. A typical melanosome has a very short thermal relaxation time (500–1100 nanoseconds), necessitating the use of short pulse duration laser to confine thermal damage.[5] For this reason, the picosecond 755 nm alexandrite laser, which originally made news in tattoo removal, is the newest laser to show promise in treating pigmented lesions.

> Sub-microsecond laser pulses (i.e. Q-switched lasers and picosecond lasers) are required to induce maximal destruction of melanosomes while avoiding damage to surrounding structures.

Background

Optimal laser treatment of pigmented lesions requires selective destruction of melanosomes, the cell organelle that is the site for synthesis, storage and transport of melanin. Melanin is the primary chromophore to be targeted when treating pigmented lesions. In order to obtain selective destruction of melanin, the pigmented lesion must be treated with a laser possessing both an appropriate energy, wavelength, and pulse duration. Regarding wavelength, melanin has a wide absorption spectrum (500–1100 nm) allowing for a multitude of lasers to effectively target these lesions. Other wavelengths not selectively absorbed by melanin may destroy pigmented tissue, but also damage non-pigmented cutaneous structures indiscriminately. Concerning pulse duration, the theory of selective photothermolysis dictates that the pulse duration must be equal to or shorter than the target's thermal relaxation time. Melanosomes possess a very short thermal relaxation time (500–1000 nanoseconds). For this reason, submicrosecond laser pulses (i.e. nanosecond and picosecond lasers) are required to induce melanosome destruction and avoid damage to surrounding structures.[5]

PROCEDURE

Pretreatment

A consultation including a history and physical should be done prior to treatment. At this visit, we recommend reviewing expectations with the patient including the anticipated need for multiple treatments, post-treatment changes and side effects which consist of erythema, swelling, transient discomfort, and possible purpura, dyspigmentation, blistering, crusting and sloughing of skin. Patients with skin types III and above need to be counseled on the increased risk for permanent dyspigmentation and the need for possible test spots or alternative treatments. Medications and topical treatments should be reviewed including the use of isotretinoin, anticoagulants, prior or current use of gold supplements or treatments, and photosensitizing agents. The patient should avoid the sun and aggressively use sunscreen with at least SPF 30 so that the skin is free of tan at the time of treatment and for at least one month after treatment. Any history of abnormal scarring should be addressed. We recommend taking pretreatment photos of the patient including photos prior to each treatment to help monitor for treatment efficacy and to help manage patient expectations. As with tattoos, pigmented lesions can be improved but often not completely erased with laser treatment. It is also important to review the cost of treatment as these procedures are often considered cosmetic and therefore not covered by insurance.

> Photos should be obtained prior to starting treatment and prior to each treatment to monitor for progress and manage treatment expectations.

General Considerations

Pigmented lesions are best categorized into epidermal, dermal, or combined epidermal and dermal processes. Epidermal pigmented lesions consist of ephelides, lentigines, café au lait macules (CALM), and seborrheic keratoses. Dermal lesions include intradermal melanocytic nevi, nevus of Ito and Ota, drug-induced hyperpigmentation and Mongolian spots (congenital dermal melanocytosis). Lastly, combined epidermal and dermal pigmented lesions include melasma, post-inflammatory hyperpigmentation, melanocytic nevi and Becker's nevi. Tattoo pigments are another area of consideration for treatment with pigment-specific lasers and may consist of metal salts, vegetable dyes, organic pigments, and plastic-based pigment which may all be targeted by specific wavelengths of light.[6]

Effective pigment-specific lasers include green-light, red-light, and near-infrared lasers. Other less-specific lasers including argon, krypton, copper, carbon dioxide, and more recently Er:YAG have been used to treat pigmented lesions, however; non-specific target destruction may lead to textural changes and/or scarring.[5] Green-light lasers (510 nm pulsed dye and 532 nm frequency-doubled Nd:YAG) have shorter wavelengths and thus penetrate more superficially into skin. Accordingly, they are most effective in treating epidermal pigmented lesions. Red-light lasers (694-nm ruby and 755 nm alexandrite) and near-infrared lasers (1064 nm Nd:YAG) with their longer wavelengths can treat dermal and combined epidermal-dermal pigmented lesions in addition to epidermal lesions. In the authors' experience, the 1064 nm Nd:YAG is less effective for epidermal lesions (Table 1). Lasers that are primarily used in skin resurfacing like the carbon dioxide and erbium:YAG lasers can also remove superficial pigmented lesions as a secondary benefit. In summary, lentigines, ephelides, and dermal melanocytoses typically respond favorably to laser treatment whereas other pigmented processes yield mixed results. Tattoo pigments have variable responses to laser treatment. The response is dependent upon the composition, depth, amount, and color of the tattoo ink, the laser wavelengths utilized, and the selected treatment protocol. Blue, black, and green tattoos are more responsive to laser treatment, while white and fluorescent colors prove more difficult.[6]

> Lentigines, ephelides, dermal melanocytoses, and blue, black, and green tattoo pigments typically respond most favorably to laser treatment.

Table 1: Selective lasers, wavelengths and pigmented lesions treated.

Laser	Wavelength	Lesions targeted
Pulsed dye	510 nm	Epidermal
Q-switched Nd:YAG	532 nm	Epidermal
Q-switched ruby	694 nm	Epidermal, dermal, and combined
Q-switched Alexandrite	755 nm	Epidermal, dermal, and combined
Q-switched Nd:YAG	1064 nm	Dermal and combined > epidermal
Picosecond	532, 755, 1064 nm	Epidermal, dermal

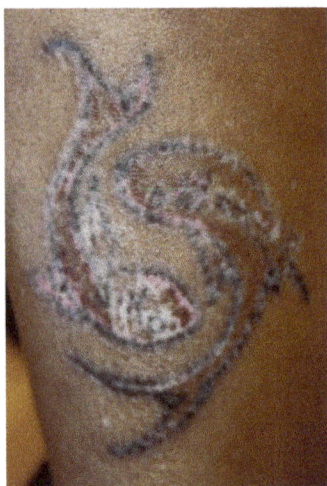

Fig. 1: Post-treatment pigment alteration.

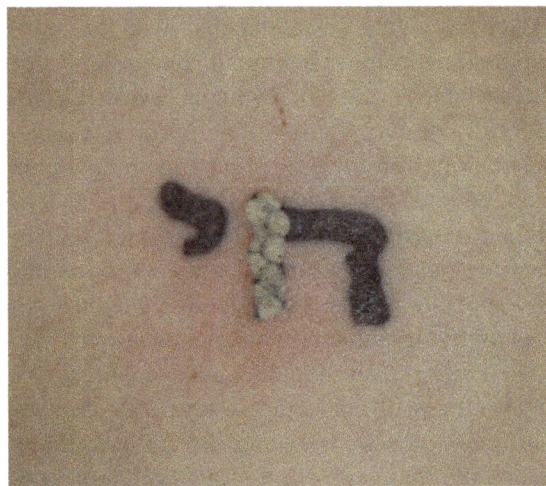

Fig. 2: Skin whitening/frosting with laser treatment.

Spot testing treatment areas may be practical prior to engaging in a full treatment. This can be performed to assess the potential for clinical improvement which is not uniformly predictable. In addition, spot tests permit an assessment of the potential for adverse events including post-inflammatory hyperpigmentation, hypopigmentation, and even depigmentation or texture change. Adverse effects are more common in patients with darker skin tones. When adverse effects occur in these patients hyperpigmentation is more difficult to treat, and permanent dyspigmentation can occur (Fig. 1). This metered approach will help ensure that the patient is happy with the result before large areas are treated.

> Spot treatment with the laser is prudent prior to treating larger or multiple lesions. This is especially important in patients with darker skin tones where risks, including permanent dyspigmentation, are more likely.

When treating pigmented lesions, the clinician should observe for a "popping/snapping sound" and tissue whitening, which is an instantly visible useful marker for effective treatment. The cause of this phenomenon is not completely understood, but likely is owed to the formation of gas bubbles in the targeted melanosome or pigment aggregates within the dermis that cause light scattering[5] (Fig. 2).

> When treating pigmented lesions with Q-switched lasers the presence of an audible snapping sound and instant tissue whitening portend effective treatment.

Post-treatment Care

After treatment of pigmented lesions, sloughing of necrotic cells typically occurs with transient hypopigmentation followed by gradual repigmentation over weeks to the constitutive skin color. This occurs as melanocytes associated with adnexal structures or surrounding skin migrate into treated areas. Studies comparing the induction of pigment injury with various laser wavelengths on guinea pig skin determined that shorter wavelengths damage pigmented cells at lower fluences, whereas longer wavelengths require more energy.[4] These findings hold true for human skin. Effective treatment of pigmented lesions can be achieved with lower fluences using lasers with shorter wavelengths. When treating tattoos, particularly in more heavily pigmented skin, in addition to the aforementioned blistering and sloughing of necrotic skin, temporary hypopigmentation can occur in treated areas. Certain tattoo pigments, particularly white (titanium dioxide) and cosmetic tattoos (ferric oxide) may paradoxically darken following laser treatment. This paradoxical darkening may respond to subsequent laser treatments or may in rare cases become permanent. Therefore it is imperative to counsel patients of this possibility and to consider performing a test spot to evaluate for treatment response.[7] During the post-treatment healing time, the authors recommend strict photoprotection for a period of at least one month. Patients are also instructed to promote wound healing with a petroleum-based lubricant. Finally, irritating chemical products, such as prescription and over-the-counter "anti-aging" creams, should be avoided completely or used with caution during the healing period.

Epidermal Pigmented Lesions

Superficial pigmented lesions including ephelides, lentigines, and macular seborrheic keratoses can be successfully treated with any of the aforementioned pigment-specific lasers.[8-10] Both green and red light lasers produce excellent results (Figs. 3A and B). However, because the shorter wavelength in green light lasers is also well absorbed by oxyhemoglobin, purpura formation may occur following laser irradiation. If the patient is averse to having short-term purpura lasting up to 10 days, the Q-switched ruby (694 nm) and the alexandrite (755 nm) produce excellent results, with a low side-effect profile and reportedly no purpura.[5] In our experience, purpura is less frequent but still can occur. Typically, one to two treatment sessions at 6–8 week intervals are

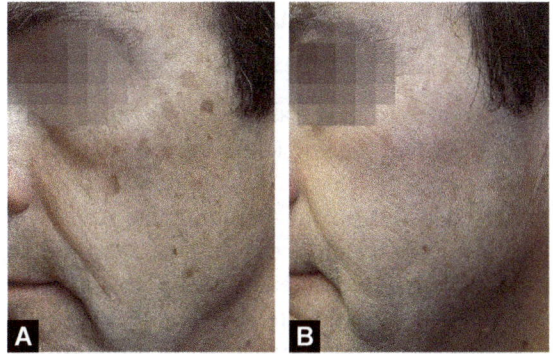

Figs. 3A and B: Before (A) and after (B) photographs following the treatment of lentigines with 532 nm Q-switched laser. *Source*: Janine Sot

necessary to achieve significant improvement; however, additional treatments may be required. Although the pigment may clear quickly, patient expectations should be tempered with the information that multiple treatments may be required and that lesions may recur with sun exposure. Ephelides tend to recur following sun exposure, whereas lentigines usually demonstrate the best long-term response to laser therapy.

> It is important to convey to patients that although there is a chance that their pigmented lesion may clear quickly with laser, multiple treatments may be necessary.

Café au lait macules (CALMs) are often more difficult to treat than the other pigmented skin lesions. Although there can be initial lightening or resolution, recurrence is common and serial treatments over months to years are often necessary.[11] The mechanism for the higher resistance seen in CALMs is not known. It has been proposed that repigmentation occurs as a result of proliferation of neighboring untreated melanocytes. Accordingly, the entire lesion should be treated at each session to reduce the likelihood of this phenomenon occurring. It is not uncommon for skip areas to be noticed after treatment. This applies not only to CALMs but also other pigmented lesions as well. These skip areas often respond after further focused therapy.

> Skip areas may be noticed after laser treatment of any pigmented lesion. These areas often respond after further focused therapy.

Mixed Epidermal/Dermal Pigmented Lesions

Laser treatment of melasma is difficult as long-term clearance is not commonly achieved.[12-13] Melasma can be categorized as epidermal, dermal, or mixed based on the predominant histologic location of pigment in these patches. As would be expected, epidermal melasma responds to laser treatment more frequently than the other types of melasma. It has been suggested that melasma's poor response to laser therapy and frequent recurrences result from the failure to control underlying etiological factors. These include continued exposure to the sun as well as non-modifiable risk factors related to genetic and hormonal factors.[5] Also of concern, laser treatment of melasma can produce hyperpigmentation or worsening of melasma itself. Given this risk and its inconsistent efficacy, employing laser therapy as a singular modality for melasma is not recommended. Rather, it should be combined with adjunctive therapeutics including sun avoidance, meticulous use of physical sunscreens such as those containing iron oxide, topical retinoids, bleaching agents, and chemical peels. Recent research has implicated a vascular component in melasma, and some studies have demonstrated improved patient satisfaction utilizing a combination of pulse dye laser in conjunction with pigmented lesion laser although others have not found therapeutic benefit in a combined approach.[14,15] Irrespective of which treatment is recommended, patients should be carefully educated to temper their expectations and test spots should be performed to assess results before the larger areas are treated.

Laser treatment for post-inflammatory hyperpigmentation is routinely disappointing. Not only does the response tend to be poor, but laser irradiation may cause worsening hyperpigmentation just as it can in melasma.[16] The poor response may be due to the inability of the laser to target melanin within melanophages.

Q-switched laser treatments for Becker's nevi achieve variable results. This is likely due to retention of pigment in adnexal structures and to the hormone dependency of these lesions as has been demonstrated by their increased androgen receptor activity.[17] Hypertrichosis is one of the primary concerns of patients with Becker's nevi, and combination of Q-switched and long-pulse laser may be required to address both components of these lesions.[5] Test spots should also be performed to assess the potential risks and benefit when treating these lesions.

Dermal Pigmented Lesions

Q-switched lasers have become the gold standard of treatment for dermal melanocytosis including nevus of Ito and Ota.[18-20] Specifically, the Q-switched ruby (694 nm), Q-switched alexandrite (755 nm), and the Q-switched Nd:YAG (1064 nm) with their longer wavelengths effectively target the deep spindle-shaped dermal melanocytes. Complete clearance can be seen in as few as 3 treatments, and clearance is typically permanent. However, the number of treatments required has been shown to be related to lesion color and extent of pigmentation.[21] More heavily pigmented blue-green nevi tend to require more treatments than brown or violet lesions. Proper eye protection (a metal shield) should be worn when the treatment of nevus of Ota is performed inside the orbital rim. To minimize the risk of corneal abrasion, the shield should be gently applied and liberally lubricated with ophthalmic ointment.

Drug-induced hyperpigmentation including blue-black pigmentation secondary to minocycline, amiodarone, and pigmentation induced by silver (argyria) have responded well to the Q-switched lasers.[22,23] It is essential that the causative drug is stopped prior to commencing laser treatment. Of note, Q-switched laser treatment has been demonstrated to cause chrysiasis confined to treatment areas in patients who have a history of parenteral gold therapy. Case reports of this phenomenon suggest that the skin discoloration is permanent.[24] The 1064 nm and 755 nm Q-switched lasers demonstrate the highest efficacy in treating most forms of drug-induced pigmentation. A test spot produces instantaneous evidence to determine the most effective wavelength and fluence. Just as with laser treatment of other conditions, multiple treatments may be required for maximal clearance. Depending upon treatment dosing and the amount of pigment being treated, post-treatment edema and treatment-related discomfort may occur.

Tattoo Removal

Q-switched laser devices have long been the gold standard for the therapeutic removal of tattoos (Table 2). More recently picosecond lasers have emerged as highly effective therapeutic adjuncts to tattoo removal. Prior to commencing a treatment regimen for tattoo removal, it is imperative to elicit a complete medical history from the patient, including the consideration of any history of hypertrophic scarring, sarcoidosis, autoimmune disease, and immunosuppression. The presence of immunosuppression may be a particularly important issue in patient selection as the patient's immune system plays a key role in clearing residual ink particles following laser treatment. For this reason, immunosuppressed patients may be at greater risk for poor healing and ink retention. One must also elicit a complete history regarding the tattoo being treated including any infections or difficulty healing following tattoo placement. A history of infections or difficulty healing may indicate an increased likelihood of occult dermal scarring concealed under the tattoo which can result in patient dissatisfaction following an otherwise successful treatment. Careful palpation of the tattoo and examination utilizing side lighting can help elucidate subtle elevations of the skin in the tattooed areas that may not be evident until the tattoo ink is removed. In the author's experience, evaluating tattoos from multiple angles and with side lighting can be useful in detecting induration. Additionally, some tattoos are placed as a cover-up for a previously regretted tattoo and in these circumstances, additional treatments will likely be required to achieve patient satisfaction. When removing a cover-up tattoo, the colors not only of the visible tattoo, but the colors of the covered tattoo will be important in determining the likelihood for successful treatment.[6,7]

Picosecond Laser

The US FDA approved the first picosecond 755 nm alexandrite laser (Cynosure; Westford, MA) in 2012 after its demonstrated success in tattoo removal. This laser requires fewer treatments to clear tattoos than traditional nanosecond quality switched (Q-switched) lasers.[25] Picosecond lasers have an ultra-short pulse duration of 550–750

Table 2: Tattoo pigments and appropriate lasers.

Tattoo color	Pigments	Most therapeutic laser
Red	Cadmium selenide (Cadmium red) Mercury sulfide (Cinnabar) Ferric hydrate (Sienna) Sandalwood Brazilwood	Q-switched Nd:YAG 532 nm
Orange	Disazodiarylide Disazopyrazolone Cadmium seleno-sulfide	Q-switched Nd:YAG 532 nm
Yellow	Cadmium sulfide (Cadmium yellow) Curcumin yellow Ochre	Q-switched Nd:YAG 532 nm
Green	Chromium oxide (Casalis green) Malachite green Lead chromate Ferro/ferric cyanide Curcumin green Phthalocyanine dyes	Q-switched Ruby 694 nm Alexandrite 755 nm
Blue	Cobalt aluminate (Cobalt blue) Azure	Q-switched Ruby 694 nm Alexandrite 755 nm Q-switched Nd:YAG 1064 nm
Purple	Manganese Aluminum	Alexandrite 755 nm Q-switched Nd:YAG 1064 nm
Black	Carbon (India ink) Iron Oxide Logwood	Q-switched Ruby 694 nm Alexandrite 755 nm Q-switched Nd:YAG 1064 nm
White	Titanium oxide Zinc oxide	No Consensus, Test spots recommended
Brown	Ferric oxide	Q-switched Nd:YAG 532 nm

picoseconds, causing both photomechanical and photothermal effects on tissue. The picosecond laser currently has FDA approval for the treatment of wrinkles, acne scarring, and removal of tattoos and pigmented lesions. Currently available Q-switched lasers have pulse durations in the nanosecond range, which have the potential to heat surrounding, unaffected skin leading to greater potential adverse effects. The rapid absorption of picosecond light energy damages the target (tattoo or melanin), reducing the amount

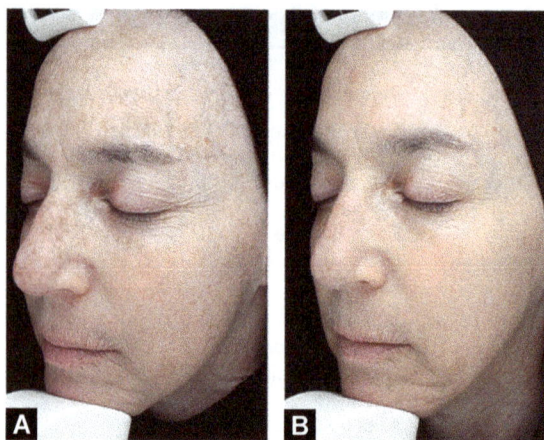

Figs. 4A and B: Before (A) and after (B) photographs following the treatment of lentigines with a picosecond laser showing moderate response.

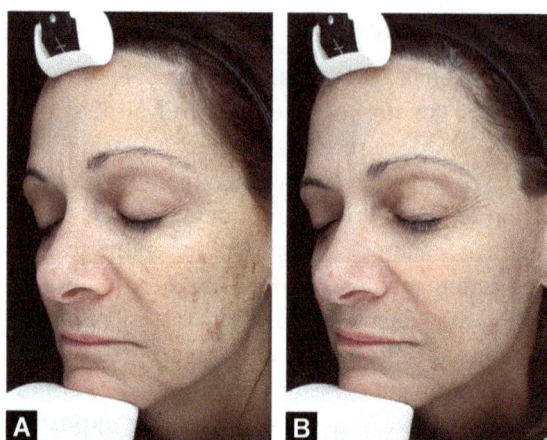

Figs. 5A and B: Before (A) and after (B) photographs following the treatment of lentigines with a picosecond laser showing dramatic response.

of remaining target (either tattoo pigment or melanin), leaving the treated skin uniform in color and texture. The new generation of picosecond lasers have efficient delivery of energy and lower thermal diffusion to surrounding tissues making them better suited to treat pigmented lesions compared to prior Q-switched lasers (Figs. 4 and 5). Because picosecond lasers have pulse durations that are approximately 100 times shorter than the commonly used QS lasers, they are closer to the thermal relaxation time of melanosomes.[26] This allows for more power to be delivered at a lower fluence, allowing for more effective treatments with fewer adverse reactions.

Although picosecond devices can be used to treat a variety of conditions, certain factors should be taken into consideration prior to commencing treatments including Fitzpatrick skin type, and current or prior treatments (including laser or other). Again, it is imperative to inquire about a history of parenteral gold therapy to prevent laser-induced chrysiasis, which theoretically could also occur with use of picosecond lasers. Regardless of the laser used, it is important that patients understand multiple sessions are required and the tattoo or pigmented lesion can typically be improved, but not erased.

ADDITIONAL TATTOO REMOVAL TREATMENT TIPS

While Q-switched (QS) lasers are the gold standard for tattoo removal, they often require mul-

tiple sessions and are costly and time consuming to the patient. QS lasers work by the theory of selective photothermolysis and the laser energy is selectively absorbed by tattoo ink particles due to the preferential wavelength and thermal relaxation time. After treating a tattoo with a QS laser, there is gentle whitening or frosting of the tattoo pigment. This prevents further penetration of laser into the skin.[1] By using the 'R20' method; the tattoo is repeatedly exposed to laser light in a single session. By giving a gap of 20 or more minutes, the frosting subsides, and the tattoo can be treated with the same or different laser parameters. The gentle whitening observed during the first pass may not be seen in subsequent passes. Utilizing this method allows for fewer treatment sessions/office visits when treating both professional and amateur tattoos.[1,2] The authors have also had good success with using the R20 method with picosecond followed by QS lasers. The disadvantages are that it can take several hours to complete and requires long wait times for the patient. Although the initial studies showed this method was safe in Fitzpatrick skin types I–IV, it has not been studied in darker skin types. There is a theoretical increased risk of blistering, scarring and pigment alteration in darker skinned patients.[2]

> Utilizing the R20 method can decrease the number of treatment sessions needed for tattoo removal.

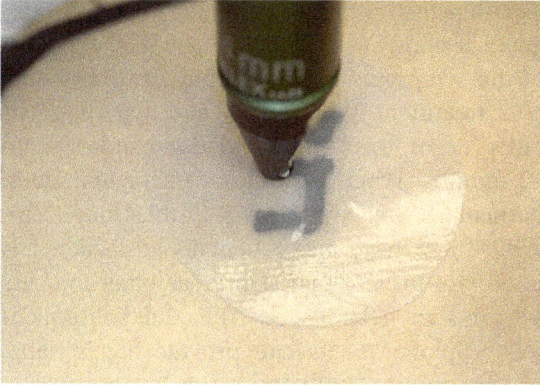

Fig. 6: Treatment through transparent perfluorodecalin (PFD) infused patch decreases pain and improves tattoo clearance.

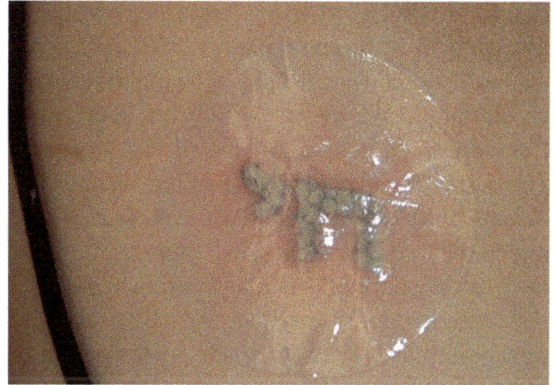

Fig. 7: Post-treatment, transparent perfluorodecalin (PFD) infused patch remains in place to improve patient comfort.

Another way to improve laser-assisted tattoo removal is to treat through a transparent perfluorodecalin (PFD) infused patch (Fig. 6). Several studies have shown more rapid tattoo clearance and less pain leading to greater patient satisfaction. The patch prevents epidermal whitening that occurs with QS and picosecond lasers. The PFD patch allows for several (around 4) passes to be done at a higher energy, rather than doing the traditional one pass, when the tattoo is treated through air.[3] The PFD infused patch can also be left in place after laser treatment of tattoos to provide increased pain relief and comfort to the patient (Fig. 7).

> Treating through a transparent perfluorodecalin infused patch can help expedite tattoo clearance and decrease pain.

Cosmetic tattoos, which often contain brightening pigments, flesh-colored, white, red, and brown tattoos can paradoxically darken with laser treatment given the reduction of titanium dioxide to titanium oxide and ferric to ferrous oxide. The authors advise doing a test spot to demonstrate the instantaneous darkening that will occur. If the patient wishes to proceed with treatment the entire tattoo is then treated with the new darkened pigment becoming the new chromophore to treat.

> White, red-brown, and cosmetic tattoos may paradoxically darken with treatment. This may resolve with further laser treatments.

BENEFITS COMPARED TO OTHER APPROACHES

Pigmented lesions can be treated using a variety of modalities including topical bleaching products, chemical peels, dermabrasion, electrodesiccation, and surgical excision. The primary benefit of laser treatment when compared to alternative approaches is related to the theory of selective photothermolysis. Controlled targeting of melanosomes is possible with minimal damage of surrounding structures.[27] This leads to excellent cosmetic results. In addition, the procedure is quick and well tolerated by patients.

Unfortunately, comparative studies between lasers and other treatment modalities for pigmented lesions are few. The comparative studies that have been performed focus on the treatment of lentigines. In one randomized controlled trial comparing three separate lasers (frequency-doubled Q-switched Nd:YAG laser, krypton laser, and 532 nm diode-pumped vanadate laser) to cryotherapy, the lasers yielded superior results. They were also preferred by 93% of patients.[28] Another study comparing the frequency-doubled Q-switched Nd:YAG laser and 35% trichloroacetic acid for treatment of facial lentigines demonstrated greater efficacy with laser therapy.[29]

Intense pulsed light (IPL) is a non-laser filtered flash lamp device that delivers a broad-spectrum pulse of light, usually in the visible spectral range of 420 to 1400 nm with varying pulse durations. Distinct from lasers, IPL uses a wider range of light resulting in absorption by a variety of chromophores. In other words, it has less selectivity. This is overcome by using cutoff filters to refine the spectrum of emitted wavelengths allowing for specific chromophore selectivity. By utilizing specific filters, various targets can be treated with the same device, making this device appealing to many clinicians. The older generation of IPL devices treated pigmented epidermal lesions, however, newer devices are more effective at treating superficial pigmented lesions, vascular lesions, acne, and unwanted hair.[30] With its ability to target multiple types of lesions, IPL is a useful tool in treating the pigmentary and vascular changes that occur in sun-damaged skin. There are a variety of IPL devices available, each with unique characteristics. Most devices have built-in cooling which helps to protect the skin from unwanted thermal damage which is also minimized using water-soluble gels. IPL devices vary in the amount of cooling, the ability to vary the pulse duration, spectral output and wavelengths, and the spot size. Not all IPL devices are created equal. It is essential to know the specifications, nuances, and capabilities of each device being used. IPL treatments are well-tolerated with relatively rare side effects when appropriately used. The most commonly occurring side effects include post-treatment discomfort, erythema, purpura, edema, blistering and crusting, which are typically mild and self-limited. Some patients experience an urticarial response in areas of targeted lesions such as lentigines (Fig. 8). Most of the symptoms resolve within 24 to 48 hours after treatment. When hypo- and hyperpigmentation occur, the dyspigmentation can last up to 12 months. When treating extensive lentigines, particularly over large areas, skip areas may occur. While these may cause patient dissatisfaction, it is important to note that skip areas often indicate an excellent response to IPL and subsequent touch-up treatments can provide highly satisfactory results (Figs. 9A to C). It is important to

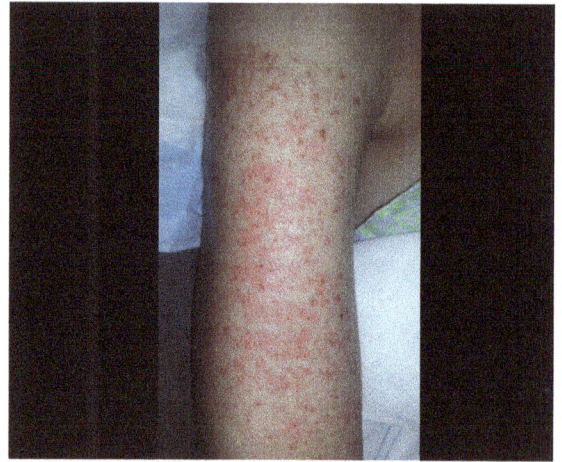

Fig. 8: Urticarial reaction to IPL treatment of lentigines.

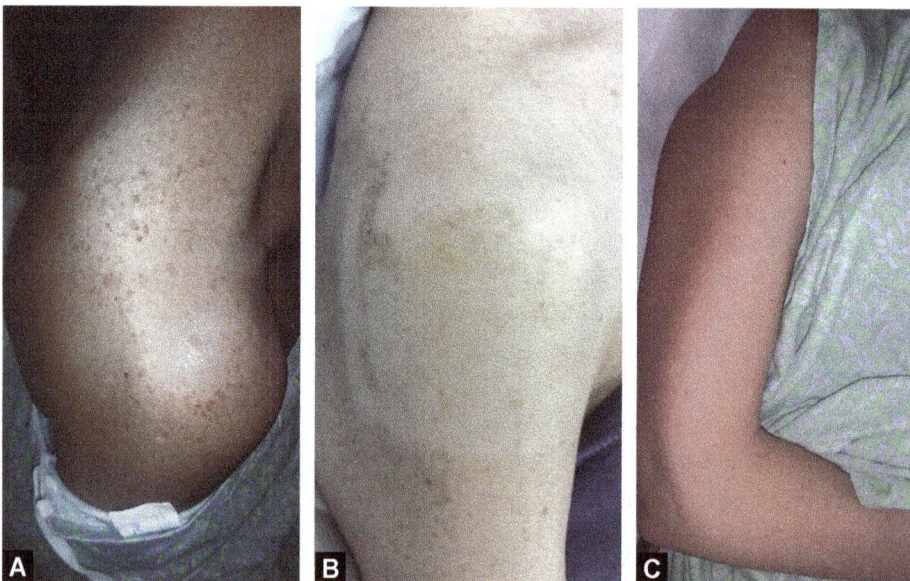

Figs. 9A to C: Before (A), after first treatment with skip areas (B), and after subsequent treatment (C) photographs showing response of extensive lentigines to IPL treatment.

consider numerous factors including skin type and skin condition in the treatment area, location and size of lesions, number of treatments, and pain tolerance. Regardless of the device used, it is essential for patients to understand that multiple treatments are required to achieve the best possible results. The clinician must be cognizant of both warning signs and treatment endpoints when using all of these devices. IPL has not proven useful in treating tattoos.

RISKS/LIMITATIONS

Although laser therapy has become one of the most effective treatment modalities for treatment of pigmented lesions, it does not come without some risks, limitations, and some controversy. While treatments are well tolerated, common side effects may include intratreatment and post-treatment discomfort, erythema, edema, purpura, dyspigmentation, texture changes, blistering and crusting/sloughing of skin. The adverse effects of post-inflammatory hyper- or hypopigmentation and possible depigmentation are important considerations as they may be permanent. Dyspigmentation is more common in darker skin types (i.e. Fitzpatrick skin type III and above) and in suntanned skin. As such, test spots should always be done first and when possible, in treating darker skin types, consideration should be given to using the longest effective wavelength of laser to minimize unwanted exposure of epidermal melanocytes. One can also consider pretreatment with topical bleaching agents. Nightly application of hydroquinone 4% cream for at least two weeks prior to treatment is a common regimen that is employed prior to laser therapy of pigmented lesions. Treating tanned patients should be avoided until they are back to their baseline pigment and post-treatment tanning and sun exposure should be avoided. As previously discussed, results in treating certain types of pigmented lesions can vary widely. Although the mechanism is not entirely understood, suboptimal results are thought to be the result of deep localization of dermal pigment, repigmentation from adnexa, or stimulation of melanocytes in the adjacent epidermis.

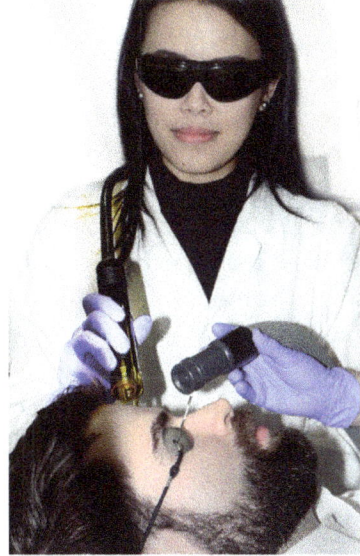

Fig. 10: A cooling unit (Synderon Zimmer®) being used in conjunction with laser of a pigmented lesion to alleviate discomfort during the treatment session.
Source: Janine Sot, Medical photographer, Cleveland Clinic Foundation, Cleveland, Ohio, USA.

Patient tolerance is also a consideration when treating any type of lesion with lasers. Some lasers are more painful than others, and this should be considered when selecting the optimal treatment modality. Cooling units, devices designed to blow cold air onto the treatment field as the laser is fired, represent a useful tool that can reduce patient discomfort during the procedure and may reduce epidermal injury thereby decreasing the risk of residual dyspigmentation. This technique is frequently employed by the authors when treating any lesion (Fig. 10). Intermittent ice application can also be a useful tool to help alleviate laser-related pain. However, caution is advised against direct ice application for extended periods during laser treatment as it can increase the risk of residual dyspigmentation. Finally, for patients who are sensitive to pain, a 30% topical lidocaine ointment can be used for a minimum of 20 minutes prior to treatment to alleviate discomfort.

Consideration should be given to the area of application as large surface areas may absorb enough lidocaine to result in systemic toxicity.

> A 30% topical lidocaine ointment applied for a minimum of 20 minutes prior to laser treatment will alleviate some discomfort.

The most controversial issues in laser treatment of pigmented lesions pertains to the use of laser in treating melanocytic nevi, both congenital and acquired. The standard of care for the treatment of melanocytic nevi is surgical excision, which allows for histologic assessment of any atypical features. Sometimes however, surgical excision of these lesions in cosmetically or functionally sensitive areas is not ideal. In these cases a variety of lasers have been employed. In the past, continuous-wave lasers including the carbon dioxide and argon were used which resulted in significant scarring. In addition, recurrences can produce lesions that clinically and histopathologically resemble melanoma (pseudomelanoma or recurrent nevus).[31] More recently, both short-pulsed and long-pulsed lasers have been used to treat melanocytic lesions with variable responses. Concern lies in the potential malignant transformation of nevomelanocytes and subsequent development of melanoma with the potential obfuscation of a classic sign of melanoma: pigment change. Laser irradiation differs compared to ultraviolet irradiation on cells in that UV exposure causes DNA damage and subsequent mutation development, whereas laser primarily induces a thermal injury. As no long-term studies have been performed, it is not known whether laser-induced thermal injury has deleterious effects on cells. One hypothesized concern is that incomplete laser-induced destruction of the superficial melanocytes in a nevomelanocytic lesion can remove the protective pigment of the lesion rendering the remainder of the lesion more susceptible to UV-induced DNA damage.[5] With this information in mind, clinicians should be cautious when using laser or light devices to treat melanocytic nevi and reserve its use for lesions in cosmetically or functionally sensitive areas where alternative treatments are unacceptable. Furthermore, patients who have undergone laser treatment of their melanocytic nevi should be observed closely for any signs of recurrence. At our institutions, we do not treat melanocytic lesions with lasers and do not recommend this practice as these lesions cannot be ideally monitored for malignant transformation after they are treated.

REFERENCES

1. Maiman T. Stimulated Optical Radiation in Ruby. Nature. 1960;187(4736):493-4.
2. Goldman L, Blaney D, Kindel D, et al. Effect of the Laser beam on the skin. Journal of Investigative Dermatology. 1964;42(3):247-51.
3. Polla LL, Margolis JR, Dover JS, et al. Melanosomes are a primary target of Q-switched ruby laser irradiation in guinea pig skin. Journal of Investigative Dermatology. 1987;89(3):281-6.
4. Dover J. Pigmented guinea pig skin irradiated with Q-switched ruby laser pulses. Morphologic and histologic findings. Archives of Dermatology. 1989;125(1):43-9.
5. Stratigos A, Dover J, Arndt K. Laser treatment of pigmented lesions: How far have we gone? Arch Dermatol. 2000;136(7):915-21.
6. Kilmer SL. Laser treatment of tattoos. Dermatol Clin. 1997;15(3):409-17.
7. Kirby W, Chen CL, Desai A, et al. Causes and recommendations for unanticipated ink retention following tattoo removal treatment. J Clin Aesthet Dermatol. 2013;6(7):27-31.
8. Kilmer S. Treatment of epidermal pigmented lesions with the frequency doubled, Q-switched, Nd:YAG laser: A controlled, single-impact, dose-response, multicenter trial. Arch Dermatol. 1994;130(12):515-9.
9. Imhof L, Dummer R, Dreier J, et al. A prospective trial comparing Q-switched Ruby laser and triple combination skin lightening cream in the treatment of solar lentigines. Dermatologic Surgery. 2016;42(7):853-7.
10. Vachiramon V, Panmanee W, Techapichetvanich T, et al. Comparison of Q-switched Nd: YAG laser and fractional carbon dioxide laser for the treatment of solar lentigines in Asians. Lasers Surg Med. 2016;48(4):354-9.
11. Grossman M. Treatment of cafe au lait macules with lasers. A clinicopathologic correlation. Arch Dermatol. 1995;131(12):1416-20.
12. Gokalp H, Akkaya AD, Oram Y. Long-term results in low-fluence 1064-nm Q-Switched Nd:YAG laser for melasma: Is it effective? J Cosmet Dermatol. 2016;15(4):420-6.
13. Hofbauer Parra CA, Careta MF, Valente NY. Clinical and Histopathologic assessment of facial melasma after low-fluence Q-switched neodymium-doped yttrium aluminium garnet laser. Dermato Surg. 2016;42(4):507-12.
14. Geddes ER, Stout AB, Friedman PM. Retrospective analysis of the treatment of melasma lesions exhibiting increased vascularity with the 595-nm pulsed dye laser combined with the 1927-nm fractional low-powered diode laser. Lasers Surg Med. 2017;49(1):20-6.

15. Eimpunth S, Wanitphakdeedecha R, Triwong-waranat D, Varothai S, Manuskiatti W. Therapeutic outcome of melasma treatment by dual-wavelength (511 and 578 nm) laser in patients with skin phototypes III-V. Clinical and Experimental Dermatology [serial online]. 2014;39(3):292-297. Available from: Academic Search Complete, Ipswich, MA. Accessed May 14, 2017.

16. Arora P, Garg V, Sonthalia S, et al. Melasma update. Indian Dermatol Online J. 2014;5(4):426-35.

17. Formigón M. Becker's nevus and ipsilateral breast hypoplasia-androgen-receptor study in two patients. Arch Dermatol. 1992;128(7):992.

18. Shah VV, Bray FN, Aldahan AS, Lasers and nevus of Ota: a comprehensive review. Lasers Medi Sci. 2016;31(1):179-85.

19. Alster TS, Williams CM. Treatment of nevus of ota by the Q-switched alexandrite laser. Dermatol Surg. 1995;21(7):592-6.

20. Geronemus R. Q-switched ruby laser therapy of nevus of Ota. Arch Dermatol. 1992;128(12):1618-22.

21. Ueda S, Isoda M, Imayama S. Response of naevus of Ota to Q-switched ruby laser treatment according to lesion colour. Br J Dermato. 2000;142(1):77-83.

22. Wiper A, Roberts DH, Schmitt M. Amiodarone-induced skin pigmentation: Q-switched laser therapy, an effective treatment option. Heart. 2007;93(1):15.

23. Wee S, Dover J. Effective treatment of psychotropic drug-induced facial hyperpigmentation with a 755-nm Q-switched Alexandrite laser. Dermatologic Surgery. 2008;34(11):1609-12.

24. Trotter M. Localized chrysiasis induced by laser therapy. Arch Dermatol. 1995;131(12):1411-4.

25. Graber E, Iyengar V, Rohrer T, et al. Laser treatment of tattoos and pigmented lesions. In: Robinson JK, Hanke CW, Siegel DM, Fratila A (Eds). Surgery of the Skin: Procedural Dermatology. 2nd ed. China: Mosby. 2010. pp. 537-48.

26. Ross E, Naseef G, Lin C, et al. Comparison of responses of tattoos to picosecond and nanosecond Q-Switched Neodymium:YAG Lasers. Arch Dermatol. 1998;134(2):167-7.

27. Anderson RR, Parrish JA. Selective photothermolysis: precise microsurgery by selective absorption of pulsed radiation. Science. 1983;4596:524-7.

28. Todd M, Rallis TM, Gerwels JW, et al. A comparison of 3 lasers and liquid nitrogen in the treatment of solar lentigines. Arch Dermatol. 2000;136(7):841-6.

29. Li Yang K. Comparison of the frequency doubled Q-switched Nd:YAG laser and 35% trichloroacetic acid for the treatment of face lentigines. Dermatol Surg. 1999;25(3):202-4.

30. Ross E, Smirnov M, Pankratov M, et al. Intense pulsed light and laser treatment of facial telangiectasias and dyspigmentation: some theoretical and practical comparisons. Dermatologic Surgery. 2006;31:1188-98.

31. Trau H, Orenstein A, Schewach-Miller M, et al. Pseudomelanoma following laser therapy for congenital nevus. The Journal of Dermatologic Surgery and Oncology. 1986;12(9):984-6.

CHAPTER 18

Intense Pulsed Light

Jessica Tran, Daniel P Friedmann, Vineet Mishra

HISTORY

Intense pulsed light (IPL) was first conceived as a therapeutic treatment for vascular lesions by Goldman, Fitzpatrick, and Eckhouse in April 1992.[1] Following clinical studies on 10 rabbit ears by Goldman in October 1992, the first research data was presented at the 6th Annual Congress of the American College of Phlebology in Orlando on February 1993 titled: "Clinical and Histologic Evaluation of the ESC Vascular Laser, Pulsed Light Source on the Dorsal Marginal Rabbit Ear Vein." In 1995, IPL therapy became cleared by the US Food and Drug Administration (FDA) for the treatment for telangiectasias of the lower limbs.[2]

Results of the first clinical study on humans were published in 1996.[3] A clearance rate of 75–100% was achieved for 79% of treated lower extremity spider veins, with more than 50% clearance in 94% of cases. In 1997, the IPL successful treatment of essential telangiectasia and therapy-resistant port wine stains were also reported.[2,4] After noticing hair loss areas treated with IPL, use of the device for hair removal began, with the first successful hair removal study using IPL reported in 1997.[5] A hair clearance rate of 60% was observed after a single treatment session in a variety of body areas. Since that time, IPL technology has also been used to treat a number of other cutaneous conditions, including acne vulgaris, rosacea, solar lentigines, poikiloderma of Civatte, melasma, and capillary malformations.[1,6]

MECHANISM OF ACTION

Intense pulsed light devices emit incoherent, noncollimated, polychromatic light in the 500–1,200 nm range (with a peak at 600 nm) produced by a filtered, xenon flash-lamp light source.[7] This broad-spectrum, high-intensity light allows for the simultaneous selective photothermolysis of melanin (400–755 nm), deoxyhemoglobin (550–560 nm), and oxyhemoglobin (540 and 575–580 nm), leading to the targeted destruction of pigmented and vascular dermal structures, respectively.[8,9] The output bandwidth of these light sources can also be modified with the use of cutoff filters to eliminate spectral output of lower and more superficially penetrating wavelengths, thereby limiting background nonspecific melanin absorption and collateral tissue damage, enhancing target selectivity, and promoting selective photothermolysis of deeper dermal vessels by longer wavelengths.[7] While certain devices have interchangeable external quartz cutoff filters for a single handpiece (M22, Lumenis Ltd., Yokneam, Israel), other IPL devices have interchangeable handpieces depending on the selective waveband desired (Nordlys, Ellipse A/S, Hørsholm, Denmark and Icon Aesthetic System, Cynosure, Inc., Westford, MA).

Moreover, deeply penetrating IPL wavelengths in the 800–1,200 nm range may stimulate dermal fibroblast activity and procollagen I/III, elastin, and collagenase expression through a combination of direct photothermal effects on the dermal matrix and chromophore-triggered cytokine and growth factor pathways.[10-14] Upregulation of transforming growth factor beta-1 and downregulation of multiple matrix metalloproteinases may lead to further photorejuvenative effects.[15-17] Although clinical studies have demonstrated histologic evidence of papillary and reticular dermal collagen production and epidermal thickening, rete ridge flattening, and diminished solar elastosis,[18-21] other studies[11,22] have shown no epidermal or dermal remodeling following IPL.

INDICATIONS

A number of prospective clinical studies have demonstrated the safety and efficacy of IPL devices for the treatment of facial photoaging, including telangiectasias, pigmentation, irregular texture, pore size, and fine lines, after 1–7 treatment sessions.[23-27] The treatment of photodamage off-the-face, such as on the neck,[28-30] chest,[28,30,31] back, or upper and lower extremities, can also lead to excellent results.

CONTRAINDICATIONS

Active infection or abnormalities localized to the treatment area (e.g. malignant lesions, scarring, or burns), photosensitivity, and/or medical conditions or medications that may impair wound healing should be ruled out prior to IPL treatment. Evidence of recent tanning, long-term excessive tanning, or sunless tanner use are common reasons to delay treatment with any IPL device, given the increased risk of epidermal injury. Likewise, darker Fitzpatrick skin types (FSTs III–V) are prone to a greater incidence of adverse events, and their treatment should be approached with significant caution. IPL treatment of patients with a FST VI is best avoided. IPL should also not be used to treat cosmetic and professional tattoos, due to the long (ms) pulse duration of IPL dramatically exceeding the ultrashort thermal relaxation time of microscopic tattoo particles, which places patients at markedly high risk of blistering, erosions, and scarring.

Although the myth of foregoing the treatment of patients who have used oral retinoids within the prior 6 months persists, one of the authors (DP Friedmann) has treated a number of patients on oral retinoid therapy without added adverse events. The treatment of pregnant patients should be discouraged; however, breastfeeding patients can be treated safely.

PREOPERATIVE CONSIDERATIONS

All patients have standardized digital photographs of their face taken with 45° soft lighting in a windowless room and written informed consent obtained upon arrival. Patients then wash the area(s) with a neutral cleanser, removing makeup or other impurities that may interfere with treatment.

Since IPL treatment is typically uncomfortable but not overtly painful, with patients often describing a stinging sensation similar to that of a snap of a hot rubber band, pretreatment topical anesthesia is generally unnecessary. Nevertheless, tetracaine-based topical anesthetics can be applied for 15–30 min prior to IPL in order to elicit background erythema and flushing in patients with erythematotelangiectatic rosacea, so as to maximize treatment. These topical anesthetics include a self-occluding 7% lidocaine/7% tetracaine cream (Pliaglis cream; Galderma Laboratories LP, Ft. Worth, TX) or compounded 7% lidocaine/7% tetracaine, 23% lidocaine/7% tetracaine, or 20% benzocaine/6% lidocaine/6% tetracaine. Of all of these options, the author (DP Friedmann) has found that compounded 23% lidocaine/7% tetracaine produces the most rapid, complete anesthetic effect. Prophylactic antiviral therapy for herpes simplex virus is ordinarily unnecessary, but may be beneficial in patients with a history of recurrent outbreaks localized to the treatment area, particularly perioral. Valacyclovir 500 mg PO BID for 3 days, starting the day prior, is sufficient in these high-risk patients.

Disposable adhesive eye shields (LASER-Aid, DELASCO, Inc., Council Bluffs, IA) are almost always used by the authors, but stainless steel or polymer-based ocular shields may also be utilized. Intraocular metal eye shields are needed only when upper or lower eyelid skin *within* the orbital rim is to be treated. Device operators and ancillary staff must wear IPL glasses at all times when the device is in use. IPL system tests and confirmation of the correct cutoff filter or handpiece are performed immediately pretreatment. A typical IPL tray setup is shown in Figure 1.

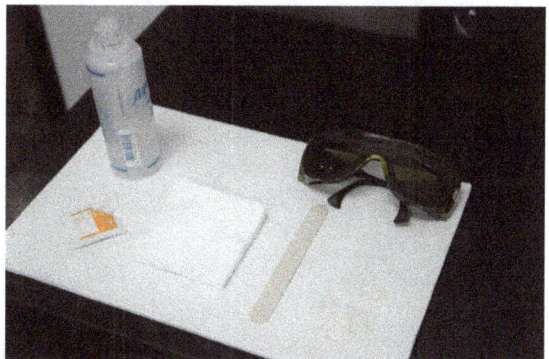

Fig. 1: Intense pulsed light (IPL) tray. [Clockwise: Ice-cold water-based ultrasound coupling gel, IPL glasses, disposable adhesive eye shields, tongue depressor (to apply gel), 4 × 4″ gauze, and an isopropyl alcohol swab].

TREATMENT

Treatment paradigms are, not surprisingly, rather similar between the numerous currently available IPL systems, with parameters individualized for each patient and the type of chromophore to be targeted. Given the large spot sizes and rapid pulse delivery of current IPL systems, a full face can be treated in 10 minutes or less. Patients often require a series of 2-6 (mean of 3) treatments spaced 3-4 weeks apart to achieve significant improvement.

The combination of an integrated chilled sapphire crystal tip, a 1 mm thick layer of cold water-based coupling gel, and periprocedural cold-air cooling provide epidermal protection and minimal patient discomfort during treatment. Cold gel is more than just a heat sink, enhancing optical coupling between the crystal and treatment area. This decreases the index of refraction of light and allows for deeper energy delivery. Water-based gel may likewise absorb potentially damaging, unnecessary near-infrared wavelengths more than 1,000 nm.[32]

Using the 35×15 mm crystal with the M22 system from Lumenis Ltd., light-skinned (FSTs I-II) Caucasian patients are treated using a 560 nm cutoff filter, with a 10-15 ms delay between double pulses (Figs. 2 and 3). Fluences of 16-18 J/ cm^2 are recommended initially for the face; however, based on clinical response, fluence may be increased by up to 10-20% with subsequent treatments until an optimal energy density is achieved. Darker skinned (FST III) Caucasian patients should be treated with a 560 nm filter, an interpulse delay of 20 ms, and fluences of 15-17 J/cm^2. Asian, Hispanic, or light-skinned African American patients with a FST III-IV require the use of a higher cutoff filter (590 nm) and longer interpulse delay (20-40 ms) in order to spare epidermal melanin (Figs. 4A and B). Dark-skinned patients (FST V) should be treated cautiously using a 695 or 755 nm cutoff filter and double to triple pulsing with low fluences (12-15 J/cm^2). Comparable settings by FST for other commonly used devices are shown in Table 1.

For lentigines, freckles, or other pigmented lesions, 3.0 ms double-pulsing is performed. Mild darkening is often noted almost immediately post-treatment (Figs. 5A and B). Using the M22, small-diameter, superficial vascular lesions such as telangiectasias are treated with a double pulse at 4.0 ms. Large caliber telangiectasias can also be safely double-pulsed at fluences of 19-26 J/cm^2 and a single pulse duration of 4-12 ms by means of a smaller 8×15 mm crystal. The treatment endpoint for vascular lesions is always transient vessel spasm (i.e. temporary vessel disappearance

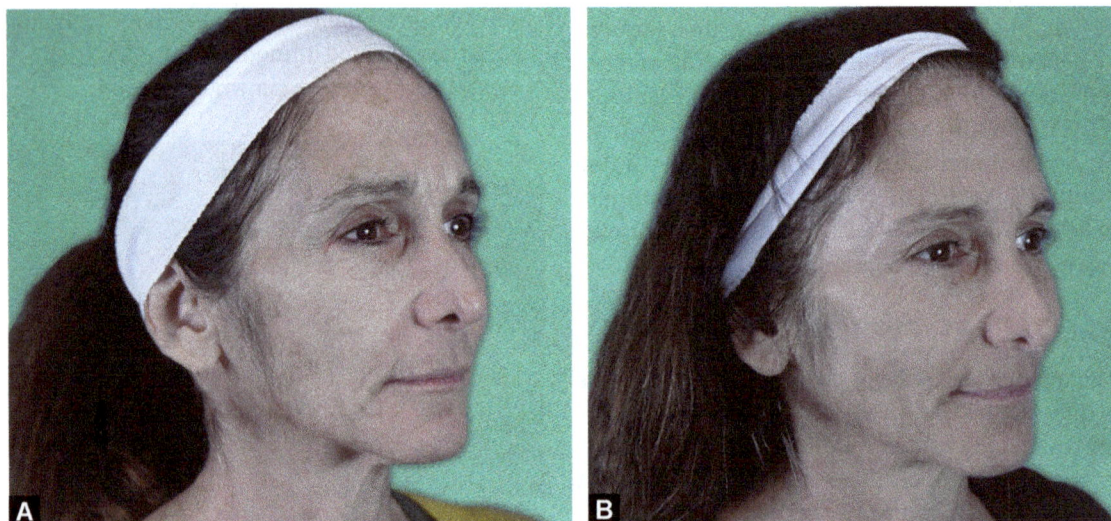

Figs. 2A and B: Before (A) and 3 months following (B) 3 monthly treatments with intense pulsed light (560 nm cutoff filter; 3 ms double pulse, 15 ms interpulse delay, and 18 J/cm^2 with 35×15 crystal to full face; 6 ms single pulse and 19 J/cm^2 with 8×15 mm crystal for fine telangiectasias).

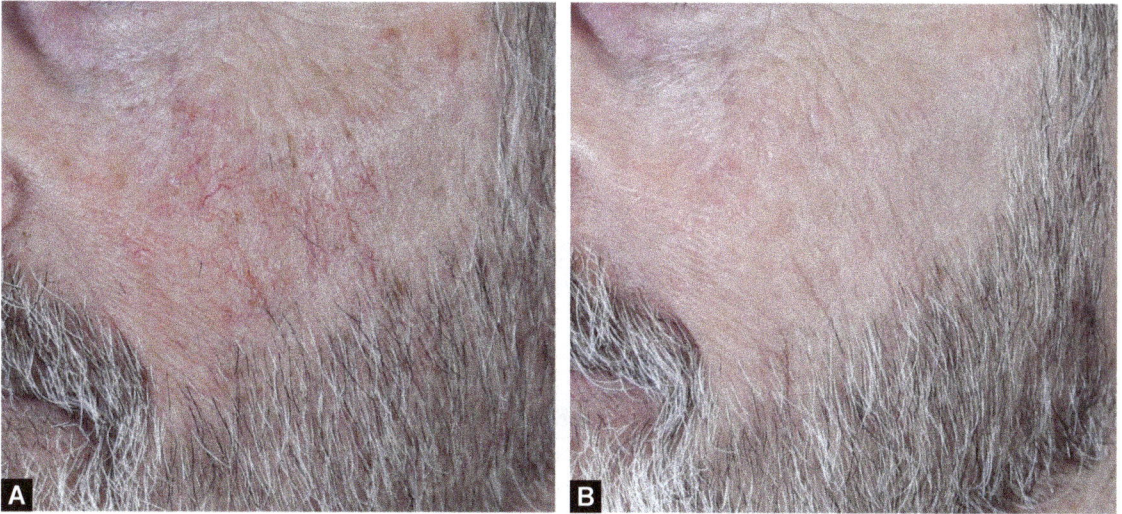

Figs. 3A and B: Before (A) and 3 months following (B) 3 monthly treatments with intense pulsed light (560 nm cutoff filter; 3 ms double pulse, 15 ms interpulse delay, and 17–18 J/cm² with 35 × 15 crystal to full face; 6–12 ms single pulse and 19–22 J/cm² with 8 × 15 mm crystal for fine telangiectasias).

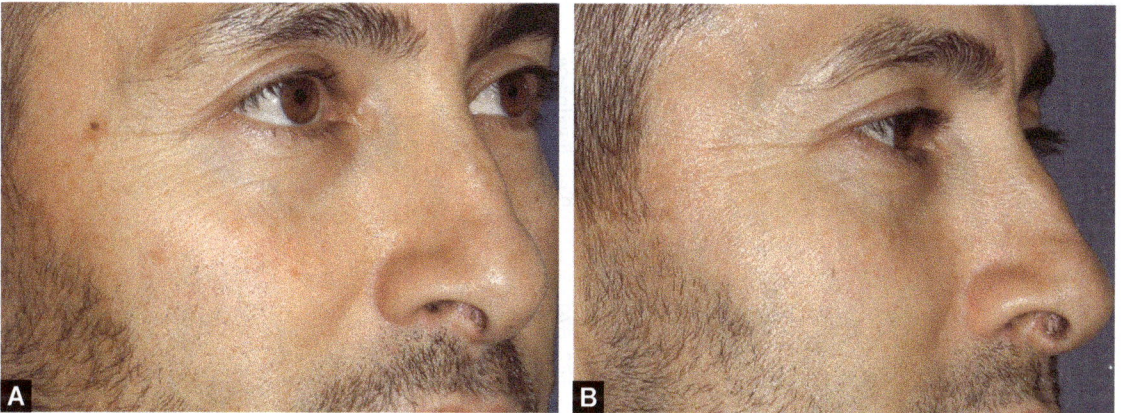

Figs. 4A and B: Before (A) and 1 month following (B) a single treatment with intense pulsed light for lentigines and fine telangiectasias of the periorbital areas and cheeks in a Hispanic male with type IV skin type (590 nm cutoff filter; 3–4 ms double pulse, 30 ms interpulse delay, and 16–17 J/cm² with 35 × 15 crystal).

or dusky discoloration). When treating vascular indications, minimal pressure should be applied against the skin with the handpiece so as to not compress the target vessels.

Since off-the-face treatments are prone to longer recovery and greater risk of adverse events, the authors also follow a simple algorithm based on facial settings, regardless of the patient skin type, indication, or device. Neck settings are obtained by decreasing the fluence by 5–10% and adding 5 ms to the interpulse delay from the treatment parameters used for the face. Moreover, fluence is decreased by 10–15% and interpulse delay increased by 5–10 ms for the chest, back, and upper/lower extremities, depending on the extent of photodamage (Figs. 6 and 7).

Post-treatment Considerations

Coupling gel is wiped away when the treatment is complete, and cold-air cooling or ice packs can be used in-office to reduce the mild burning sensation that may persist for 10–15 min post-treatment. A broad-spectrum physical (zinc oxide or titanium dioxide) sunscreen is also applied prior to departure. Since IPL treatments are noninva-

Table 1: Commonly used pulsed light devices for rosacea (R), telangiectasias (T), and lentigines (L).

	Nordlys (Ellipse A/S, Hørsholm, Denmark)	Palomar Icon (Cynosure, Inc., Westford, MA)	M22 (Lumenis Ltd., Yokneam, Israel)
FST I-II (Caucasian)	R: PR, 1.5 ms single pulse, 5–7 J/cm² T: PR, 13 ms, 13 J/cm² L: VL, 2.5/10/2.5 ms*, 10–14 J/cm²	R: Max G, 15–20 ms, 38–44 J/cm+ T: Max G, 10–15 ms, 40–42 J/cm² L: MaxG, 20–30 ms, 40–42 J/cm² or MaxYs, 15–20 ms, 23–40 J/cm²	R: 560 nm, 4/10–15/4 ms, 16–18 J/cm² T: 560 nm, 4–12 ms, 19–26 J/cm² L: 560 nm, 3/10–15/3 ms, 16–18 J/cm²
FST III (Caucasian)	R: PR, 1.5 ms, 4–6 J/cm² T: PR, 10 ms, 10 J/cm² L: VL, 2.5/10/2.5 ms, 4–6 J/cm²	R: Max G, 15–20 ms, 38–44 J/cm² T: Max G, 10–15 ms, 40–42 J/cm² L: MaxG, 20–30 ms, 40–42 J/cm² or MaxYs, 15–20 ms, 23–40 J/cm+	R: 560 nm, 4/20/4 ms, 15–17 J/cm² T: 560 nm, 4–12 ms, 19–25 J/cm² L: 560 nm, 3/20/3 ms, 15–17 J/cm²
FST III-IV (Asian, Hispanic, or light-skinned African American)	R: VL, 1.5 ms, 5–7 J/cm² T: VL, 15 ms, 13 J/cm² L: VL, 2.5/10/2.5 ms, 3–5 J/cm²	R: Max G, 20 ms, 36–40 J/cm² T: Max G, 20 ms, 36–40 J/cm² L: MaxG, 25-30 ms, 30–36 J/cm² or MaxYs, 20 ms, 20–30 J/cm²	R: 590 nm, 4/20–40/4 ms, 14–16 J/cm² T: 590 nm, 4–12 ms, 14–20 J/cm² L: 590 nm, 3/30–40/3 ms, 14–16 J/cm²
FST V	N/A	N/A	R: 699 or 755 nm, 4 ms triple pulse with 30–40 ms delays, 12–15 J/cm² T: 699 or 755 nm, 4/30–40/4 ms, 12–15 J/cm² L: 699 or 755 nm, 3 ms triple pulse with 40 ms delay, 12–15 J/cm²

PR: 530–755 nm handpiece; VL: 555–950 nm handpiece; MaxG: 500–670/870–1,200 nm handpiece; MaxYs: 525–1200 nm handpiece
VL handpiece: 555–950 nm
*Double pulse settings listed as 2.5/10/2.5 ms, indicating a 2.5 ms double pulse with 10 ms interpulse delay
Dark-skinned patients (FST V) should be treated cautiously using a 695 or 755 nm cutoff filter and double to triple pulsing with low fluences (12–15 J/cm²).
For lentigines, freckles, or other pigmented lesions, 3.0 ms double-pulsing is performed.
Using the M22, small-diameter, superficial vascular lesions, such as telangiectasias are treated with a double pulse at 4.0 ms. Large caliber telangiectasias can also be safely double-pulsed at fluences of 19–26 J/cm² and a single pulse duration of 4–12 ms by means of a smaller 8 × 15 mm crystal.

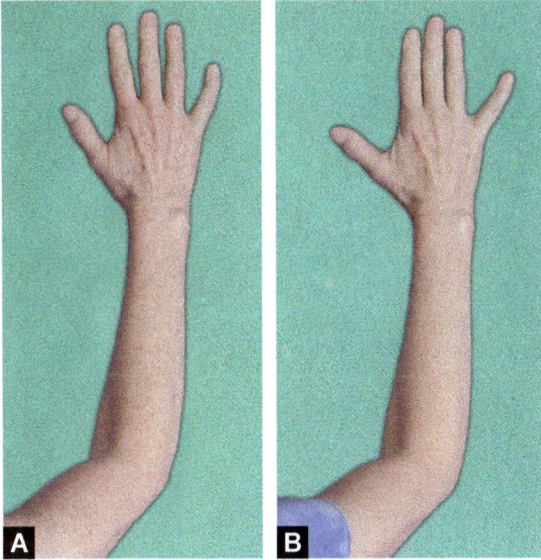

Figs. 5A and B: Mild darkening and erythema localized to lentigines evident minutes after an intense pulsed light treatment of the dorsal upper extremities (A) compared to baseline (B). Treatment parameters included a 560 nm cutoff filter, 3 ms double pulse, 15 ms interpulse delay, and 16 J/cm².

ultraviolet exposure is expected are encouraged in order to maintain optimal results.

BENEFITS COMPARED TO ALTERNATIVE APPROACHES

Intense pulsed light therapy is often recognized for its broad functionality and efficiency in treating various dermatological conditions. Unlike lasers, which are capable of only emitting one wavelength (or extremely narrow range of wavelengths), an IPL device emits a very broad spectrum of wavelengths, giving it the unique ability to treat multiple chromophores simultaneously. IPL devices also have the added benefit of targeting larger areas compared to other modalities due to its larger spot size. This characteristically decreases needed treatment time while also allowing clinicians to limit the number of pulses per treatment.[6] IPL has also been shown to cause less treatment discomfort and post-treatment edema than 595 nm or 532 nm laser devices in split-face studies, as well as far less risk of post-treatment purpura than the former.[33,34] Nevertheless, other studies have found superior clearance of facial telangiectasias and lentigines with a 595 nm pulsed-dye laser than IPL.[35,36] Compared to an erbium:YAG laser micropeel, IPL also leads

sive and require minimal recovery, patients can thereby proceed with normal life activities immediately postprocedure. Subsequent semiannual to annual maintenance treatments and strict sun protection with reapplication every 2 hours when

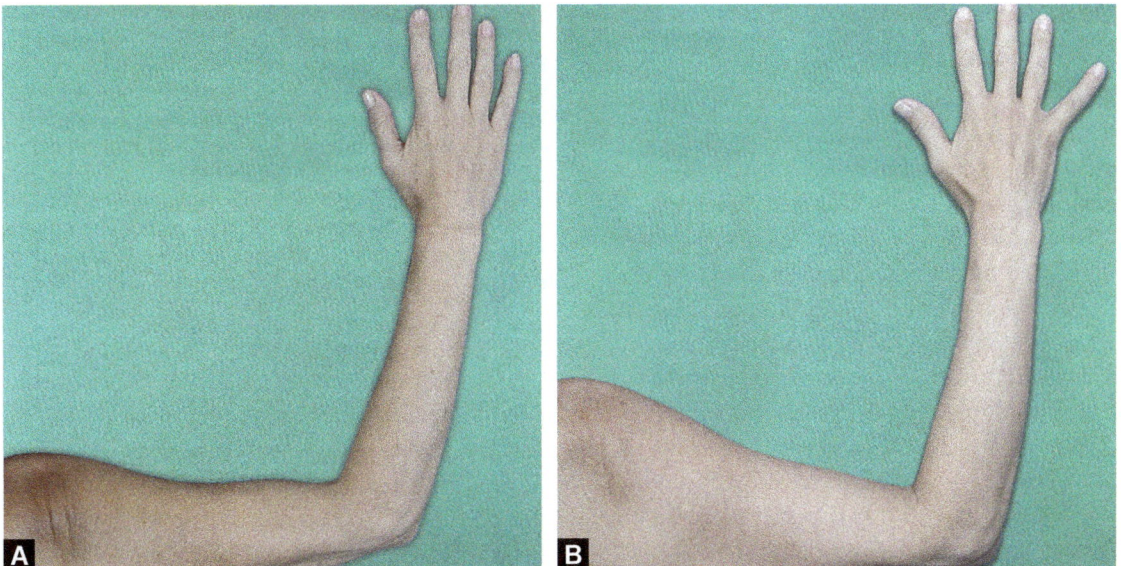

Figs. 6A and B: Before (A) and 1 month following (B) three treatments with intense pulsed light to dorsal upper extremities (560 nm cutoff filter; 3 ms double pulse, 20 ms interpulse delay, and 14–17 J/cm² with 35 × 15 crystal).

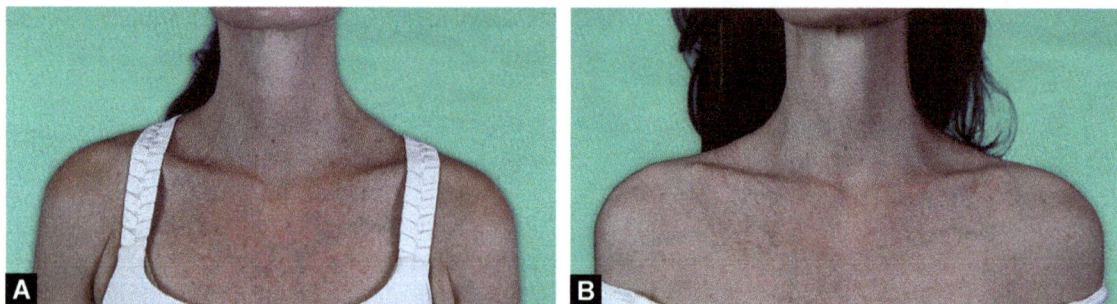

Figs. 7A and B: Before (A) and 1 month following (B) three treatments with intense pulsed light to extensive photodamage of the neck, chest, and shoulders (560 nm cutoff filter; 3–3.5 ms double pulse, 20 ms interpulse delay, and 14–17 J/cm^2 with 35 × 15 crystal).

to equivalent results with far less downtime.[37] Although IPL and a Q-switched 1064 Nd:YAG device led to equivalent improvement in skin texture and pore size, IPL treatment was faster but was not as effective for skin tone.[38]

Although sclerotherapy is the gold standard for reticular (feeder) and telangiectatic (spider) veins of the lower extremities, IPL may be a valuable adjunct therapy for refractory or noncannulable (≤0.3 mm) telangiectasias following sclerotherapy. Patients with an allergy to sclerosing agents (extremely rare), needle phobia, or who refuse to wear graduated compression stockings may also benefit from IPL therapy.[39]

RISKS/LIMITATIONS

Adverse events from IPL treatment are commonly mild and self-limited. The most common expected adverse event is erythema, which usually resolves within hours to 3 days and can be masked with green-tinted makeup. A subset of patients may develop edema for 24–72 hours following initial full-face treatment. Postprocedure topical steroid use for erythema and edema is rarely necessary. Coffee ground crusting of pigmented lesions is expected but may not develop for several days to a week and resolves by 2 weeks post-treatment. Purpura formation is very rare with IPL but can occur with the use of overly short pulse durations or 515 nm wavelength filters, resolving within 2–5 days. Given that IPL can permanently damage dark-colored terminal hairs, IPL treatments are generally avoided in hair-bearing skin of the male beard area without prior informed consent.

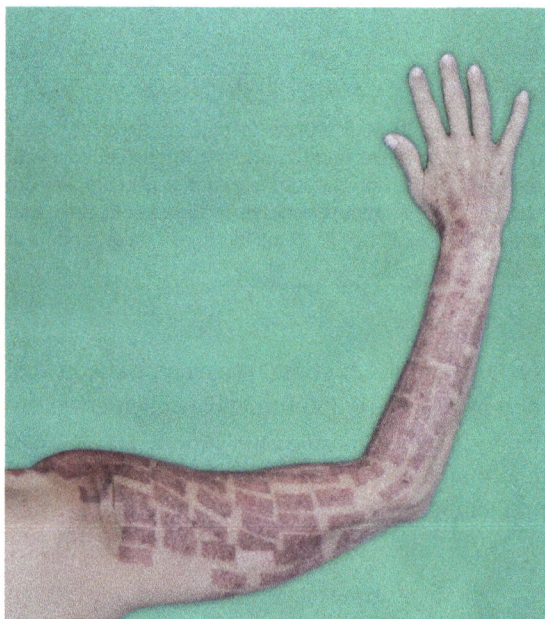

Fig. 8: Severe erythematous reticular footprinting (striping) with a few scattered superficial erosions following initial intense pulsed light treatment of the patient in Figure 6. Potential causes include significant sun exposure in the days prior to treatment or the unintentional use of a 515 nm (instead of a 560 nm) cutoff filter. Two further treatments with nearly the same fluences and identical interpulse delays led to no further striping. The patient experienced no long-term sequelae of this adverse event.

The striping of untreated areas between reticular footprints may occur with the use of aggressive treatment parameters, as well as the use of normal (but relatively inappropriate) settings in tan or dark-skinned patients (Fig. 8).[7,40] Employing a 10% overlap between pulses minimizes reticular footprinting. If it occurs, it can be easily corrected with subsequent (often more conservative) treatment of the interspersed untreated areas, typically with the IPL crystal rotated 90°.

Excessive overlapping, exorbitant fluences, poor epidermal cooling, and/or insufficient delay between sequential pulses, particularly in tan or dark-skinned individuals, may lead to dyspigmentation, blistering, and scabbing.[40] Nevertheless, the safety of IPL treatment in darker skin types (IV–V) has been well documented.[20,41] Scarring due to inappropriate treatment parameters or technique is exceedingly rare.

CONCLUSION

Intense pulsed light technology has proven to be a safe, multifaceted, and effective treatment option for multiple pigmentary and vascular conditions of the skin with minimal downtime. As the use of IPL devices widens and our understanding of the technology expands, the range of applications for this modality continues to grow.

REFERENCES

1. Wat H, Wu DC, Rao J, et al. Application of intense pulsed light in the treatment of dermatologic disease: a systematic review. Dermatol Surg. 2014;40: 359-77.
2. Raulin C, Weiss RA, Schönermark MP. Treatment of essential telangiectasias with an intense pulsed light source (PhotoDerm VL). Dermatol Surg. 1997;23:941-5.
3. Goldman MP, Eckhouse S. Photothermal sclerosis of leg veins. ESC Medical Systems, LTD Photoderm VL Cooperative Study Group. Dermatol Surg. 1996;22:323-30.
4. Raulin C, Hellwig S, Schönermark MP. Treatment of a nonresponding port-wine stain with a new pulsed light source (PhotoDerm VL). Lasers Surg Med. 1997;21:203-8.
5. Gold MH, Bell MW, Foster TD, et al. Long-term epilation using the EpiLight broad band, intense pulsed light hair removal system. Dermatol Surg. 1997;23:909-13.
6. Goldberg DJ. Current trends in intense pulsed light. J Clin Aesthet Dermatol. 2012;5:45-53.
7. Goldman MP, Weiss RA, Weiss MA. Intense pulsed light as a nonablative approach to photoaging. Dermatol Surg. 2005;31:1179-87.
8. Ross EV, Smirnov M, Pankratov M, et al. Intense pulsed light and laser treatment of facial telangiectasias and dyspigmentation: some theoretical and practical comparisons. Dermatol Surg. 2005;31:1188-98.
9. Steinke JM, Shepherd AP. Effects of temperature on optical absorbance spectra of oxy-, carboxy-, and deoxyhemoglobin. Clin Chem. 1992;38:1360-4.
10. Cao Y, Huo R, Feng Y, et al. Effects of intense pulsed light on the biological properties and ultrastructure of skin dermal fibroblasts: potential roles in photoaging. Photomed Laser Surg. 2011; 29:327-32.
11. El-Domyati M, El-Ammawi TS, Moawad O, et al. Intense pulsed light photorejuvenation: a histological and immunohistochemical evaluation. J Drugs Dermatol. 2011;10:1246-52.
12. Feng Y, Zhao J, Gold MH. Skin rejuvenation in Asian skin: the analysis of clinical effects and basic mechanisms of intense pulsed light. J Drugs Dermatol. 2008;7:273-9.
13. Iyer S, Carranza D, Kolodney M, et al. Evaluation of procollagen I deposition after intense pulsed light treatments at varying parameters in a porcine model. J Cosmet Laser Ther. 2007;9:75-8.
14. Luo D, Cao Y, Wu D, et al. Impact of intense pulse light irradiation on BALB/c mouse skin-in vivo study on collagens, matrix metalloproteinases and vascular endothelial growth factor. Lasers Med Sci. 2009;24:101-8.
15. Huang J, Luo X, Lu J, et al. IPL irradiation rejuvenates skin collagen via the bidirectional regulation of MMP-1 and TGF-β1 mediated by MAPKs in fibroblasts. Lasers Med Sci. 2011;26:381-7.
16. Wong WR, Shyu WL, Tsai JW, et al. Intense pulsed light effects on the expression of extracellular matrix proteins and transforming growth factor beta-1 in skin dermal fibroblasts cultured within contracted collagen lattices. Dermatol Surg. 2009; 35:816-25.
17. Wong WR, Shyu WL, Tsai JW, et al. Intense pulsed light modulates the expressions of MMP-2, MMP-14 and TIMP-2 in skin dermal fibroblasts cultured within contracted collagen lattices. J Dermatol Sci. 2008;51:70-3.
18. Hernández-Pérez E, Ibiett EV. Gross and microscopic findings in patients submitted to nonablative full-face resurfacing using intense pulsed light: a preliminary study. Dermatol Surg. 2002;28: 651-5.
19. Patriota RC, Rodrigues CJ, Cucé LC. Intense pulsed light in photoaging: a clinical, histopathological and immunohistochemical evaluation. An Bras Dermatol. 2011;86:1129-33.
20. Li YH, Wu Y, Chen JZS, et al. A split-face study of intense pulsed light on photoaging skin in Chinese population. Lasers Surg Med. 2010;42:185-91.
21. Goldberg DJ. New collagen formation after dermal remodeling with an intense pulsed light source. J Cutan Laser Ther. 2000;2:59-61.
22. Prieto VG, Sadick NS, Lloreta J, et al. Effects of intense pulsed light on sun-damaged human skin, routine, and ultrastructural analysis. Lasers Surg Med. 2002;30:82-5.

23. Trelles MA, Allones I, Velez M. Nonablative facial skin photorejuvenation with an intense pulsed light system and adjunctive epidermal care. Lasers Med Sci. 2003;18:104-11.

24. Bitter PH. Noninvasive rejuvenation of photodamaged skin using serial, full-face intense pulsed light treatments. Dermatol Surg. 2000;26:835-42.

25. Goldberg DJ, Cutler KB. Nonablative treatment of rhytids with intense pulsed light. Lasers Surg Med. 2000;26:196-200.

26. Bjerring P, Christiansen K, Troilius A, et al. Facial photorejuvenation using two different intense pulsed light (IPL) wavelength bands. Lasers Surg Med. 2004;34:120-6.

27. Sadick NS, Weiss R, Kilmer S, et al. Photorejuvenation with intense pulsed light: results of a multi-center study. J Drugs Dermatol. 2004;3:41-9.

28. Rusciani A, Motta A, Fino P, et al. Treatment of poikiloderma of Civatte using intense pulsed light source: 7 years of experience. Dermatol Surg. 2008;34:314-9.

29. Vanaman M, Fabi SG, Cox SE. Neck rejuvenation using a combination approach: our experience and a review of the literature. Dermatol Surg. 2016;42:S94-S100.

30. Weiss RA, Weiss MA, Beasley KL. Rejuvenation of photoaged skin: 5 years results with intense pulsed light of the face, neck, and chest. Dermatol Surg. 2002;28:1115-9.

31. Wu DC, Friedmann DP, Fabi SG, et al. Comparison of intense pulsed light with 1,927-nm fractionated thulium fiber laser for the rejuvenation of the chest. Dermatol Surg. 2014;40:129-33.

32. Weiss RA, Weiss MA, Goldman MP. Intense pulsed light and nonablative approaches to photoaging. In: Goldman MP, Weiss RA (Eds). Advanced Techniques in Dermatologic Surgery. New York, NY: Taylor & Francis Group; 2006. pp. 299.

33. Galeckas KJ, Collins M, Ross EV, et al. Split-face treatment of facial dyschromia: pulsed dye laser with a compression handpiece versus intense pulsed light. Dermatol Surg. 2008;34:672-80.

34. Butler EG, McClellan SD, Ross EV. Split treatment of photodamaged skin with KTP 532 nm laser with 10 mm handpiece versus IPL: a cheek-to-cheek comparison. Lasers Surg Med. 2006;38:124-8.

35. Jørgensen GF, Hedelund L, Hædersdal M. Long-pulsed dye laser versus intense pulsed light for photodamaged skin: a randomized split-face trial with blinded response evaluation. Lasers Surg Med. 2008;40:293-9.

36. Kono T, Groff WF, Sakurai H, et al. Comparison study of intense pulsed light versus a long-pulse pulsed dye laser in the treatment of facial skin rejuvenation. Ann Plast Surg. 2007;59:479-83.

37. Hantash BM, De Coninck E, Liu H, et al. Split-face comparison of the erbium micropeel with intense pulsed light. Dermatol Surg. 2008;34:763-72.

38. Huo MH, Wang YQ, Yang X. Split-face comparison of intense pulsed light and nonablative 1,064-nm Q-switched laser in skin rejuvenation. Dermatol Surg. 2011;37:52-7.

39. Meesters AA, Pitassi LHU, Campos V, et al. Transcutaneous laser treatment of leg veins. Lasers Med Sci. 2014;29:481-92.

40. Greve B, Raulin C. Professional errors caused by lasers and intense pulsed light technology in dermatology and aesthetic medicine: preventive strategies and case studies. Dermatol Surg. 2002; 28:156-61.

41. Munavalli GS, Weiss RA, Halder RM. Photoaging and nonablative photorejuvenation in ethnic skin. Dermatol Surg. 2005;31:1250-60.

PART 6

Tips and Tricks: Photodynamic Therapy

— Allison R Cruse, Dylan Harrell, Jeremy D Jackson

CHAPTER 19

Photodynamic Therapy

Allison R Cruse, Patrick C Carr, Dylan Harrell, Jeremy D Jackson

> *"Photodynamic therapy is today's leading non-surgical miracle for aging skin, acne, and skin cancer"*
>
> —Kimberly Moskowitz

HISTORY OF PHOTODYNAMIC THERAPY

Photodynamic therapy (PDT) was first described in the early 1900s. Oscar Raab, a German medical student observed that paramecium cultures exposed to acridine dye in conjunction with light died, while paramecium exposed to either acridine or light alone survived. His professor expounded on this observation and used a combination of topical eosin and white light to treat skin tumors while further demonstrating the role of oxygen in such photosensitization reactions. The term "photodynamic action" was created to describe this phenomenon. In 1913, photosensitization by hematoporphyrin was reported. This discovery was later improved upon with the development of hematoporphyrin derivative (HPD), a synthetic porphyrin mixture with better affinity for tumor tissue and stronger phototoxicity than crude hematoporphyrin.[1]

Despite these advancements, PDT's potential for tumor eradication was not fully realized until a series of investigations on humans performed in the 1970s by Dougherty and colleagues. A series of skin cancers were successfully treated with HPD and red light from a xenon arc lamp.[1,2] There were, however, major limitations in the treatment of skin cancer with HPD. Most notably patients developed persistent skin photosensitization.

The introduction of porphyrin precursors such as topical 5-aminolevulinic acid (ALA) in 1990 was a significant milestone in the development of PDT skin cancer treatment because photosensitization typically resolves in 24 hours.[1,3] Topical ALA plus blue fluorescent light was approved by the US Federation of Drug Administration (FDA) for the treatment of actinic keratoses (AKs) in 1999 followed by the approval of topical methyl aminolevulinate (mALA) plus red light for the treatment of AKs in 2004.

MECHANISM

Photodynamic therapy involves the interaction of light, oxygen, and a photosensitizer, which is a molecule that localizes to target cells and can be activated by the light source. Once exposed to the appropriate wavelength of light, the photosensitizer is activated from its ground state to its excited state. When the photosensitizer returns to its ground state, the energy is released in the form of oxygen free radicals, which leads to damage of intracellular organelles and cell death.[4]

Photosensitizers

Two photosensitizers are currently approved by the FDA for the treatment of dermatologic conditions: (1) ALA, and (2) mALA. Once absorbed, these inactive molecules are converted into protoporphyrin IX, an active photosensitizing compound, by the heme biosynthetic pathway. These photosensitizers pass easily through abnormal keratin and are more easily taken up by abnormal or malignant cells than by normal cells.[4]

In the United States, ALA is approved as a 20% topical solution (Levulan® Kerastick®) in combination with blue light for the treatment of AKs of the face and scalp. In 2016, the FDA approved a 10% gel formulation of ALA (Ameluz®) in combination with a red light source for lesion-directed and field-directed treatment of AKs of the face and scalp. mALA (Metvixia®), a methylated derivative of ALA, is approved in a 16.8% cream formulation in combination with red light for the treatment of AKs of the face and scalp. Although available in Europe (Metvix®), mALA is no longer commercially available in the United States. While mALA has increased lipophilicity compared with ALA allowing for deeper skin penetration, studies have shown there is no difference in efficacy between ALA and mALA in the treatment of AKs and basal cell carcinoma (BCC).[42]

Light Sources

Several light sources are available for PDT, though only two are approved by the FDA. Protoporphyrin IX has a strong absorption peak in the blue wavelength region of the visible light spectrum (405–420 nm), as well as the red wavelength region (635 nm). Longer wavelengths correlate with deeper tissue penetration. While blue light, which has a shorter wavelength than red light, is sufficient for treatment of thin AKs, red light provides a deeper clinical effect and is better suited for deeper lesions, such as sebaceous hyperplasia, Bowen's disease, or BCC.[4,5]

> For the treatment of deeper lesions such as sebaceous hyperplasia, Bowen's disease, and basal cell carcinoma, a red light source is recommended because of its greater tissue penetration.

ACTINIC KERATOSES

Actinic keratoses are rough, scaly lesions in chronically sun-exposed areas with the potential to progress to squamous cell carcinoma (SCC). The conversion rate ranges from 6% to 20% over 10 years, and approximately 65% of all primary SCCs arise in lesions previously diagnosed as AKs.[6] Actinic keratoses can be effectively treated with cryotherapy, chemical peels, curettage, or topical treatments such as 5-fluorouracil (5-FU), imiquimod, ingenol mebutate, and diclofenac. PDT with ALA or mALA is approved for the treatment of AKs of the face and scalp. PDT has been shown to have a 14% better chance of clearance of thin AKs of the face and scalp at 3 months compared with cryotherapy alone.[7] PDT with blue light has also been reported to not only be more effective than treatment with 5-FU but better tolerated as well.[8] Additionally, treatment with PDT has an improved cosmetic outcome when compared with cryotherapy and 5-FU.[9] Although approved for the treatment of AKs of the face and scalp, PDT is also commonly used clinically to treat AKs of the upper extremities. In general, response rates are greater for the face than the scalp.[10] Treatment response on the upper extremities is greatly reduced.[11]

Multiple PDT regimens have been used for the treatment of AKs. Modifications have been made to improve response rates and decrease adverse side effects. In general, the steps in performing PDT for AKs include:

1. "Degreasing" the treatment area with alcohol or acetone.
2. The photosensitizer (ALA or mALA) is applied to the specific lesions and often the general area for field cancerization.
3. An incubation period ranging from 30 minutes to 4 hours is allowed before placing the patient under the chosen light source.
4. The patient is placed under the chosen light source for a specific amount of time (16 minutes and 40 seconds for the Blu-U® light source).
5. The area is then washed with soap and water and sunscreen is liberally applied.
6. The patient is advised to follow strict sun avoidance for 40 hours after the treatment.

While there is great variability in the clinical use of PDT, most of this variability is related to incubation times, pretreatment mechanisms, and light sources.

Incubation Times

Photodynamic therapy was originally approved by the FDA for the treatment of AKs after a 14–18-hour incubation period. Although effective, this long incubation time is not practical in clinical use. Shorter incubation periods of 1–3 hours are commonly used and can still be effective for clearance of AKs. These shorter incubation periods also decrease the reported pain associated with PDT therapy. Pariser and colleagues showed that incubation of 1-hour after application of ALA showed similar efficacy as 2- and 3-hour incubation periods. Patients who were incubated for 1-hour had decreased incidence and severity of side effects including edema, erythema, stinging, and burning. A repeat PDT treatment 8 weeks later using a 1-hour incubation period showed similar lesion clearance to the FDA-approved 14–18-hour incubation period (79% vs 83.4%).[12]

> 1-hour incubation will maintain efficacy while decreasing adverse side effects like edema, erythema, stinging and burning.

> Two treatments of PDT, 8 weeks apart, will increase efficacy.

Pretreatment

Adequate penetration and absorption of the photosensitizer is important in effective treatment with PDT. PDT is approved for the treatment of minimally to moderately thick AKs. Hyperkeratotic AKs respond less to PDT than nonhyperkeratotic lesions. Although approved for treatment of AKs on the face and scalp, PDT is often used to treat AKs on the extremities. However, the efficacy of PDT on the extremities is lower than that on the face and scalp. Several techniques for pretreatment of AKs have been used in efforts to improve penetration of the photosensitizer and increase the efficacy of PDT.

Curettage is the most common technique used to remove hyperkeratotic scale before application of the photosensitizer. It is an inexpensive and effective way to enhance treatment of thicker lesions.[13] Other methods that can be used for pretreatment include microdermabrasion, microneedling with dermarollers, and ablative fractional laser. Although ablative fractional laser has been shown to be most effective in improving efficacy, it is not as readily available and involves high costs that may be prohibitive.[13,14] The use of topical retinoids for 1–2 weeks prior to PDT can also be an effective pretreatment that improves treatment efficacy, particularly to the upper extremities.[15]

> Curettage of thicker lesions prior to application of the photosensitizer is an inexpensive technique that improves efficacy.

Two other effective and inexpensive pretreatment techniques are—(1) occlusion and (2) temperature elevation. These techniques are particularly helpful for treatment of the upper extremities. Occlusion with plastic wrap after application of the photosensitizer can improve treatment responses with PDT (Figs. 1A to C). Patients reported increased erythema and pain with occlusive pretreatment but still tolerated the treatment well.[14]

> Occlusion with plastic wrap (Saran™ or Glad® Press'n Seal®) after application of the photosensitizer improves efficacy of PDT when treating the upper extremities.

Increased temperatures increase the synthesis of protoporphyrin IX after the application of ALA or mALA. This can result in improved efficacy of PDT. After application of the photosensitizer, the arms are occluded with plastic wrap. Heating pads are then wrapped around the upper extremities and turned to medium setting for a 1-hour incubation (Fig. 2). Heating pads should not be used in patients with any impaired sensory or vasomotor function, such as patients with peripheral vascular disease or diabetes. Although usually tolerated, there is an increase in pain during treatment and erythema after treatment.[11]

> The use of heating pads during incubation results in increased temperatures and increased efficacy of PDT treatments on the upper extremities.

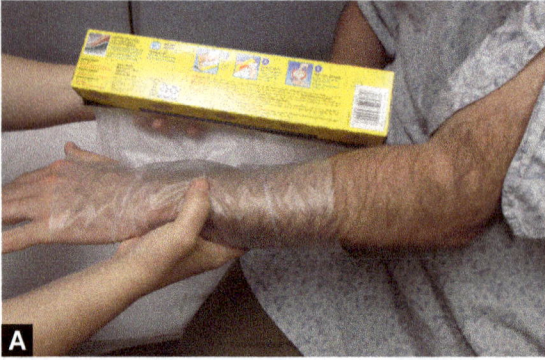

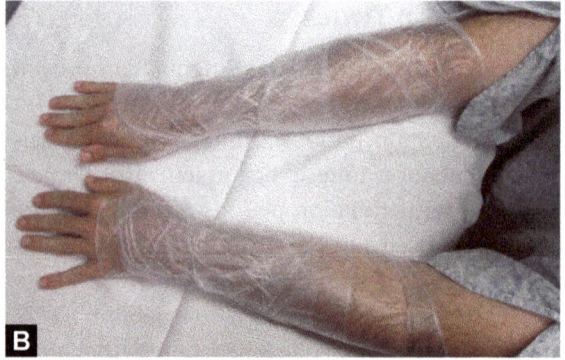

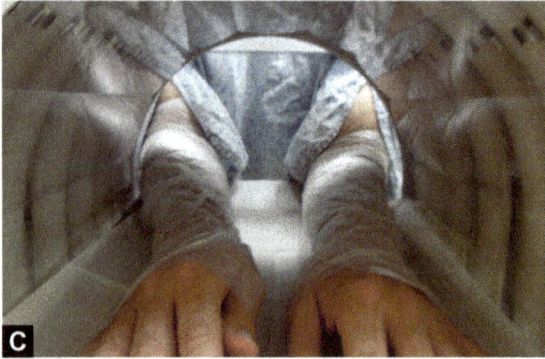

Figs. 1A to C: After application of topical ALA (Levulan®) to the forearms and dorsal hands, Glad® Press'n Seal® is wrapped around the treated areas for occlusion during the incubation and treatment period.

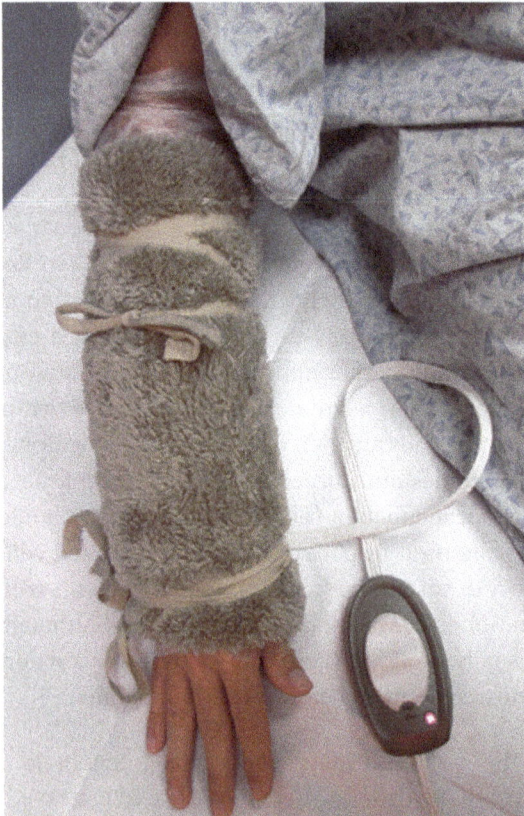

Fig. 2: A heating pad is wrapped around the forearm and turned to medium setting for a 1-hour incubation period.

Daylight Photodynamic Therapy

Photodynamic therapy using natural daylight was first described in 2008. It has been found to be as effective in treating AKs on the face and scalp as conventional PDT using a blue or red light source. Daylight PDT does not require the longer incubation periods or the availability of an artificial light source. Daylight PDT is as effective as conventional PDT but is better tolerated with less pain reported. The protocol involves application of the photosensitizer and exposure to daylight within 30 minutes of application. The patient should be exposed to natural sunlight for 2 hours. After 2 hours of exposure, the patient should wash off the treated area with soap and water. Sunscreen should be applied after washing the area, and the patient should remain indoors the remainder of the day and avoid sun exposure for the next 48 hours. Similar pretreatment techniques as discussed for conventional PDT may be used to enhance the response. Daylight PDT is a good option for patients who did not tolerate conventional PDT.[16,17]

PDT using natural daylight is as effective as PDT using artificial light sources but is better tolerated with less associated pain.

DECREASING ADVERSE SIDE EFFECTS

Studies have shown that the tolerability to PDT is high. Pain during PDT is the most common limiting side effect, and erythema and edema are common side effects after treatment. Expectations should be given to patients in pretreatment counseling (Fig. 3). At 4 weeks after treatment with ALA and Blu-U®, all erythema and edema should resolve.[18] In this author's experience, most erythema and edema resolve 5–7 days after treatment. Strategies to decrease pain and other side effects, such as erythema and edema have previously been discussed. Daylight PDT and 1-hour incubation times both have been shown to decrease pain and erythema. Although they increase efficacy, pretreatment techniques such as occlusion and temperature elevation increase pain and erythema and may need to be avoided in patients who have concerns or previous experience with pain with PDT. The use of a handheld fan during treatment can be helpful in decreasing pain during the procedure (Figs. 4A and B). Cold air analgesia is a preferred approach to pain management during PDT and has been shown to also decrease erythema and edema following treatment. Nonsteroidal anti-inflammatory drugs (NSAIDs) have been shown to be effective in management of pain following PDT.[19] In our experience, the liberal use of petroleum jelly for 5 days following PDT improves pain and reduces erythema.

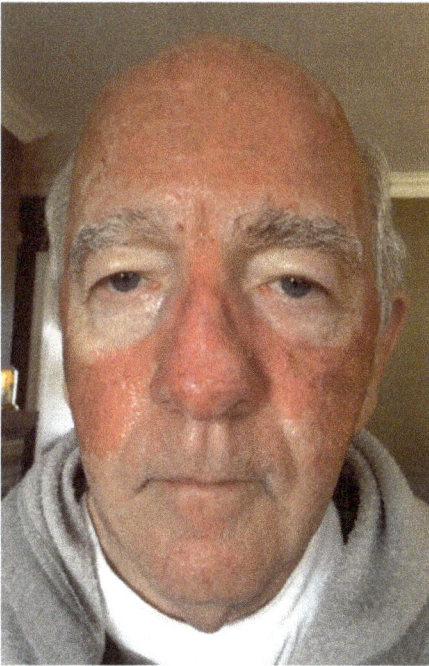

Fig. 3: Expected result 4 days after treatment with photodynamic therapy-5-aminolevulinic acid (PDT-ALA). Patients should be counseled appropriately about post-treatment expectations.

> Pain during treatment with PDT is the most common limiting side effect and can be mitigated by the use of a handheld fan during treatment.

> Erythema and edema after PDT treatment is often short-lasting but can be managed with use of NSAIDs and topical petroleum jelly. Patients should be counseled about post-treatment expectations.

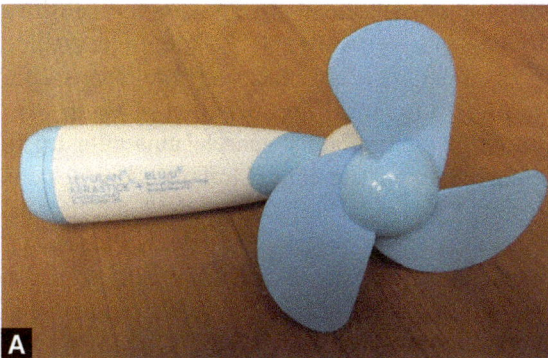

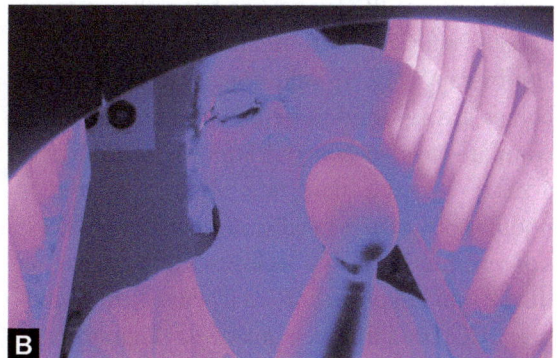

Figs. 4A and B: The use of a handheld fan, such as those provided by Levulan® Kerastick®, can be helpful in decreasing pain during treatment with photodynamic therapy (PDT).

Squamous Cell Carcinoma

The treatment options for SCC are based on metastatic potential. There are multiple treatment options for low risk cutaneous SCC, whereas surgical excision is required for invasive cutaneous SCC. PDT can be effective in treating SCC in situ (Bowen's disease), but it is ineffective in treating invasive SCC.[5,20] ALA-PDT has been shown to be more effective than 5-FU in treating Bowen's disease with a complete response rate of 88% vs 67% with 5-FU. After 1 year of follow-up, complete clinical clearance rates were 82% vs 42% with 5-FU. An incoherent light source was used in the red light range for this study. A larger study using mALA and red light showed similar cure rates of Bowen's disease (93% complete response; 74% cure at 1 year).[5] PDT also offers less scarring and an improved cosmetic profile when compared to cryotherapy or 5-FU.[21]

> PDT is an option for treatment of SCC in situ (Bowen's disease). Cure rates of Bowen's disease with PDT compare favorably to other non-surgical therapies.

Basal Cell Carcinoma

Treatment options for BCC include excisional surgery, Mohs micrographic surgery, electrodesiccation and curettage, radiation, cryotherapy, laser surgery, imiquimod, 5-FU, vismodegib, and PDT. The use of PDT to treat BCCs has been studied extensively. PDT is very effective at treating superficial BCCs and has been shown to be equally efficacious in treatment compared to cryotherapy (Fig. 5). Additionally, cosmetic outcomes are reported to be better with PDT when compared to cryotherapy.[22] Superficial BCCs have a more favorable cure rate when compared to nodular BCCs (87% vs 53%, respectively).[5] PDT is not recommended to treat lesions that are deeper than 2 mm but pretreatment by curettage of nodular BCCs can improve outcomes.[23] Light sources in the visible red light range were used in these studies.

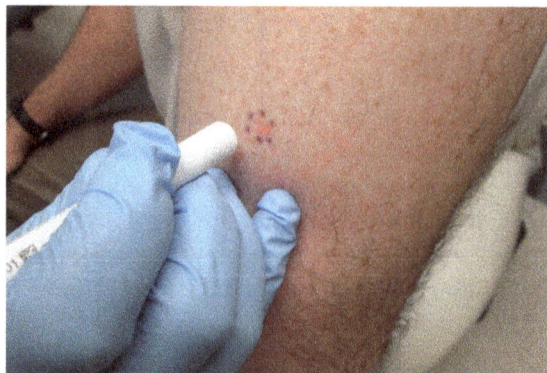

Fig. 5: Application of topical 5-aminolevulinic acid (ALA) (Levulan® Kerastick®) to a typical superficial basal cell carcinoma (BCC).

> PDT is an effective treatment option for treating superficial BCCs, but is less effective in the treatment of nodular BCCs. The choice of appropriate lesions is important when deciding whether to treat BCC with PDT therapy. Thicker lesions and morpheaform BCCs are less likely to respond to PDT.

OTHER USES OF PHOTODYNAMIC THERAPY

Acne Vulgaris

With growing concerns about antibiotic resistance and side effects from isotretinoin, PDT offers a relatively safe method for treating acne vulgaris. PDT is effective in the treatment of acne because it selectively targets the pilosebaceous unit and decreases the number of *Propionibacterium acnes*. *P. acnes* naturally makes porphyrins as a by-product of its metabolism, so it is very sensitive to light-based treatments.[24,25] High intensity blue light alone, in the absence of any photosensitizer, can lead to clinical improvement of up to two-thirds of inflammatory acne lesions after up to eight treatment sessions.[24] Inflammatory lesions respond better to PDT than comedonal lesions. For best results, one study concluded that long-term remission was associated with incubation periods of 3 hours or more. A red light source, due to its deeper penetration, is more likely to destroy sebaceous glands, resulting in higher response rates.[26]

Sebaceous Hyperplasia

Sebaceous hyperplasia is a benign condition often seen on the face of older patients. Because of the accumulation of porphyrins in sebaceous glands, PDT is a possible treatment option. There is evidence that PDT therapy with a 1-hour incubation period is sufficient to clear sebaceous hyperplasia regardless of light source. Multiple treatments are often needed. Combined treatment with PDT and ablative laser or pulsed-dye laser is reported to be more effective than PDT alone in the treatment of sebaceous hyperplasia.[25]

LESS COMMON USES

Photodynamic therapy has been shown to be effective in treating other conditions, such as cutaneous T-cell lymphoma, hidradenitis suppurativa, actinic cheilitis, verruca vulgaris, and Leishmaniasis.[4,27] Nail diseases, such as nail psoriasis and onychomycosis have been studied using PDT. PDT alone was not effective in treating nail psoriasis but when combined with tazarotene, did show better response than treatment with tazarotene alone. PDT has shown some effectiveness in the treatment of onychomycosis but further studies are needed.[25]

Because it is inexpensive and has relatively low side effects, the use of PDT for multiple cutaneous conditions continues to be investigated. It is an effective treatment option for the clinician for actinic keratoses, Bowen's disease, and superficial BCCs. There continues to be innovative ideas in order to make therapy more effective and more tolerable. Hopefully, using some of these tips will improve your clinical outcomes using PDT.

REFERENCES

1. Ackroyd R, Kelty C, Brown N, et al. The history of photodetection and photodynamic therapy. Photochem Photobiol. 2001;74(5):656-69.
2. Dougherty TJ. Photoradiation therapy for the treatment of malignant tumours. Cancer Res. 1978;36:2628-35.
3. Kennedy JC, Pottier RH. Endogenous protoporphyrin IX, a clinically useful photosensitizer for photodynamic therapy. J Photochem Photobiol B. 1992;14:275-92.
4. Wan MT, Lin JY. Current evidence and applications of photodynamic therapy in dermatology. Clin Cosmetic Investig Dermatol. 2014;7:145-63.
5. Szeimies RM, Morton CA, Sidoroff A, et al. Photodynamic therapy for non-melanoma skin cancer. Acta Derm Venereol. 2005;85:483-90.
6. Criscione VD, Weinstock MA, Naylor MF, et al. Actinic keratoses: natural history and risk of malignant transformation in the Veterans Affairs Topical Tretinoin Chemoprevention Trial. Cancer. 2009;116:23-30.
7. Patel G, Armstrong AW, Eisen DB. Efficacy of photodynamic therapy vs other interventions in randomized clinical trials for the treatment of actinic keratoses: a systematic review and meta-analysis. JAMA Dermatol. 2014;150(12):1281-8.
8. Smith S, Piacquadio D, Morhenn V, et al. Short incubation PDT versus 5-FU in treating actinic keratoses. J Drugs Dermatol 2003;2(6):629-35.
9. Gupta AK, Paquet M, Villanueva E, et al. Interventions for actinic keratoses. Cochrane Database Syst Rev. 2012;12:CD004415.
10. DUSA Pharmaceuticals. (2016). Levulan® Kerastick®. [online] Available from https://www.accessdata.fda.gov/drugsatfda_docs/label/2010/020965s007lbl.pdf. [Accessed April, 2017].
11. Willey A, Anderson RR, Sakamoto FH. Temperature-modulated photodynamic therapy for the treatment of actinic keratosis on the extremities: a pilot study. Dermatol Surg. 2014;40(10):1094-102.
12. Pariser DM, Houlihan A, Ferdon MB, et al. Randomized vehicle-controlled study of short drug incubation aminolevulinic acid photodynamic therapy for actinic keratoses of the face or scalp. Dermatol Surg. 2016;42(3):296-304.
13. Bay C, Lerche CM, Ferrick B, et al. Comparison of physical pretreatment regimens to enhance protoporphyrin IX uptake in photodynamic therapy: a randomized clinical trial. JAMA Dermatol. 2017.
14. Taub AF, Schieber AC. New methods for the clinical enhancement of photodynamic therapy. J Drugs Dermatol. 2015;14(11):1329-24.
15. Galitzer BI. Effect of retinoid pretreatment on outcomes of patients treated by photodynamic therapy for actinic keratosis of the hand and forearm. J Drugs Dermatol. 2011;10(10):1124-32.
16. Philipp-Dormston WG, Sanclemente G, Torezan L, et al. Daylight photodynamic therapy with MAL cream for large-scale photodamaged skin based on the concept of 'actinic field damage': recommendations of an international expert group. J Eur Acad Dermatol Venereol. 2016;30(1):8-15.
17. Ibbotson S, Stones R, Bowling J, et al. A consensus on the use of daylight photodynamic therapy in the UK. J Dermatolog Treat. 2016;27:1-8.

18. DUSA Pharmaceuticals. Blu-U®. [online] Available from https://www.accessdata.fda.gov/cdrh_docs/pdf/P990019B.pdf. [Accessed April, 2017].

19. Wang B, Shi L, Zhang YF, et al. Gain with no pain? Pain management in dermatological photodynamic therapy. Br J Dermatol. 2017.

20. Morton CA, Szeimies RM, Sidoroff A, et al. European guidelines for topical photodynamic therapy part 1: treatment delivery and current indications–actinic keratoses, Bowen's disease, basal cell carcinoma. J Eur Acad Dermatol Venereol. 2013;27(5):536-44.

21. Bath-Hextall FJ, Matin RN, Wilkinson D, et al. Interventions for cutaneous Bowen's disease. Cochrane Database Syst Rev. 2013;(6):CD007281.

22. Basset-Seguin N, Ibbotson SH, Emtestam L, et al. Topical methyl aminolaevulinate photodynamic therapy versus cryotherapy for superficial basal cell carcinoma: a 5 year randomized trial. Eur J Dermatol. 2008;18(5):547-53.

23. Christensen E, Mørk C, Foss OA. Pretreatment deep curettage can significantly reduce tumour thickness in thick basal cell carcinoma while maintaining a favourable cosmetic outcome when used in combination with topical photodynamic therapy. J Skin Cancer. 2011.

24. Elman , Slatkine M, Harth Y. The effective treatment of acne vulgaris by a high-intensity, narrow band 405-420 nm light source. J Cosmet Laser Ther. 2003;5(2):111-7.

25. Megna M, Fabbrocini G, Marasca C, et al. Photodynamic therapy and skin appendage disorders: a review. Skin Appendage Disord. 2017;2(3-4):166-76.

26. Sakamoto FH, Lopes JD, Anderson RR. Photodynamic therapy for acne vulgaris: a critical review from basics to clinical practice: part I. Acne vulgaris: when and why to consider photodynamic therapy? J Am Acad Dermatol. 2010;63(2):183-93.

27. Kim JE, Kim SJ, Hwang JI, et al. New proposal for the treatment of viral warts with intralesional injection of 5-aminolevulinic acid photodynamic therapy. J Dermatolog Treat. 2012;23(3):192-5.

Index

Page numbers followed by b *refer to box,* f *refer to figure, and* t *refer to table*

A

Acanthosis 34
Acid-fast bacilli 23
Acne
    scars, treatment of 168f
    vulgaris 202
Acral skin 36
Acrochordons 62
Actinic cheilitis 139, 203
Actinic keratoses 62, 139, 150f, 198, 203
Adenocystic carcinoma 105
Adenoma, sebaceous 24
Adnexal carcinoma 105
Adson forceps 71f
Allergic contact dermatitis 12, 24
Alopecia 33
    nonscarring 37
Aluminum 179
    chloride 43f, 46f
        solution 65
American Academy of Dermatology 146
American College of Micrographic
        Surgery and Cutaneous
        Oncology 101
Aminolevulinic acid 197
Anesthesia 62, 66, 68
    techniques 116
Apocrine carcinoma 105
Argyria 178
Arthropod bites 12
Aspergillosis 24
Atrophy 34
Autoimmune disease 35

B

Bacillary bacterial colonies 24
Back squeeze 81
    maneuver 82f
Basal cell carcinoma 24, 36, 37, 82f, 96,
        105, 109, 202
    pigmented 24
    sclerotic 67
    superficial 42f, 62
    typical superficial 202f
Basal cell nevus syndrome 105
Basaloid cells 24
Becker's nevi 178
Bees pattern, swarm of 24
Betadine 102
Bichloroacetic acid 87, 92f
Bilobed flap
    original 131f
    Zitelli modification of 131f

Biopsy
    excisional 41
    porokeratosis 35f
    technique 37, 60f
    with curettage, feathering of 68f
Bishop Harmon forceps 71
Black dot ringworm 6
Blastomycosis 24
Bleeding 123
Botryomycosis 24
Bowen's disease 202, 203
Bowenoid papulosis 139
Budding spores 24
Bullous impetigo 23
Bullous pemphigoid 12, 24, 26, 31
Bumpy dermal edema
        development 161f
Buried vertical mattress suture 76, 112
Burns 187
Burow's graft 131f
Burow's triangle 131f
Burrow ink test 14

C

Cadmium
    selenide 179
    seleno-sulfide 179
    sulfide 179
Café au lait macules 175, 177
Candida albicans 5
Candidiasis 9, 24
Carbon 179
    dioxide 95
Carcinoma
    mucinous 105
    sebaceous 105
Cells 23
    acantholytic 23, 24
    atypical 24
    inflammatory 23
    necrotic 24
    nonkeratinocytic 24
    nonnevoid 24
Cellulitis, compartmental 123
Cervix, benign erosions of 87
Chemical
    matricectomy 121
    nail avulsion 118
Cherry angioma 159, 160f
Chest, extensive photodamage of 192f
Chicago sky blue stain 9f
Chickenpox 26
Chlorhexidine 102
Chromium oxide 179

Cleft palate 170f
Clitoris 91
Cobalt aluminate 179
Cold agglutinin disease 144
Collagenized stroma 24
Contact dermatitis, irritant 24
Cornoid lamella 34
Cosmetic tattoos 181
Crusted scabies, scaling plaques of 17
Cryoglobulinemia 144
Cryosurgery 139, 142, 143, 144
    dermatologic 139
    history of 140
    principles behind 140
    treatment 148t
Cryotherapy 66, 121, 139
    matricectomy 121
C-suture 53f
Cyst 87, 109
    borders of 55f
    excision of 55
    punch excision of 55f

D

Darier disease 24
Daylight photodynamic therapy 200
Deep sutures 76
Dental syringe 115
Dermal melanocytosis, congenital 175
Dermal pigmented lesions 178
Dermatitis
    herpetiformis 12, 31
    seborrheic 12
Dermatofibroma 24, 41
Dermatofibrosarcoma protuberans 105
Dermatophyte infection 9
    superficial 3
Dermatosis papulosa nigra 62, 66
    curettage of 67f
Dermoscopy 18
Diabetic neuropathy 119
Dichloroacetic acid 87, 88, 93f, 94f
    treatment 87
Dichotomous branching 24
Diffuse eczematous papules 12f
Digital mucous cysts 121
Digital myxoid cyst treatment 121
Digital nerve block 116, 117
Dimethyl sulfoxide 3, 5, 7f, 9f
Diphenhydramine 68
Direct fluorescent antibody 26
Disazodiarylide 179
Disazopyrazolone 179
Distal interphalangeal joint 117

Distal nail avulsion 118
Distal subungual onychomycosis 4, 4*f*
Dorsal nasal rotation flap 129*f*
Double action nail nippers 115
Double trephine punch 54, 55
    method 54
    technique 54*f*, 59
Dynamic cooling device 155, 157
Dysplastic nevus 109

E

Ear lesions, cryosurgery of 145
Ecchymosis 164*f*
    postprocedural 163, 164*b*
Eccrine carcinoma 105
Ectopic sebaceous glands 91
Electrodesiccation 62-65
Electrofulguration 64
Electrosurgery matricectomy 121
Elliptical excision 109
Eosinophils 24
Ephelides 175
Epidermal
    disk 34
    pigmented lesions 177, 178
Epidermis, full-thickness necrosis of 24
Epidermolysis bullosa acquisita 31
Epinephrine 63*f*, 117
Epitheliocytes, necrotic 24
Erbium: yttrium aluminum garnet laser
        96, 166
Erythema 48, 162
    annulare centrifugum 4
    multiforme 24, 25*f*
Erythematous reticular footprinting,
        severe 192*f*
Erythroplasia of Queyrat 24
Excess potassium hydroxide,
        removing 8*f*
Eyebrows 126, 127*f*
Eyelids 76

F

Facial
    molluscum 95
    tumors 105
Fascial structures, use of 83
Feathering technique 45
Felon 123
Ferric
    cyanide 179
    hydrate 179
    oxide 177, 179
    subsulfate 47
Fibrin filaments 24
Fibroblasts 24
    spindle-shaped 24
Fibroxanthoma, atypical 105
Fitzpatrick skin 156, 173, 180, 187
Flaccid blister 37
Flap donor site, scarring of 133

Fordyce spots 91, 92*f*
Fungal
    elements 9*t*
    infections, superficial 4*f*
    type 9

G

Genodermatoses 22, 24
Giant cells, multinucleated 23, 25*f*, 26
Ginkgo biloba 156
Gland, sebaceous 91, 93*f*
Glass slide and cover slip 15
Glove technique 115
Glucose transporter 1 158
Granular immunoglobulin G 35
Granules, pigmented 24
Grossing technique 59
Guarnieri bodies 23

H

Hailey-Hailey disease 24
Hand-foot-mouth disease 23
Hemangiomas 146, 158
    proliferating 159
    superficial 159
Hematoma 114*f*
Hematoporphyrin derivative 197
Hemorrhagic bullae 149*f*
Hemostasis 47*f*, 112
Henderson-Patterson bodies 23, 65
Herpes
    infection 22, 25*f*
    polymerase chain reaction 25
    simplex 23
        disseminated 25*f*
        vesicopustules 22*f*
Hidradenitis suppurativa 203
Histiocytoma, malignant fibrous 105
Horizontal mattress suture 80, 81*f*
Horny cysts 24
Hovert technique 34, 34*f*
Human papillomavirus 66
Hyperkeratosis 13*f*, 24
Hyperkeratotic disorders 13*f*
Hyperpigmentation, postinflammatory
        156, 159
Hyperplasia, sebaceous 87, 88, 91, 92,
        94*f*, 203
Hypertrichosis 178
Hyphae 9
Hypopigmentation, postinflammatory
        150*f*

I

Immune disorders 22, 24
Impetigo 12
Infantile hemangiomas 158
    laser treatment 159*b*
Infectious diseases 22, 23

Ingrown nails 87
Instrument tamponade 53, 53*f*
Intense pulsed light 155, 186, 187*f*, 188*f*
Iron oxide 179
Island pedicle flap 128*f*
Isopropyl alcohol swab 187*f*

J

Joint stiffness 124

K

Keratinocytes
    acantholytic 23
    necrotic 24
    pigmented 24
Keratinous cyst, small 145*f*
Keratosis, seborrheic 24, 46*f*, 62, 66,
        87, 175
Keratotic papule 46*f*
Knee bend 83
Koilocytes 24

L

Labia majora 91
Large macrophages, cytoplasm of 24
Large oval lesions, excision of 56
Laser
    beam profile, square-shaped 167*f*
    hypertrophic scars 163
    treatment 163
Lead chromate 179
Leiomyosarcoma 105
Leishman-donovan bodies 24
Leishmaniasis 24, 203
Lentigines 175, 180*f*, 182*f*, 190*t*
    treatment of 177*f*, 180*f*
Leprosy 23
Lesions, dermal pigmented 178
Leukemias 144
Leukocytes 24
Leukocytoclastic vasculitis 36, 37
Leukoplakia 139
Lichen planus 4, 24
    erosive 26
Lichenoid tissue reaction 34
Lidocaine 42, 56, 63*f*, 116
Light electrodesiccation 66*f*
Linear IgA bullous dermatosis 31
Lipoma 109
    excision of 56
    multiple painful 56
    punch excision of 57*f*
Lips, herpes simplex of 22*f*
Liquid nitrogen 140
Luer-lock syringe 115
Lupus erythematosus 33, 35, 37
Lymphangitis 123
Lymphocyte 24
    predominance 24

Lymphomas 144
Lymphoproliferative disease 144

M

Malassezia furfur 5
Malignant lesions 187
Manganese 179
Mantle cells 24
Mastocytoma 24
Mastoid interpolation flap 133
Maximal skin tension lines 110
Mayo stand 42
Melanocytes 140
Melanocytic lesion 120
Melanocytic nevi 24
Melanocytoses, dermal 175
Melanoma 24, 109, 147
Melasma, laser treatment of 178
Melolabial interpolation interpolation
        flap 1133
Mercury sulfide 179
Merkel cell carcinomas 24, 105, 147
Methanol burner 5
Methyl aminolevulinate 197
Meticulous intraoperative
        hemostasis 126
Microcystic adenexal carcinoma 105
Microscope 5, 15
Mohs map 103
Mohs micrographic surgery 67, 101,
        113, 126
Mohs surgery 80, 101, 104, 105,
        105*b*, 106
Molluscum contagiosum 23, 62, 65, 95
    curettage of 66*f*
Mongolian spots 175
Monochloroacetic acid 87
Monsel's solution 47, 65
Montgomery tubercles 91
Mosquito hemostat 115
Mucormycosis 24
Myeloma, multiple 144*f*

N

Nail
    avulsion 117
        partial 119*f*
        techniques 118*f*
    clippings 122
    diseases 203
    dystrophy 120, 123
    matricectomy 120
    matrix
        biopsy 119
        excisional 120
    plate elevator 115
    procedures 115, 116
        history of 115
    spatula 116
    splitter 115
Neck, extensive photodamage of 192*f*

Needle driver 70
    jaws 71*f*
Neodymium-doped yttrium aluminum
        garnet 155
Neutrophil predominance 24
Nevoid cells
    atypical 24
    dermal type 24
    epidermal type 24
Nodular basal cell carcinoma 62
Nodules
    multiple 13
    subdermal 36
Nonsteroidal anti-inflammatory
        drugs 201

O

Onychocryptosis 117
Onycholysis 4*f*
Onychomycosis 4*f*
Oral therapy 158
Osteitis, terminal 123
Osteomyelitis 123
O-z flap 128

P

Paget cells 24
Paget's disease 24
    extra-mammary 105
    pigmented mammary 24
Pain 123
Palm, pigmented lesion of 36
Palmar direction 117
Palms and soles, hyperkeratosis of 13*f*
Panniculitis 36, 37, 54, 54*f*
Papules, erythematous 25*f*
Paramedian forehead flap 133
Parapsoriasis 4
Patient observer self-assessment
        scale 112
Pemphigus
    foliaceus 24
    herpetiformis 24
    vulgaris 24
Pencil technique 64*f*
Perfluorodecalin 181
    transparent 181*f*
Periodic acid-schiff 9
    stain 10, 10*f*, 122
Peripheral vascular disease 119
Photodynamic therapy 197, 201*f*, 202, 203
Photodynamic therapy, history of 197
Photosensitizers 197
Phthalocyanine dyes 179
Picosecond laser 179
Pigmented lesion lasers 174
Pityriasis versicolor 5*f*
Plantar direction 117
Plastic jaeger lid plate 145*f*
Poikiloderma of civatte 160
Poikilokaryosis 24

Polydioxanone 72
Polymerase chain reaction 26
Porokeratosis 34, 36
Porphyria cutanea tarda 31
Port-wine stain 157*f*
    birthmarks 155, 156
    laser treatment 159*b*
Potassium hydroxide 3, 4*f*, 7*f*, 9, 122
    preparation 3, 6*f*, 7*f*
    solution, application of 8*f*
Potassium titanyl phosphate 155
Potato peeler technique 64*f*
Povidone-iodine 102
Proper scraping technique 6*f*
Prophylactic antibiotics 101
Propionibacterium acnes 202
Proximal nail
    avulsion 117
    matrix 119*f*
Pseudohyphae 24
Pulsed dye laser 155, 159-161, 162*f*
    treatment 157*f*, 160*f*, 161*f*, 163*f*, 164*f*
Punch biopsies 51, 54*f*, 59
Punch incision 57*f*
Pustular dermatoses 22*f*
Pyogenic granuloma 62

Q

Q-switched ruby laser 174

R

Raynaud's disease 144
Raynaud's syndrome 144
Reflex sympathetic dystrophy 124
Rheumatoid arthritis 144
Rhombic flap 130, 130*f*
Rhytides, treatment of 169*f*
Rieger dorsal nasal rotation flap 128, 129*f*
Ropivacaine 116, 123
Rosacea 160, 190*t*
Rotation flap
    bilateral 129*f*
    unilateral 128*f*
Rule of halves 127*f*

S

Salicylic acid 66
Sanguinaria canadesis 101
Sarcoma, pleomorphic 105
Sarcoptes scabiei 12, 16
    infestation 12
Saucerization 41
    approaches 59
    biopsies 41, 59
    technique 48, 59
Scabies 12, 12*f*, 13
    diagnosis of 14
    mite 17*f*
    preparation 12
    treatment of 18*t*

Scabietic nodules 17
Scalp
    alopecia 34*f*
    wound, closure of 83*f*
Scalpel dermabrasion 46
Scarring 187
    alopecia 37
Scars 162
    treatment of 163*b*
Scleroderma 144
Sclerotherapy 121
Seborrheic keratosis
    curettage of 67*f*
    treatment of 66
Sentinel lymph node biopsy 105
Septate hyphae 24
Sertoli rosettes 24
Shave and saucerization techniques 41
Shoulder
    extensive photodamage of 192*f*
    flexion 81
        maneuver 82*f*
Skin
    biopsy 10*f*, 37*t*
    cancer, non-melanoma 105
    disease 23, 23*t*
    graft
        full-thickness 125, 132*f*
        split-thickness 131
    hooks 71
        single- and double-pronged 116
    lesions 62*t*
        pigmented 22, 24
    whitening 176*f*
Smooth jaws 71*f*
Sole, pigmented lesion of 36
Spencer suture scissors 72*f*
Spider angiomas 159, 160*b*
Spongiotic dermatitis 22, 24
Spores 9, 24
Squamous cell carcinoma 24, 36, 62,
        104, 109, 142, 143*f*, 202
    cutaneous 105
    in-situ 62
Standard punch biopsy technique 51
Staphylococcal scalded skin
        syndrome 23, 26
Staphylococcus aureus 113
Stevens-Johnson syndrome 24, 26
Stratum corneum 10*f*
Streptocytes 24
Striae distensae 162
Subepidermal blistering diseases 31

Surgery, dermatologic 109
Suture 72
    absorbable 73*t*
    grasp trailing end of 78*f*
    needle 74
    nonabsorbable 72, 74*t*
    running subcuticular 80, 80*f*
    scissors 72
    superficial 79
    thread 72
Suturing technique 76
Syncytial nuclei 23
Systemic lupus erythematosus 144

T

Tadpole cells 24
Tattoo pigments 179*t*
Tattoo removal 179
    treatment tips 180
T-cell lymphoma, cutaneous 4, 203
Telangiectasia 160, 162*b*, 190*t*
    over right nasal ala 162*f*
    residual 159
Tense blister 37
Tinea
    capitis infection 9
    corporis 4, 4*f*
    faciei 4*f*
    versicolor 9, 10*f*
Tissue
    adhesives 75
    necrosis 123
Titanium oxide 179
Toluidine blue stain 103
Tongue
    blade 145*f*
    depressor 187*f*
Topical 5-aminolevulinic acid,
        application of 202*f*
Toxic epidermal necrolysis 24, 26
Trichloroacetic acid 87
Trichophyton tonsurans 3, 5
Tuberculosis 23
Tumors 22, 24, 105
    recurrent 105
Tyler technique 33*f*
Tyson's glands 91
Tzanck cells 24
Tzanck preparation 21, 25*f*
    techniques 23*t*
Tzanck smear 21, 22, 22*t*, 26, 27
    utility of 22
Tzanck test, modified 23

U

Ulceration 159
Ulcers, nonhealing 109
Upper cutaneous lip 133*f*

V

Vagal reactions 123
Vaginal mucosa 91
Vandenbos procedure 120
Varicella 12
    zoster 23
Vascular lesion lasers 155
    surgery of 155
Verrucae 66, 87
Verrucae vulgaris 62, 203
Verrucous hyperplasia 34
Vertical mattress suture 80, 81*f*
Vesicopustules, herpes simplex
        cluster of 22*f*
Vitamin E 156

W

Waldenström's macroglobulinemia 144
Warts 24, 66
White onychomycosis, superficial 4
Wound
    care 122
    closure 112
        materials 72
    management 104

X

Xanthelasma 87-89, 90*f*
    lesions 96
    palpebrarum 89
Xeroderma pigmentosa 105

Y

Yellow papules, patch of 93*f*

Z

Zinc
    chloride 101
    oxide 179
Z-plasties 130

EU GSPR Authorised Reprsentative
Logos Europe, 9 rue Nicolas Poussin
1700, La Rochelle, France
Phone: +33 (0) 6 67 93 73 78
E-mail: contact@logoseurope.eu

www.ingramcontent.com/pod-product-compliance
Lightning Source LLC
Chambersburg PA
CBHW081555220326
41598CB00036B/6685